Redesigning Health Care for Children with Disabilities

Redesigning Health Care for Children with Disabilities

Strengthening Inclusion, Contribution, and Health

by

Heidi M. Feldman, M.D., Ph.D.
Ballinger-Swindells Professor of Developmental and Behavioral Pediatrics
Neonatal and Developmental Medicine
Pediatrics
Stanford University School of Medicine
Palo Alto, CA

Baltimore • London • Sydney

·P A U L·H·
BROOKES
PUBLISHING CO.®

Paul H. Brookes Publishing Co.
Post Office Box 10624
Baltimore, Maryland 21285-0624
USA

www.brookespublishing.com

Typeset by Cenveo Publisher Services, Baltimore, Maryland.
Manufactured in the United States of America by
Sheridan Books, Inc., Chelsea, Michigan.

Cover photo © Veer/Denys Kuvaiev.

Library of Congress Cataloging-in-Publication Data

Feldman, Heidi M.
Redesigning health care for children with disabilities : strengthening inclusion, contribution, and health / by Heidi M. Feldman.
p. ; cm.
Includes bibliographical references and index.
ISBN 978-1-59857-234-6—ISBN 1-59857-234-2
I. Title.
[DNLM: 1. Comprehensive Health Care. 2. Disabled Children. 3. Delivery of Health Care. 4. Inservice Training—methods. 5. Patient Care Team. W 84.5]

RC570
362.3—dc23 2013009479

British Library Cataloguing in Publication data are available from the British Library.

2017 2016 2015 2014 2013

10 9 8 7 6 5 4 3 2 1

Contents

About the Author

Heidi M. Feldman, M.D., Ph.D., holds the Ballinger-Swindells Endowed Professorship in Developmental and Behavioral Pediatrics at Stanford University School of Medicine and serves as the Medical Director of the Mary L. Johnson Developmental-Behavioral Pediatrics Clinical Programs at Lucile Packard Children's Hospital. She earned a Ph.D. in developmental psychology at the University of Pennsylvania in 1975. Her dissertation research was indicative of her early interest in children with disabilities; in collaboration with fellow graduate student Susan Goldin-Meadow, she conducted a study on how children who were deaf, born to hearing parents, and educated in the oral tradition learned to communicate. With an irrepressible desire to serve and understand children with disabilities, she decided to go to medical school at the University of California, San Diego School of Medicine, earning an M.D. degree in 1979. She then completed pediatric residency training at the University of California, San Diego Medical Center in 1982. Her primary mentor was Martin J. Stein, M.D., who demonstrated the power of the biopsychosocial model of pediatrics. Her fellowship training at the Children's Hospital Boston in 1983–1984 was an individualized program. She studied under three productive pioneers in the emerging field of developmental-behavioral pediatrics: Melvin D. Levine, M.D., who focused on the assessment and treatment of children with high-prevalence neurodevelopmental disorders; T. Berry Brazelton, M.D., who studied child development with an emphasis on infants; and Eli H. Newberger, M.D., who explored the causes and treatments of child abuse.

In 1984, Dr. Feldman joined the faculty at the University of Pittsburgh and worked at the Children's Hospital of Pittsburgh. She initially served as the Director of the Child Development Unit, an interdisciplinary team that served children with disabilities. In a major restructuring in 1993, the unit joined the Division of General Academic Pediatrics to integrate developmental-behavioral pediatrics with primary care pediatrics, adolescent medicine, and child abuse services into a single division. Dr. Feldman served as Division Chief from 1993 to 2001.

A seminal event in Dr. Feldman's career was the creation of the University, Community, Leaders, and Individuals with Disabilities (UCLID) Center at the University of Pittsburgh. In response to a request for proposals from the Maternal and Child Health Bureau of Health Resources and Services Administration in the U.S. Public Health Service, a diverse group of colleagues from across the campus and hospitals of the University of Pittsburgh successfully prepared a grant proposal to launch the Leadership Education in Neurodevelopmental Disabilities program at the University of Pittsburgh. Dr. Feldman was the Project Director of the UCLID Center from 1995 to 2006; it brought together university faculty and students, community leaders, and individuals with disabilities. The center trained advanced professionals from 11 disciplines, hosted workshops and conferences, created model programs, and advocated for comprehensive and high-quality services for children with disabilities and their families.

In 2006, Dr. Feldman moved to Stanford University School of Medicine to assume her current position. She continues to conduct research on language and cognition in children with health care conditions that put language learning at risk. She is an active teacher. She teaches an undergraduate course; is a research mentor to medical and graduate students and to postdoctoral fellows; and provides professional training for developmental-behavioral pediatrics fellows, medical residents and fellows from a variety of disciplines, and practicing pediatricians throughout the country and the world. She advocates for children and for children with disabilities through projects funded by First 5 San Mateo County and by participation in the Board of Directors of Abilities United in Palo Alto, California.

Dr. Feldman has held several leadership positions nationally in the American Academy of Pediatrics. She is past President of the Society for Developmental and Behavioral Pediatrics and former Chair of the Sub-Board of Developmental-Behavioral Pediatrics of the American Board of Pediatrics. She is also one of the editors of the premier textbook in the field of developmental-behavioral pediatrics. In 2012, she received the prestigious C. Anderson Aldrich Award of the American Academy of Pediatrics, which honors physicians who make lasting contributions to the field of child development.

Dr. Feldman is also a dedicated yoga enthusiast and certified yoga teacher.

Prologue

For many of you entering a health profession, a substantial portion of your professional life will be dedicated to providing care for individuals with disabilities and related conditions. For those of you who have been practicing for some time, unless you have subspecialized, you may be noticing a steady shift toward increasing numbers of individuals with disabilities in your practice. The Institute of Medicine reports that "chronic illness," a compilation of many different specific diseases and disorders, is the fastest growing category of health conditions in the United States and Western world (Institute of Medicine, 2001).

Providing health care to individuals with disabilities is less dramatic and may be considered less glamorous than working in other health care settings, such as the operating room, intensive care unit, or emergency department. The surgeons, intensivists, and other health professionals in those settings can now prolong life for many individuals who not so long ago might have succumbed to their illness or injury. Unfortunately, the survivors are often left with a myriad of long-lasting consequences that are not nearly as well understood or cared for as the acute precipitating event. The long-term care of those individuals falls to an interdisciplinary team of health professionals from medicine, nursing, therapeutic disciplines, social work, and education. Although the subsequent interventions may not cure residual conditions, health care services and supports to these individuals can make vast improvements in their lives, in the lives of their families, and in the society at large. It is possible to heal even if you cannot cure.

Providing health care to children with disabilities is my occupation. Actually, it's my passion. I am a developmental-behavioral pediatrician. When I began my career in pediatrics, developmental-behavioral pediatrics was a small, diverse interest group that was just beginning to differentiate from general pediatrics. Since the 1970s and accelerating since the 1980s, the field has burgeoned into a well-established, thriving subspecialty of pediatrics. Growth within the profession has been fueled by intense general interest in the conditions that developmental-behavioral pediatricians diagnose and treat—attention-deficit/hyperactivity disorder and autism, for example. It has been aided by shifting social attitudes and passage of legal protections. It has become a critical component of comprehensive care of children with disabilities. In the course of my own career, I have had the distinct pleasure of working with thousands of children and their families. This book represents the core, the essence of what I have learned, over more than 30 years.

The book focuses on health care for *children* with disabilities. Why focus on children? First, the population has grown exponentially in size since the 1970s. However, changes in health care delivery have not kept pace with changes in medical interventions and in demographics. Second, national surveys confirm that many children fail to get supports and services that would be helpful to them (Newacheck & Kim, 2005; U.S. Department of Health and Human Services, 2008). Families struggle to negotiate the complexities of a fragmented, poorly coordinated, overly bureaucratic, and insensitive set of financially and personally expensive services. Even after yeomen work to obtain services, the services often fail to meet the needs of the children or the family. Finally, childhood is a time of life when the forces of human development are propelling children to dramatic change. They acquire new skills and knowledge and become increasingly active and independent members of the community. All children develop, learn, and transform. Just as society takes advantage of the forward momentum of children's lives and the plasticity of their young nervous system in providing education at young ages, it makes sense to capitalize on their developmental status in providing additional supports and services if they have disabilities.

Health care systems require fundamental reform in order to serve children—and by extension adults—with disabilities. The traditional model for care of children with disabilities was aimed at improving the child's health by preventing or curing conditions if at all possible, and otherwise at reducing signs or symptoms of the conditions or providing corrective interventions. If children with disabilities lived in the community with their family rather than in institutions or state hospitals, it was assumed that health was a prerequisite for them to participate in selective and segregated settings, such as special education classes or sheltered workshops. If children excelled in those settings, then they were offered opportunities to be included in the broader social network.

This book proposes turning that old paradigm on its head. It describes three fundamental pillars in health care for children with disabilities in the order of priority. The first pillar is inclusion. Inclusion is a fundamental right for children and adults with disabilities (General Assembly of the United Nations, n.d.). Inclusion counters the sordid history of neglect and maltreatment that prevailed for millennia. Inclusion is not a specific classroom or school or job. It is a social attitude, welcoming individuals with disabilities into all aspects of community life, and a set of legal protections to ensure that folks do the right thing. The second pillar is contribution. A focus on contribution means that within their social contexts, children receive education, support, accommodations, and encouragement to participate. It is not sufficient for society to accept children with disabilities as passive observers or to restrict them to narrow roles that limit their opportunities and possibilities; they deserve equality of opportunity. The third pillar is health. Health is defined broadly, not simply as the absence of illness, injury, or pain, but rather a state of physical, mental, and social well-being (World Health Organization, 1946). Health care works closely with other community resources and policies, such as education and social service, to encourage and support inclusion and contribution. Health care interventions should deliberately and explicitly promote an individual's full social participation. When health care interventions are proposed, whether they are surgeries, medications, therapies or psychotherapies, durable medical equipment, or simply counseling and answering questions, the target outcomes of the intervention should be made explicit. Those target outcomes should connect in a transparent way to inclusion and contribution.

This change in the direction of priorities may seem minor at first. However, it could ultimately lead to major shifts in how health care for children with disabilities is delivered. Making the priorities explicit could alter what families choose for their children's care. I recently evaluated a 4-year-old boy with cerebral palsy who was able to walk independently over long distances but could speak only about 100 words with poor intelligibility. When I asked his mother and father to each tell me their main goal for their son at that time, his father stated improved communication, and his mother stated improved gait. Together, as I reflected with them, they realized that his ability to communicate more effectively was far more pertinent to his long-term function than his ability to walk more smoothly. Insisting on health care in the service of inclusion and contribution would affect how the interdisciplinary team advises families and communicates among its members. In an era of limited resources, these priorities may even influence what services health insurance will cover.

The book is organized into four sections. The first introduces the population of children with disabilities. It expands on why they are an important focus and on the complexity of their health care. The second section focuses on the overall goals of health care: inclusion, contribution, and health, in that order. The third section provides strategies and tools that support a new approach to health care. Chapter 7 promotes function-focused care. Chapter 8 encourages the development of comprehensive and integrated health care plans. Chapter 9 discusses the role of family in the processes and recommends that families play a central role in creating and owning the comprehensive and integrated care plans. Chapter 10 recognizes the burden of these responsibilities on families and promotes care coordination to support their efforts. The fourth section describes how to move the system in the proper direction through education, research, and policy.

Throughout the book you will meet various children, families, and professionals. I have learned so much throughout the years by listening to the stories of the children and families I serve. Their personal tales are an important counterweight to facts and figures in academic literature. Therefore, I wanted to bring to you some of these stories for your consideration. Some of the vignettes are compilations of several children. In those about real children, I have changed the children's names and have also simplified or modified many of the details of their lives in order to respect their confidentiality. I have also interviewed adult leaders and parents. When I use their full name and quote them directly, I have solicited their permission to tell their story.

Health care delivery is in a state of flux. Patients and families can gain access to information and pressure their clinicians for particular treatments or services. Health care clinicians need skills to guide the families and negotiate what make sense for a child. Health care costs have skyrocketed. Employers who contribute premiums for health insurance in the United States, insurance companies, and health policy makers are all interested in reducing the costs of care. The Affordable Care Act of 2010 [PL 111-148] includes many provisions to improve quality and safety while reducing costs. It is quite challenging to be an active clinician and have the time and energy to participate in the change process. It is my sincere hope that this book stimulates health professionals, those just emerging into their professional roles or those in practice for many years, to engage in the reform process in order to ensure that their distinctive perspectives are included and to guarantee that children have positive clinical and functional outcomes.

REFERENCES

General Assembly of the United Nations. (n.d.). *The universal declaration of human rights.* Retrieved from http://www.un.org/en/documents/udhr/index.shtml

Institute of Medicine, Committee on Quality of Health Care in America. (2001). *Crossing the quality chasm: A new health system for the 21st century.* Washington, DC: National Academies Press.

Newacheck, P.W., & S.E. (2005). A national profile of health care utilization and expenditures for children with special health care needs. *Archives of Pediatrics and Adolescent Medicine, 159*, 10–17.

U.S. Department of Health and Human Services, Health Resources and Services Administration, Maternal and Child Health Bureau. (2008). *The National Survey of Children with Special Health Care Needs Chartbook 2005–2006.* Rockville, MD: U.S. Department of Health and Human Services.

World Health Organization. (1946). *Preamble to the Constitution of the World Health Organization.* Retrieved from http://www.who.int/about/definition/en/print.html

Acknowledgments

Throughout my life, I have had the great fortune to have many exceptional teachers and colleagues. To keep this section short, I will name just a few, although my gratitude extends beyond this list. My parents, Sylvia and Joe, were my first great teachers. My father, in particular, instilled in me a deep respect for medicine that propelled me into the field of pediatrics. My husband, Jay McClelland, has been a model of intelligence and integrity in every aspect of life. I appreciate his support and patience while I wrote this book. My daughters, Mollie McClelland and Heather Greening, may see me as their teacher, but now the lessons flow in all directions.

One of the inspirations for this book is my great colleague from Children's Hospital of Pittsburgh, William I. Cohen, M.D. (1946–2009). Bill was an extraordinary physician whose kindness and compassion were legendary among the families of children with Down syndrome in Western Pennsylvania, across the United States, and around the world. Bill taught and exemplified family-centered practice. His teachings continue to guide me, and I miss him very much.

The faculty, students, staff, and community partners of the UCLID Center at the University of Pittsburgh were key influences in the development of the ideas I present here. George McClomb, Ph.D., Co-Director of the UCLID Center, broadened my thinking about disability and demonstrated new ways to collaborate with partners in the community. Stephen J. Bagnato, Ed.D., emphasized the importance of authentic and functional assessments for children. Jennifer Angelo, Ph.D., Thomas F. Campbell, Ph.D., M. Kathleen Kelly, Ph.D., PT, and Cheryl Messick, Ph.D., were extraordinary therapists who elaborated on the ideas of function as the primary focus of intervention. Rebecca Kronk, RN, Ph.D., and Susan Van Cleve, RN, DVP., were exemplary nurses on the team. Charlene A. Trovato, Ph.D., taught us all about leadership. Lucy Spruill, M.S.W., and Paul W. O'Hanlon, J.D., were among the many community partners whose frank feedback and unfailing support pushed me and the UCLID Center to understand disability from the person's perspective. Rob Oliver was a dedicated staff member whose unflappable good cheer was remarkable given how much effort it took for him to get to work. Thank you all. I hope I have faithfully presented the ideas that we worked on together.

At Stanford University School of Medicine, I want to acknowledge my colleagues in Neonatal and Developmental Medicine and Developmental-Behavioral Pediatrics. Irene M. Loe, M.D., once a fellow and UCLID trainee, is now a colleague who continues the lineage. Anne M. DeBattista, M.S.N., RN, Lynne Huffman, M.D., Lucy Crain, M.D., Cheryl Goldfarb-Greenwood, RNC, M.N., CNS, and Brian Tang, M.D., form a powerful team that is trying to put the ideas expressed in this book into action. In Palo Alto, California, I have had the privilege to sit on the Board of Directors of Abilities United, a community-based organization that serves individuals with disabilities and is now making inclusion and contribution the strategic vision for the organization.

My sincere thanks go to Dianna Ploof, Ed.D., who critiqued an earlier version of the entire manuscript. I met Dianna in about 1986 and we worked together on many different projects over the years. She has always opened my eyes and my heart. Her insights and edits were invaluable. I would also like to extend my appreciation to Stephen Plocher and Johanna Cantler of Paul H. Brookes Publishing Co. for their confidence in me and their wise guidance.

Finally, I want acknowledge the children and families whom I have had the privilege to serve. They have shared their lives openly with me. I am filled with awe at the strength, dedication, flexibility, and creativity that I witness time and time again. I hope I have captured their truth and that it inspires others as it has taught me.

To colleagues, partners, trainees, and friends from the UCLID Center at the University of Pittsburgh. Our collective work germinated the concepts I present here.

I

Disabilities

1

What Are Disabilities?

Ashley

Ashley was born 4 months prematurely, weighing 540 grams (1 pound, 3 ounces). At first, she was quite ill, unable to breathe on her own, eat by mouth, or fight infections effectively. She needed x-rays, blood tests, intravenous injections, and blood transfusions. After 4 months of intensive neonatal care, she gradually improved and was ready for discharge home. Her family expected that discharge would be the end of this long ordeal.

Her parents quickly learned that despite the optimistic predictions of the staff, Ashley still faced many different challenges. As an infant, she developed respiratory difficulties that landed her in the emergency department on several occasions; she took medications daily to allow her to breathe without effort. She had persistent feeding difficulties, poor weight gain, and poor growth. The pulmonologist who managed her respiratory problems recommended that the family consult a gastroenterologist. The gastroenterologist referred them to a dietician. The dietician in turn suggested they visit an occupational therapist who specialized in feeding issues. The occupational therapist referred them to a psychologist, convinced that some of Ashley's feeding issues were what she called "behavioral." Eventually, Ashley began to gain weight and grow, in the 5th percentile of the growth charts.

Ashley's care became a bit more organized when she connected with the High Risk Infant Follow-up program at the hospital of her birth when she was 10 months old (6 months of age corrected for the degree of prematurity). When she was 16 months of age (12 months corrected for the degree of prematurity), the program team confirmed her parents' observations that gross motor development was slow. When she reached 24 months of age, they diagnosed her with cerebral palsy and developmental delays. They helped the family to arrange for a visit to a child neurologist and for weekly physical and occupational therapy. Ashley obtained light plastic braces to keep her ankles flexible and a walker to encourage ambulation. She was also deemed eligible for publicly financed early intervention services, first receiving weekly home-based therapeutic and developmental services and then going to a center-based program two mornings a week. At age 3 years, she made the transition to special education programs. She was assigned to a classroom of typically developing peers and also received the services of speech-language pathologists, special educators, and occupational and physical therapists in one-on-one private sessions. She took therapeutic horseback riding, warm water swimming lessons, and music classes. By kindergarten, she was able to walk independently without support.

At grade-school age, Ashley was hard working and very friendly. She had two best friends with whom she played at school and at home on weekends. However, despite average intelligence, she experienced learning problems, difficulties with focus and concentration, and excessive worries. She received in-class tutoring as well as special education services in the school's resource room. During middle school and high school, she intermittently saw mental health professionals who prescribed medications to improve focus, then psychotherapy to control anxiety.

Ashley graduated from high school with her classmates. She enrolled in a small, liberal arts college known for its support of students with learning disabilities. Her goal was to become an early childhood educator.

The child in the vignette, Ashley, one of many children you will meet in this book, was born prematurely and developed multiple disabilities. Her medical conditions lasted throughout her childhood and adolescence; required many health and related services; and affected basic functions, including breathing, eating, mobility, and learning. What makes this particular case poignant is that her parents, and indeed the professionals who worked with the family during her neonatal hospitalization, implicitly conceptualized prematurity as a short-term health condition. The team of doctors, nurses, therapists, and other providers used modern equipment, potent medications, and complex interventions to support the infant until her lungs, stomach, and brain developed sufficiently to take over basic functions. However, they did not discuss with her parents the predictable warning signs that this child might experience difficulties with other functions and require continued elevated health care services beyond the initial hospital stay, or if they did, the parents did not fully understand. The parents later said that they did not feel properly prepared for the complications that arose. Plans for subsequent care were generated piecemeal, involving many different specialists as specific problems arose. The experience for the child and her parents was chaotic and overwhelming.

Ashley's case is not unusual for a child born prematurely. Since the 1980s, advances in medical science and technology have dramatically changed the survival statistics for premature infants. As of 2013, in the United States and other developed countries, the vast majority of these small infants survive (Behrman, Butler, & Committee on Understanding Premature Birth and Assuring Healthy Outcomes, 2007). However, even when treated optimally in the newborn period, they may experience subsequent health problems that require medications; emergency room and hospital visits; and intense vigilance on the part of their parents, caregivers, and teachers. They may, like Ashley, develop limitations in basic life functions, such as respiration or feeding. Approximately one in five of the very low birth weight subgroup is eventually diagnosed with major disabilities, such as visual impairment, hearing loss, cerebral palsy, or intellectual disability (Behrman et al., 2007). These children may, like Ashley, need regular occupational, physical, and/or speech-language therapy; medical equipment, such as braces, walkers, or hearing aids; medications; and/or operations to align the eyes or to relieve muscle tightness. Approximately one in two children born preterm and very low birth weight develops learning disabilities by the time they reach school age (Aylward, 2002). Even children without formal diagnoses experience challenges in learning. Many are also diagnosed with mental health conditions during their school years or adolescence, including attention-deficit/hyperactivity disorder (ADHD) or anxiety (Bhutta et al., 2002). They require the support and service of multiple professionals within the health, mental health, and education systems. High-risk infant follow-up programs have been developed to identify the needs of the survivors at the youngest possible age and to support their families as they seek educational and therapeutic services. Unfortunately, in many places, these programs follow children born preterm only until the preschool years, even though problems may not be evident until later and will likely persist throughout childhood. The good news is that with supports and services, many children successfully graduate high school, find employment, have rich friendships, enjoy their independence, and experience a positive quality of adult life, as did Ashley in the opening vignette (Saigal & Doyle, 2008; Saigal & Streiner, 2009).

Ashley's health care needs are not unique to children who have been diagnosed with cerebral palsy. Rather, they are similar to those of children with different medical conditions, including genetic and chromosomal disorders, such as Down syndrome; neurological conditions, such as seizure disorder; and complex health conditions, such as congenital heart disease. Although it is easy to appreciate the differences, it is also important to recognize the commonalities across them, particularly in terms of limitations in functioning and needs for supports and services. Health care professionals from different disciplines need a shared framework for serving children with disabilities, like Ashley and the others, according to their functional and support needs, regardless of the specific health condition that leads to disability.

DEFINITIONS OF DISABILITY

A variety of definitions for disability are available. They vary on the basis of the purposes they are intended to serve and differ in implications regarding access to health services, educational programs, or civil rights. Three generic approaches are based on the presence of 1) a chronic condition, 2) functional impairment, and 3) elevated need for services (McPherson et al., 1998).

For the purposes of this book, the three generic approaches are fused into one definition with three core features. Each feature reflects a continuum, and all are influenced by physical, social, attitudinal, and political contexts. I list the core features first, then describe and explain in more detail. (See the commentary on p. 7 for alternative definitions.)

1. Disabilities are long-term physical, developmental, behavioral, or emotional conditions.
2. As a result of these conditions, individuals typically require increased levels of support and services.
3. As a result of these conditions, individuals experience challenges in their ability to function within the environment.

The first core feature requires that the conditions persist for long periods. Many short-term conditions require additional health services and affect functioning but are not considered disabilities. Consider, for example, pregnancy, which requires frequent visits to the obstetrician or midwife and may adversely affect sleep, eating, or mobility. Nonetheless, pregnancy is not classified as a disability, not only because it is a highly prevalent and predictable event in the lives of women but also because it lasts only 9 months. Similarly, a broken bone may require multiple visits to the orthopedist and physical therapist and may limit mobility for several months. It also is not typically considered a disability because of its short-term nature. The definition of *long-term* varies in different references; the usual threshold for long-term is a duration of 1 year.

It is important to recognize that although a disability lasts for a year or more, its manifestations may change over time. In conditions like muscular dystrophy, the disability is progressive, with function declining over time. In Ashley's case, respiratory and feeding difficulties resolved early in life, whereas learning and mental health issues emerged with age. Even conditions categorized as nonprogressive may change throughout the lifespan.

The second core feature is that disabilities require increased levels of support and/or services. Increased supports and services include routine care from medical subspecialists, long-term use of medication or therapy, modifications to the environment, or special equipment and other accommodations. Consider, for example, whether extremes of stature should be classified as a disability. Individuals who are very short or very tall may have long-term and distinctive life experiences as a result of their stature. However, if they do not require increased services, then their height can be considered an individual difference but not a disability. However, if their stature is associated with abnormalities of bones and other structures and requires long-term health care from medical subspecialists, such as orthopedists, then the level of service is beyond that of the majority of the population. Similarly, if individuals require equipment, such as a scooter for mobility or major accommodations to be successful in the workplace, then their stature requires increased supports. In the latter cases, the condition is a disability. Admittedly, the boundary between individual characteristics and disabilities is not always clear.

The third core feature is that disabilities represent a challenge to functioning in the environment. Hearing impairment limits the ability to detect auditory information in the environment and may also impair the ability to learn through verbal input. Muscular dystrophy compromises mobility and ultimately breathing. In some cases, increased levels of treatments, supports, and services may permit adequate function in the environment that would not be possible otherwise. For example, if a child with a hearing impairment receives and uses hearing aids, then she may no longer have functional limitations in sensory experiences or in learning. She is still classified as having a disability because her function requires the use

Commentary
Alternative Definitions of Disability

Definitions of disability vary on the basis of the purposes they are intended they serve. Three alternative definitions of disability from U.S. public policy demonstrate how the definition determines the size of the population and the rights, supports, and services that they receive.

The Social Security Administration defines disability for purposes of determining who is eligible to receive benefits (Social Security Administration, 2011):

- *The Individual cannot do work that he or she did before;*
- *The Social Security Administration decided that the individual cannot adjust to other work because of the medical condition(s); and*
- *The disability has lasted or is expected to last for at least 1 year or to result in death.*

This restrictive definition limits the number of individuals qualifying for benefits. In applying its definition, the Social Security Administration has had to modify the definition for children because children do not work. The Social Security Administration also tied the definition of disability to lists of medical conditions that frequently limit functioning. It may exclude individuals with limited functional capacity who do not have a medical diagnosis on this list. Relying on lists of health conditions to establish disability results in more restrictions among children than among adults because children are more likely to have rare conditions that do not make it on the list.

The Individuals with Disabilities Education Act (IDEA; PL 101-476), the law governing rights to special education services, defines disability for the purpose of determining who is eligible for special education services (National Dissemination Center for Children with Disabilities, 2011):

- *Mental retardation, hearing impairments (including deafness), speech or language impairments, visual impairments (including blindness), serious emotional disturbance, orthopedic impairments, autism, traumatic brain injury, other health impairments, or specific learning disabilities*
- *Who, by reason thereof, needs special education and related services.*

Again, listing the disabilities in order to establish who has a disability may unfairly exclude individuals with comparable levels of need who do not fall within one of the categories.

The Americans with Disabilities Act (ADA; PL 101-336) is civil rights legislation the purpose of which is to allow all people to have equal opportunities to participate in the economic and social life of their community. ADA therefore seeks a broad and inclusive definition. It does not distinguish between type, severity, or duration of the disability (U.S. Equal Employment Opportunity Commission, 2009):

- *A physical or mental impairment that substantially limits one or more of the major life activities of such individual*
- *A record of such impairment*
- *Being regarded as having such an impairment*

The definition emphasizes the limits on a person's ability to function in major life activities, such as learning, walking, communicating, and self-care. Despite this broad definition, a case law narrowed the scope of the legislation. A reauthorization of the law in 2008 was designed to broaden the category of individuals who receive the protections in this law.

of the hearing aid. Similarly, the young man with muscular dystrophy who obtains a wheelchair may retain mobility. He nonetheless qualifies as an individual with a disability because his mobility is facilitated through the use of adaptive equipment.

According to this three-pronged definition, Ashley's condition met the criteria for disability. The health and functional consequences of prematurity lasted throughout her childhood, meeting the criterion of persistence. She had many conditions that required increased levels of medical and educational service and support, including her respiratory condition, neurological injuries, learning problems, and mental health issues. She required consultation from many health professionals and rehabilitation specialists. She also used special education services at school. In her case, many basic functions—breathing, eating, walking, and learning—were affected, although with the increased supports and services she obtained, the actual functional limitations she experienced decreased over time. They did not prevent graduation from high school, attendance at college, opportunities for professional employment, or full participation in her community.

Disability as a Spectrum

Disabilities are part of the spectrum of life experience that spans between capability or competency and limitation. Mild disabilities require minimal additional service or supports and affect only one or two functions or affect them to a mild degree. For example, after preterm delivery, approximately half of the children develop low-severity disabilities, such as learning disorders and attention deficits, that increase the level of educational support that they require and may compromise their abilities

Commentary
Disability as a Spectrum

For each of the three defining features of disability, a continuum exists. The duration may be 1 year or a lifetime. Supports and services may be intermittent or intensive and lifelong. Functional impairment may affect one domain or multiple domains.

Whether a condition qualifies as a disability is not simply related to the duration of the health condition, the need for supports and services, and the degree of limitation in function. It is also importantly related to characteristics of the individual's physical environment, the beliefs and attitudes that exist in the social environment, access to health care, public policy definitions, and personal motivation to remain active and engaged. For example, an individual with severe hearing impairment who communicates via sign language may have a disability in many environments but not within a community of others who are deaf. The environment places demands on children that may exceed their abilities; within that context the child has a disability.

to learn, communicate, participate socially, or progress through school. Approximately 20% develop major disabilities, including cerebral palsy, hearing or vision impairment, intellectual disability, or seizures (Bhutta et al., 2002; see the commentary at the bottom of p. 8.).

Disabilities may be present from birth or may be acquired later in life. Newborns with recognizable patterns of physical features may be diagnosed with Down syndrome, for example. Other conditions, even those considered genetic or congenital, such as autism or cerebral palsy, may not present until the functional limitations become apparent. Disabilities may be caused by illnesses or accidents that occur at any time of life. Aging often gradually leads to the development of disabilities. The U.S. Census Bureau reports that over 80% of adults 90–100 years old have a disability (U.S. Census Bureau, 2011).

Traditional health care systems are not particularly well prepared to identify and care for individuals with disabilities, including children. Though many of the complications that Ashley experienced could have been anticipated, her family experienced minimal counseling or planning for such issues. Her care was reactive and fragmented. Given how prevalent disabilities are, it is essential to develop proactive and effective systems of health care for people with disabilities. Creating appropriate and responsive systems of health care and related service is a potential contribution to many diverse people; any individual might be one car accident or one decade away from acquiring disabilities. Improving systems of care for people with disabilities not only helps those who currently have disabilities but also prepares for those who may do so in the future. Acknowledging that disability might touch almost anyone in some way enables these systems to be created with generosity and compassion.

Terminology

Language is important for framing thoughts about disability. In this book, I have sought to use terms that are accurate, respectful, and acceptable to the people about whom I am writing. I want to steer clear of euphemisms and circumlocutions as well as avoid terms that have acquired negative connotations.

Person-First Language *Person-first language* is the preference of individuals with disabilities to emphasize that the disabling condition is but one feature of an individual (Snow, 2009–2010). In English, person-first language places the individual in the first position and the disability in the second position. The term *children with disabilities* is preferred over *disabled children*, and *child with Down syndrome* is preferred over *Down syndrome child*. Similarly, where possible, for similar reasons, it is also preferable to state that a person *has* a disability than to state that a person *is* disabled. For example, "a child has a hearing impairment" is preferable to a "child is hearing impaired or deaf." This linguistic approach serves as a reminder that a person is much more than his or her disability. It encourages avoidance of stereotyping and the treatment of each individual according to his or her unique characteristics. (See the commentary at the top of p. 10 for more information on language.)

Long-Term Conditions Throughout the book, I refer to the disorders that lead to disability as *long-term conditions*. The customary term for persistent adverse health problems is *chronic illness* or *chronic conditions*. Although a chronic illness or condition is simply one that is expected to last more than 1 year,

Commentary
Preferred Terminology About Disabilities

In addition to the use of person-first language, there are preferred ways of describing individuals with disabilities. The language used should reflect the lived experience of the individual and should honor the individual's preferences.

On the left of the table below are terms to avoid, and on the right are terms that are preferable. Try to figure out why the term on the left is inappropriate.

Avoid these terms	*Use these terms*
1. The boy suffers from cerebral palsy.	*1. The boy has cerebral palsy.*
2. The girl is afflicted with seizures.	*2. The girl experiences seizures.*
3. The child is wheelchair bound.	*3. The child uses a wheelchair for mobility.*
4. The teen is confined to a wheelchair.	*4. The teen uses a wheelchair for mobility.*
5. The baby had a birth defect.	*5. The baby was born with a physical difference.*
6. The child is mentally retarded.	*6. The child functions in the range of intellectual disability.*
7. He's a "special ed" kid.	*7. He receives special education services.*

the word *chronic* has unfortunately acquired negative connotations as severe, unremitting, or hopeless. Yet, children with these conditions may have mild to moderate symptoms that wax and wane or change over time. With appropriate treatment, such symptoms need not compromise these children's potential in terms of occupation, social relationships, or happiness. The vignette that opened this chapter is a case in point.

Increased Support and Service Needs This book substitutes the term *increased support and service needs* for the term *chronic care*. Again, to some, the term *chronic care* has accrued negative connotations implying expensive, excessive, or hopeless interventions. Although long-term care may be expensive, if administered appropriately as in opening vignette, it is neither excessive nor fruitless. It is this care that allows individuals to engage with others, work, and contribute to their community. Another term that gained currency since about 2000 is *complex care*. It usually refers to health care that involves multiple subspecialists and many different treatment modalities. Care for individuals with disabilities may or may not become complex.

***Use of the Term* Special** An important term in the litereature is *children with special health care needs*. This term was first used by the U.S. federal government in the Omnibus Budget Reconciliation Act of 1989 (PL 101-239) and later amended to include both children and youth. *Special health care needs* was chosen as a broad term that integrates long-term illness and disability. In the 1990s, the Maternal and Child Health Bureau Division (MCHB) of Services for Children with Special Health Care Needs set out to establish a clear definition of children with special health care needs that could be used for planning community services for children with long-term conditions. The MCHB convened an interdisciplinary work group of professionals, planners, and parents to create a definition for the term. The result is as follows:

> Children with special health care needs are those who have or are at increased risk for a chronic physical, developmental, behavioral, or emotional condition and who also require health and related services of a type or amount beyond that required by children generally. (McPherson et al., 1998, p. 138)

The work group clarified that the increased risk could be medical, such as "very low birth weight, the presence of certain metabolic deficiencies, and the existence of some chromosomal abnormalities" or social, such as "extreme poverty, absence of social support, and child abuse or neglect" (McPherson et al., 1998, p. 138). Enhanced service included specialized and/or enhanced medical and nursing services (e.g., physician subspecialists), therapeutic services (e.g., physical, speech, and occupational therapies), family support services (e.g., family counseling or care coordination), equipment and supplies (e.g., durable medical equipment and assistive devices), and related services (e.g., early intervention, special education). The advantage of a broad and inclusive definition, including children at risk rather than just those with a documented condition, is that it facilitates public health planning.

In this book, I try to minimize use of the term *special* because it connotes that children with disabilities are somehow different, separate, or distinctive in terms of their health care or education needs (Snow, 2009). The use of the term *special class* to denote a classroom where children were separated from the educational and social environments of others their age reinforced this word association and became a pejorative term among schoolchildren. Many of the services used by this group of children with disabilities are not at all special; they may be used by anyone for some period. For example, children with broken bones might use physical or occupational therapy or durable medical equipment, such as crutches or scooters. Immigrants with an accent that differs from those of American English might choose to use the services of a speech-language pathologist, although they do not qualify as having a disability.

Disability After considerable refection, I chose to retain the term *disability*. Other options, such as *challenges* or *limitations*, reflect the experience of some, but not all, individuals with long-term conditions and also seem euphemistic. Politically active individuals with disabilities who work for civil rights self-define as members of the Disability Rights movement. *Disability pride* is a term chosen by advocates with disabilities as an expression that reflects a demand for respect rather than pity. The term *disability* further connects the work here with a large body of research and public discourse.

Disability versus Handicap The terms *handicap* or *handicapped* are not appropriate in reference to individuals or groups. Rather, these terms are reserved for situations in which time, resources, or conditions disadvantage individuals such that they cannot participate in society to their full potential. The United Nations (UN) made the following distinction:

> The term "handicap" means the loss or limitation of opportunities to take part in the life of the community on an equal level with others; it describes the encounter between the person with a disability and the environment and is not a feature of the individual in isolation. Use of the term emphasizes shortcomings in the environment and in organized activities in society that prevent persons with disabilities from participating on equal terms. (United Nations Department of Economic and Social Affairs, Division for Social Policy and Development, 2006, p. 1)

In horse racing and golf, a handicap refers to the advantages or disadvantages of time or points given to contestants to equalize their chances of winning. In the world of disability, a handicap is an environmental disadvantage that increases inequality. For example, individuals who are visually impaired are handicapped by the inability to obtain large print books, voice-activated software, or other services and supports that give them access to the world of print. Individuals who use wheelchairs for mobility are handicapped by the absence of curb cuts and ramps. A person is not handicapped; the environment may be handicapping.

Disability versus Disease Disability must be distinguished from disease, illness, and sickness. *Disease* refers to the biomedical condition, often defined in terms of its underlying cause or causes. *Illness* refers to the subjective feelings of pain, compromised health or well-being, or anxiety related to the disease. *Sickness* refers to how society interprets the personal condition or the social role the person plays when experiencing ill health (Wikman, Marklund, & Alexanderson, 2005). Disease, illness, and sickness often co-occur or emerge together. For example, a person acquires a severe infection (the disease). That individual feels ill and takes the day off from work or school. Her employer acknowledges that she is sick and allows her to use sick leave or paid time off rather than dock her pay. However, it is possible to have a disease, such as hypertension, without feeling ill or being viewed as sick. It is also possible to be considered sick without feeling ill; society may require quarantine for an individual with an infectious disease even though the person does not experience any problems from their infection.

Disabilities are neither illnesses nor sicknesses and may not be distinctive biomedical conditions at all. For example, visual impairment and blindness can be caused by any one of a wide range of disorders, from malformations of the eye to infectious diseases. Similarly, cerebral palsy is a condition with a wide range of biomedical causes, such as premature birth, traumatic brain injury, or stroke. Most important, children who have cerebral palsy may not interpret their condition as illness, despite the need for medical treatment. They can be entirely healthy—feeling, eating, and sleeping well and having a rich and meaningful life—in the presence of their disability and may not want to be labeled and treated as sick by society when they feel perfectly well. Disabilities may be visible or invisible. (See the commentary below.)

Commentary
Visible and Invisible Disabilities

Often disabilities that meet the three-pronged definition are visible to others. In Ashley's case, Ashley's muscle stiffness, awkward gait, and use of equipment to improve mobility made her disability apparent to others. Individuals with Down syndrome may be recognizable from a constellation of physical features, including upslanting eyes, small ears, small jaw, short stature, and low muscle tone. Sensory impairments may be obvious on the basis of the appearance of the eyes or ears or on the basis of the equipment an individual uses to access sensory information, such as hearing aids or magnifying glasses. However, many disabilities are invisible to others and are therefore called hidden disabilities. *Ashley had two hidden disabilities: 1) learning disabilities that required educational support and service and limited her ability to learn, and*

2) mental health problems that required mental health services and affected her ability to interact with others and progress through the educational system.

The severity of a disability is not correlated with its physical manifestations. Hidden disabilities may have substantial impact on an individual's function in his or her environment. Epilepsy is one example. The repeated seizures that characterize this illness may affect a child's concentration, persistence, and learning abilities. The medications that reduce seizure frequency further contribute to fatigue and learning difficulties. Arthritis and other joint diseases are another example. Arthritis may be invisible to others but may seriously limit mobility or cause significant pain that limits endurance. Damage to the inner ear is not externally obvious but causes profound vertigo, resulting in limitations in walking and dizziness whenever the eyes move quickly, such as during reading.

Visible disabilities are more likely than hidden disabilities to generate negative attitudes of the general public. However, children with hidden disabilities may also encounter negative attitudes if they fail to meet social or academic expectations. In either case, an unfavorable attitude in the community can have significant, lasting effects on the experience of a person with a disability, restricting opportunities and contributing to negative self-concept.

Disability as Characteristic or Trait Many individuals with disabilities conceptualize their issues as characteristics or traits, not illnesses or sickness resulting from disease. They view their sensory or motor limitations as one of many individual characteristics, such as having tall or short stature, or having blue or brown eyes. If health care professionals say or imply that someone's disability is an illness, then there may be a breakdown of communication with the person they aim to serve. It is extremely important to be attentive to how each person defines himself and his condition. Many individuals who are deaf may conceptualize their hearing loss as a shared life experience, resulting in a distinctive language (sign language), as well as distinctive patterns of behavior, values, beliefs, and attitudes. Together, for these individuals, the shared features create community and culture. Others with hearing impairment who do not use sign language and do not share cultural features may define themselves very differently.

EXAMPLES OF DISABILITIES

Disabilities may be defined by their underlying cause or pathological condition or by the predominant functional limitation. In either case, there may be wide variation in the nature and/or severity of the disabilities.

Categorized by Underlying Cause

Identifying disabilities on the basis of cause may be helpful to parents and to the team caring for a child with disability. Parents appreciate having an understanding of the cause of their child's difficulties. Knowing the cause may improve prognosis or lead to specific biomedical approaches to treatment.

- Chromosomal abnormalities are conditions in which the individual has extra chromosomal material, is missing a major part of a chromosome, or has a significant rearrangement of genetic material. An example of extra chromosomes is Down syndrome, in which the individual has a third copy of chromosome 21. An example of missing chromosomal material is Turner syndrome, in which the individual is missing an X chromosome, or cri du chat, a condition in which the individual is missing part of Chromosome 5.

- Genetic conditions represent differences at the level of individual genes or small collections of genes. Tay–Sachs disease is an autosomal recessive genetic disorder, meaning that each parent contributed one copy of the abnormal gene to the child. *Copy number variant* is a term used to indicate that genetic material is deleted or duplicated. Velocardial facial syndrome and Williams syndrome are two of many conditions caused by genetic deletions. A small percentage of cases of autism are associated with copy number variants on different chromosomes (Glessner et al., 2009).
- Congenital malformations may lead to disabilities. For example, children with complex congenital heart diseases that require early surgical repair are at risk for neurodevelopmental disorders from multiple factors, including abnormal perfusion of the brain before birth (Limperopoulos et al., 2010) and complications of the surgery and postsurgical management (Kussman et al., 2010; Newburger et al., 2008).
- Infectious diseases, particularly those that directly or indirectly affect the central nervous system, may lead to disabilities. The extent of disability is associated with the type of infection, its severity, and its susceptibility to treatment. For example, meningitis is inflammation of the covering of the brain that may cause neural injury with resulting cognitive, motor, or sensory impairments. Children who are born with HIV/AIDS, a viral infection, may experience problems with mobility and learning, particularly if untreated.
- Injuries also cause disabilities. The injuries can result from motor vehicle accidents, falls, accidental trauma of other types, or nonaccidental trauma.

Categorized by Domain of Function

Disability may also be categorized according to the major domain of function that is affected. This method has the advantage of suggesting the types of services and supports that may be required because of the affected domain. However, given the complexity of the conditions, this categorization obscures the fact that many individuals have more than one disability.

- *Mobility limitations*: Cerebral palsy is defined in terms of limitations in the ability to move and control movements, often accompanied by disturbances of muscle tone and strength, and is caused by an injury to the developing brain early in life. Although the injury is permanent, the manifestations of the condition may vary over time and development. Spina bifida is a condition in which the spinal column and surrounding bony structures fail to close completely. The degree of mobility limitation is related to the location along the spine that was affected; when the spinal defect is low, in the sacral area, the symptoms are milder than when the spinal defect is higher, in the lumbar or thoracic areas.

- *Learning disability*: In the United States, the term *learning disability* has been defined in federal law as problems in learning out of proportion with what would have been expected on the basis of intellectual abilities and educational opportunities. Learning disabilities, thus defined, may include problems with reading, writing, and mathematics. However, in the United Kingdom, *learning disability* is used more broadly for any situation in which the function of learning is limited. There, the term includes what is in the United States labeled as *intellectual disability* and was formerly called *mental retardation*. The definition of intellectual disability has three components: limitations in adaptive function, including learning, communicating, taking care of oneself, and interacting with others; low scores (at least near two standard deviations below the mean) on a test of intellectual function; and onset in the developmental period.
- *Communication disorders*: Communication disorders encompass difficulty comprehending what is said and producing spoken language. Hearing loss may cause a disorder of verbal language and leave the ability to create and comprehend manual-gestural language intact. Intellectual disability may cause delays and disorders of communication, generally commensurate with abilities in other domains of function. Autism is characterized by qualitative differences in communication skills.
- *Sensory disorders*: Sensory impairments are a diverse set of problems sensing environmental stimuli with one of the five major senses, converting the information into nervous signals, and passing the signals to the brain for accurate interpretation of objects and events in the world. Vision and hearing impairment are more prevalent in developing countries than in the United States in part because of limited access to appropriate treatments (World Health [WHO] Organization, 2012).

IMPLICATIONS FOR FAMILIES OF CHILDREN WITH DISABILITIES

The care of a child with a long-term condition that results in a need for increased services and supports has profound implications for the family as well as for the child. In the past, many children with disabilities were separated from their families and shunted to nursing homes and state hospitals for their entire lives. Their families struggled with the emotional consequences of their decisions, even though professionals advised them to carry out such plans. The deinstitutionalization movement, beginning in the 1960s, has transformed the expectations for children and their families. New technologies, such as home ventilation systems, have allowed children, even those with very complex medical needs, to be free from lives in hospital settings. The care of these children now falls primarily to the family.

As Ashley's case so clearly demonstrates, caring for children with disabilities at home brings its own set of challenges and complications. (See the commentary on p. 16.) Parents and caregivers are responsible for all of the routine aspects of raising children, including feeding, personal hygiene, providing shelter, and attending to their emotional needs. They are also responsible for meeting the increased support and service needs, including taking the child to health care visits, administering medications, advocating for the child with schools, as well as doing their share of the therapies and treatments. The care of a child or youth with disabilities often requires a revision of the usual family roles, not only those of the parents and caregivers, but also those of siblings and extended family. The care may have a major financial impact on the family, either because it is expensive or because an adult decides to give up employment outside the home in order to facilitate the provision of care.

Parents typically experience considerable stress and strong emotions when their child develops a serious health problem or is diagnosed with a developmental disorder. Parents may experience depressive symptoms, although the rates of clinical depression among parents of children with disabilities are still under debate

Commentary
Ashley's Family

Ashley's parents were a constant and supportive presence in her life from the moment of her birth. During the initial hospitalization, they alternated between elation that she was hanging on and dread that one of the many downturns she experienced could cause the tiny infant to expire. They were avid learners when the nursing staff taught them procedures for home care. They took notes about follow-up appointments and medications. Nonetheless, they felt ill prepared to support their young child with disabilities.

Ashley's mother took an extended maternity leave from her teaching position in order to visit the hospital daily and participate fully in her child's care. After the baby was home for 2 months, her mother attempted to return to work, but the numerous required health care visits took priority. She felt the need to spend more time with her older child, who had her own challenges during Ashley's prolonged neonatal hospitalization. The parents ultimately decided that it would be best for their family for Ashley's father to continue working outside the home and for her mother to concentrate on working inside the home.

The family income dropped; they struggled to meet the mortgage payments. Only a few friends or family members ever volunteered to care for Ashley to give the parents a break. The parents had little time for themselves, and they began to feel isolated and overwhelmed. When Ashley started early intervention services in a center-based program, it was a relief. When her mother went with her to the cheery center, she was able to meet other mothers of children with long-term health care needs and disabilities. These women and their children and spouses became an important part of the family's social circle. The group remained close even after the children graduated from preschool and went off to different elementary schools. The parents shared information about the availability of recreational programs and the quality of educational programs.

When Ashley entered high school, her mother was ready to return to the workforce. She accepted a position as the family advocate at the early intervention program that Ashley had attended as a toddler. She was an instant success on the job because she could truly identify with the parents whom she served. Luckily, the hours were flexible, so she could continue to drive Ashley to her many therapeutic and recreational activities. When Ashley graduated from high school, her parents joked that they too should have received a diploma for all they had learned about disability and community supports.

(Bailey, Golden, Roberts, & Ford, 2007). They may also experience fear, worry, disappointment, and guilt, even when the condition does not result from any of their own actions. Unfortunately, parent and family needs may be overlooked by professionals whose exclusive focus is the child during the evaluations (Head & Abbeduto, 2007).

Serious breakdowns in family function occur more frequently in families of children with disabilities than in the general population. Rates of child abuse and neglect are higher for children with disabilities than for children with no apparent disabilities in the United States (Hudson & Giardino, 1996) and worldwide (United Nations Secretary General's Report on Violence Against Children & Thematic Group on Violence against Disabled Children, 2005). For this reason, public programs that include home visiting and enhanced social support are important components of a comprehensive approach to children with disabilities.

While it is easy to imagine the negative impact on the family of caring for a child with severe health needs or disability, it is important to recognize that many parents also find meaning in this life experience and use successful coping strategies to mitigate the effects of stress. Ashley's mother eventually used her experiences to define a new career path for herself, one that capitalized on all that she had gone through. Research has shown that a mother's ability to perceive positive family consequences of the child's disability and to maintain higher positive emotion in their daily activities is associated with healthy family adjustment (Trute, Benzies, Worthington, Reddon, & Moore, 2010). Siblings also may experience both positive and negative reactions to their brother or sister. Surprisingly, siblings of children with severe health conditions or disabilities do not necessarily experience depression or behavior problems. Moreover, brief psychoeducational interventions can increase siblings' knowledge of the child's disorder, their feelings of connectedness to their sibling, and their perceptions of self-competence (Lobato & Kao, 2005).

The changes in family life occur within a cultural context. Different cultures have distinctive attitudes, beliefs, and practices regarding disabilities. Family members may feel enormous support from their community, or they may feel shame or guilt. Interventions that encourage positive attitudes and beliefs about disability are often as important as access to health care, support for the family, and accommodations in the environment for improving the life experience of the child and the family.

SUMMARY

Disabilities are long-term conditions that require elevated supports and services because of limitation in function or the possibility of limitations in function without adequate supports and services. Definitions vary as a function of the purpose of the definition and the underlying conceptual framework. Disability is not a distinct category but rather a continuum that affects a large portion of the population. When it occurs in childhood, disability affects not only the child but also the entire family, particularly when the family assumes responsibility for the ongoing care of the child. The situation brings stress to the family and may also bring benefits and meaning to parents, siblings, and others. The availability of high-quality supports and services within the health care system and the community brings maximal benefit to the child and to the family.

Exercises

1. Generate a list of terms that have been used to label individuals with disabilities, including the unflattering terms that are no longer unacceptable. For each term on the list, generate an acceptable and respectful alternative.
2. Think about individuals with disabilities who are well known to the public, either because they are public figures, artists, actors, or even fictional characters. How are they presented in the media or in art? How does their presentation reflect the attitudes, beliefs, and values of the culture? For example, President Franklin D. Roosevelt had mobility limitations from polio. How is he depicted in the statue in the Roosevelt Memorial in Washington, D.C.?
3. Remember individuals with disabilities whom you met early in your life. How did you get to know them? How did you become aware of their disabilities? How did you think about those individuals at the time? How did it affect their participation in your family, class, or social group? How do you think about them now?
4. Consider your own work or educational setting. From a physical and social perspective, how welcoming is the setting to individuals with disabilities? Imagine people with different kinds of disabilities; what modifications in the environment might increase their participation in this setting?
5. At the time of this writing, New York City was debating whether all new taxicabs brought into the system should be "handicap accessible." Consider arguments for and against the position.
6. Calculate the number of professionals that Ashley, in the vignette, was likely to encounter during a year when she was an infant, preschooler, and school-age child. Consider the implications of these health care visits on the child, such as attendance at school. Consider how such visits influence family life in her home.

2

Why Focus on Children with Disabilities?

Proposed Budget Cuts

In 2011, Jerry Brown had just been elected Governor of California, and the state was billions of dollars in deficit. As he looked throughout the budget to find cuts to reduce the projected deficit, he targeted In-Home Supportive Services (IHSS) and Medi-Cal, California's Medicaid program, for huge reductions. IHSS supports low-income seniors and individuals with disabilities so they can live independently in their own homes. Governor Brown proposed to reduce the number of hours recipients could receive care (or cut the pay for the providers); eliminate domestic services, such as housework, shopping, meal preparation, cleaning, and laundry; and reduce the number of individuals eligible to receive IHSS. Combined, those changes would have saved the state approximately $486 million (Disability Rights California, 2011). The proposed cuts brought to public attention the large number of recipients of these services: 436,000 individuals, most of whom are ill and/or have a disability, many of whom are elderly. Their care providers earned approximately $9–$12 an hour, a particularly low wage for regions of California with high costs of living (Disability Rights California, 2011). Several lawmakers from both major political parties quickly recognized that the proposal was short-sighted and not fiscally sound. Many people denied IHSS services would end up in hospitals and nursing homes, incurring far higher state expenses than those for in-home services. The state would quickly spend more than what it had saved on this program. Within a few months, quietly, the amount of reduction for these programs was drastically lowered. The final proposed cuts were less than one third of the original proposal (Disability Rights California, 2011).

Society at large and its representatives in government and in the media are often unaware of the number of individuals with disabilities living among us. Many people have little appreciation for the life experiences of these individuals and the role of supports and services in their lives. At critical moments, such as the 2011 California budget crisis described in the opening vignette, the public suddenly becomes aware of this population. As reflected in the vignette, knowing the number of individuals with disabilities, the supports and services they use, and the costs of these supports and services is important to public policy makers, health insurance companies, and clinicians, as well as individuals with disabilities and their families.

In this book, the focus is on children with disabilities. There are several differences between adults and children that are important to keep in mind throughout the discussion.

- A higher proportion of rare conditions among children compared with adults
- Changes in the manifestations of disability as a function of the child's age and developmental status
- Greater neural plasticity during childhood than at older ages
- The possibility of improvement in function on the basis of developmental change
- The dependency of children on their families for care and for financing
- The potential of investing in children to improve their outcomes
- The potential of investing in children to reduce future health care expenditures

This chapter describes three major reasons to focus on health care of children with disabilities: prevalence, complexity of care, and costs. Though it may seem straightforward to calculate how many children have disabilities, it is actually quite challenging. For this reason, the discussion begins with a tutorial about how data on care are gathered. Then, I describe the rates of disability among children. It is even trickier to capture the complexity of care and its costs. For this reason, the discussion includes the working assumptions that go into the estimates of cost.

Although this chapter has many facts and figures, it is far more critical to appreciate in general the methods used to generate the data and the overall trends regarding prevalence and costs than to remember the specifics. The specifics are likely to vary over time, whereas the overall patterns are likely to remain stable as long as the health care system remains unchanged. It is the trends that should inform clinical practice, public health, and public policy.

PREVALENCE

Table 2.1 shows the prevalence rates of disabilities in several developed and developing countries. It shows that developed countries have higher rates of disability than developing countries and that countries that use survey methodology have higher rates than countries that use census data. Do the variations represent differences in the actual prevalence of disability across countries or differences in how prevalence is measured? To address this issue requires considering why and how the number of individuals with disabilities within a society is calculated.

Table 2.1. Prevalence of disabilities in developed and developing countries

Based on census data			Based on data from surveys		
Country	Year	Percentage	Country	Year	Percentage
United States	2000	19.4	New Zealand	1996	20.0
Canada	2001	18.5	Australia	2000	20.0
Brazil	2000	14.5	Uruguay	1992	16.5
United Kingdom	1991	12.2	Zambia	2006	13.1
Poland	1977	10.0	Ecuador	2005	12.1
Ethiopia	1984	3.8	Nicaragua	2003	10.3
Mexico	2000	2.3	Germany	1992	8.4
India	2001	2.1	China	1987	5.0
Bangladesh	1982	0.8	Italy	1994	5.0
Kenya	1987	0.7	Egypt	1996	4.4

From Mont (2007, March). *Measuring disability prevalence* (SP Discussion Paper No. 0706). Washington, DC: The World Bank; reprinted by permission.

Reasons for Generating Prevalence Data

The prevalence rates of disability—that is, the proportion of individuals within the population who have disabilities—are key for governments, service organizations, and businesses to consider as they develop policies, programs, and products that serve this population. High prevalence rates generate a sense of urgency with regard to the development and implementation of specific policies, programs, and products. Prevalence data serve initially as baseline measures and later as outcome measures regarding such policies or programs and can be used in an iterative process of quality improvement. Variations of prevalence rates as a function of social or economic disadvantage suggest targeted efforts for reducing the rates of disability among vulnerable populations and may suggest models for improving access to care to eliminate disparities. Variations in prevalence as a function of geographic distribution may suggest environmental factors that cause or contribute to the development of disabilities.

Prevalence data allow health care, education, and social service sectors to plan for supports and services for individuals with disabilities. For example, if the prevalence of disabilities among infants and young children is on the rise, then universities need to prepare by training more teachers to support these children, and states might institute policies that encourage students to consider careers in education. If the prevalence of disability is uneven throughout a country or state, then the data enable decisions about where to deploy professionals to meet the greatest need.

Methods for Generating Prevalence Data

In the United States and many other developed or developing countries, estimating disability prevalence is very challenging. The first issue is choosing the definition of disability used to generate the prevalence figures. Broad inclusive definitions, such as that used by the Americans with Disabilities Act (ADA) of 1990 (PL 101-336), result in higher estimates of disability prevalence than narrow definitions, such as that used by the Social Security Administration (Chapter 1).

A second challenge is determining the best source of data. Medical records focus on the diseases and their treatments and not generally on the functional consequences. The presence of disability cannot be reliably inferred from a diagnosis because many conditions are associated with a wide range of functional consequence. The U.S. Department of Education tracks the number of children

Table 2.2. Prevalence of 3–5-year-old children accessing IDEA, Part B in the United States and outlying areas as a function of eligibility criteria and year, fall 2000 through fall 2005

Eligibility criterion	2000	2001	2002	2003	2004	2005
Specific learning disabilities	17,497	14,685	14,831	14,464	14,102	12,065
Speech or language impairments	309,792	302,801	316,652	331,624	333,664	330,043
Intellectual disability	24,439	23,533	22,574	22,482	22,750	22,759
Emotional disturbance	6,909	6,365	6,004	5,841	5,888	5,789
Multiple disabilities	9,746	8,235	8,538	8,491	8,452	8,515
Hearing impairments	7,751	7,240	7,237	7,490	7,849	7,846
Orthopedic impairments	10,139	9,743	9,638	9,069	8,606	8,201
Other health impairments	11,115	12,642	13,392	14,934	12,994	13,135
Visual impairments	3,320	3,118	3,130	3,261	3,328	3,424
Autism	14,064	16,252	19,108	22,872	26,056	30,305
Deafness–blindness	207	211	240	248	256	236
Traumatic brain injury	817	960	999	953	1,061	1,077
Developmental delay	184,777	213,966	225,641	239,293	257,511	260,692
All disabilities	600,573	619,751	647,984	681,022	702,517	704,087

Reprinted from U.S. Department of Education, Office of Special Education Programs, Data Analysis System (DANS). (2006). *OMB# 1820-0043: Children with disabilities receiving special education under part B of the Individuals with Disabilities Education Act, 1996–2005*. Retrieved from https://www.ideadata.org/tables29th5Car_1-9.htm

receiving special education services, all of whom have disabilities (see Table 2.2 and Table 2.3). However, these data are an underestimate of the true prevalence of disability in the child population because they count only children identified as belonging to one of 13 categories deemed by federal law as eligible for special education. In addition, public education records may miss children outside the public school system, including students in private schools, children receiving homeschooling, and adolescents who have dropped out of school.

The most accurate method for calculating prevalence of disability is simply to ask individuals directly about their life experience via census or survey questions (Mont, 2007). Using the census has the advantage that the entire population is assessed; the prevalence can be calculated and not merely estimated. However, census questions tend to be short, such as "Do you have a disability?" These questions tend to generate low rates of disability (Mont, 2007), explaining some of the variation seen in Table 2.1. Reasons for the discrepancies are subject to speculation: for some, the term *disability* may arouse feelings of shame or stigma; for others, it may connote a serious condition, different from the mild or moderate limitations they experience or see their child experience. The U.S. Census included more questions in the 2000 Census than in the 1990 Census to allow individuals to report on their functional abilities. (See the commentary on p. 23.)

Surveys typically allow longer or more detailed questions than census forms. An interviewer can follow up if a respondent does not understand a question or if

Table 2.3. Prevalence of 6–21-year-old children and youth accessing IDEA, Part B in the United States and outlying areas as a function of eligibility criteria and year, fall 2000 through fall 2005

Eligibility criterion	2000	2001	2002	2003	2004	2005
Specific learning disabilities	2,881,587	2,878,319	2,878,554	2,867,069	2,839,295	2,780,218
Speech or language impairments	1,093,436	1,093,222	1,110,858	1,128,102	1,149,573	1,157,215
Intellectual disability	613,437	605,026	591,721	582,624	567,633	545,492
Emotional disturbance	474,316	477,838	482,024	484,548	484,457	472,384
Multiple disabilities	122,946	128,724	130,819	132,746	133,366	133,914
Hearing impairments	70,810	71,225	71,962	72,002	72,599	72,387
Orthopedic impairments	72,975	73,712	73,956	68,184	65,355	63,127
Other health impairments	293,963	341,266	392,951	452,708	512,219	561,028
Visual impairments	26,004	25,836	26,079	25,875	26,058	25,996
Autism	79,586	98,589	118,846	141,140	166,491	193,637
Deafness–blindness	1,318	1,608	1,600	1,664	1,702	1,592
Traumatic brain injury	14,873	20,754	21,487	22,526	23,263	23,509
Developmental delay	28,612	45,250	58,265	66,259	74,368	79,070
All disabilities	5,773,863	5,861,369	5,959,122	6,045,447	6,116,379	6,109,569

Reprinted from U.S. Department of Education, Office of Special Education Programs, Data Analysis System (DANS). (2006). *OMB# 1820-0043: Children with disabilities receiving special education under part B of the Individuals with Disabilities Education Act, 1996–2005*. Retrieved from https://www.ideadata.org/tables29th5Car_1-9.htm

an answer is unclear or incomplete. The best survey questions focus on basic functions and social participation. As Mont (2007) pointed out, "Do you have difficulty walking?" may detect limitations in mobility caused by a wide range of conditions, including cerebral palsy, polio, amputation, heart disease, or asthma. A related question is, "Does your child have a health condition that limits him or her from

Commentary
U.S. Census Questions About Disabilities

The U.S. Census Bureau (2000) asked two questions about disability:

16. Does this person have any of the following long-lasting conditions:

- *a. Blindness, Deafness, or severe vision or hearing impairments?*
- *b. A condition that substantially limits one or more basic physical activities such as walking, climbing stairs, reaching, lifting, or carrying?*

17. Because of a physical, mental or emotional condition lasting 6 months or more, does this person have any difficulty in doing any of the following activities:

- *a. Learning, remembering, or concentrating?*
- *b. Dressing, bathing, or getting around inside the home?*
- *c. (ANSWER IF THIS PERSON IS 16 YEARS OLD OR OVER) Going outside the home alone to shop or visit a doctor's office?*
- *d. (ANSWER IF THIS PERSON IS 16 YEARS OLD OR OVER) Working at a job or business?*

attending school or performing at the level of the majority of other students?" Such questions, stated in simple and matter-of-fact terms, are unlikely to generate negative feelings in the respondents.

The survey method also has several limitations. Surveys rely on personal report without validation from other sources, such as medical or educational records. Surveys of function do not necessarily connect disability with underlying health conditions and therefore cannot contribute to understanding etiological factors. Surveys must sample a cohort from the entire population. Depending on the method, biases can be introduced. For example, if the survey contacts respondents via telephone, then anyone without a telephone is missed.

Prevalence Rates

In the United States, the Survey of Income and Program Participation (SIPP), a representative survey of the civilian, noninstitutionalized population, estimates that 54.4 million Americans, or 18.7% of the population, have a disability and that 35 million, or 12%, have a severe disability (Brault, 2008). The chance of having a disability increases with age, from less than 10% for people 15 years of age or younger, to about half of the elderly population (Kaye, 2013).

The National Health Interview Survey estimates the prevalence of any developmental disability in U.S. children ages 3–17 years old in 1997–2008 was 13.87% (Boyle et al., 2011). The prevalence of disabilities among children increased between 1999 and 2008 from 12.84% to 15.04%.

WHO estimates that, worldwide, 650 million people live with disabilities of various types. The worldwide prevalence is increasing as a result of several factors: population growth; increases in the survival of individuals with long-term conditions; survival of individuals with serious injuries, such as those due to car accidents, falls, and war; and the aging of the population. Eighty percent of the world population of individuals with disabilities, particularly children, live in low-income countries (WHO, 2011).

In summary, the rates of disability in the United States and worldwide—both in the young and in the total population—are high. Therefore, it is exceedingly important to provide outstanding policies, programs, and products and to develop effective systems of care.

COMPLEXITY

Surprisingly, no metric for the complexity of health conditions or their impact is in standard use in the health care system. Such a measure would be very useful at the clinical and public health levels. For example, if a child's health care was deemed complex by a reliable metric, then the time scheduled for a health care visit for that child could be increased over the usual time allotted to care for an otherwise healthy child. If two hospitals had very different rates of mortality or morbidity within the same service line, the complexity metric could help regulators to determine whether differences could be explained by differences in the complexity of the cases. Monitoring the complexity of care required for different groups or at different locations could also improve planning and distribution of services. Adjusting reimbursement rates for health care as a function of complexity would also be extremely useful for encouraging care providers and hospitals to assume responsibility for patients with complex needs. Reimbursement for visits or hospital stays are determined by the diagnosis and procedures only, regardless of the patient's associated health care issues, even though such issues may make additional uncompensated time with the patient necessary. The complexity measure might allow corrections in the reimbursement process.

Other fields of science have generated metrics of complexity. In computer science, complexity refers to the resources, including time, processes, or memory, required to solve problems. In engineering, complexity indicates the amounts of communication required, such as the number of gates in a circuit. In industry, complexity refers to operation times in the assembly process (Hinckley & Barkan, 1995). Individuals with disabilities utilize health care and related services to a greater extent than do individuals with no apparent disabilities. With regard to the other definitions of complexity, high utilization of services within health care is analogous to increased amounts of resources, communication, and time, all of which contribute to a higher chance of error.

Sources of Complexity

As health care providers have become increasingly specialized in Western medicine, children with disabilities have come to use a large number of different providers. For example, ophthalmologists may treat only disorders of the retina or cornea instead of the entire eye. If an individual has both a retinal detachment and cloudy cornea, that person may need to go to two different ophthalmologists who may or may not communicate with each other. Similarly, among therapists, occupational therapists may focus either on fine motor skills or on feeding disorders. So, individuals who need extensive services usually need many different health care providers, each of whom makes a relatively narrow contribution to the broad set of supports and services. The clinicians have their own offices and schedules and do not share systematic approaches to communication with one another. For these reasons, the care of individuals with disabilities is prone to fragmentation and poor coordination. (See Carly's story in the commentary on p. 26.)

A further contribution to complexity is that individuals with disabilities often experience more than one disability. Among adults with a single disability, 44% also have a second disability (Institute of Medicine, 2001). Among children with a single disability, 28% also have a second disability (Maag, 2000). Complexity increases with each additional disability; each additional condition brings its own issues and care requirements.

Evidence of Complexity

Children with extensive health care needs use a wide range of services and supports. Table 2.4 shows the proportion who need each of the various health services. Almost all of these children use medication; approximately half use subspecialty care. One in four use mental health services, and one in five use physical, occupational, or speech-language therapy.

Individuals with disabilities use health care services and supports at higher rates than those of the general population. Table 2.5 compares hospital days, physician visits, and other types of services among children with disabilities with those of children without disabilities. Some services, such as home health care, are rarely used among children without disabilities, whereas they are well utilized among children with disabilities.

Table 2.4. Diversity of health services for children with extensive health care needs

Health services	Percentage of children with special health care needs receiving the service
Prescription drugs	86.4
Preventive dental care	81.1
Routine preventive care	77.9
Specialty care	51.8
Eyeglasses/vision care	33.3
Mental health care	25.0
Other dental care	24.2
Physical, occupational, or speech therapy	22.8
Disposable medical supplies	18.6
Durable medical equipment	11.4
Hearing aids/hearing care	4.7
Home health care	4.5
Mobility aids/devices	4.4
Substance abuse treatment	2.8
Communication aids/devices	2.2

Reprinted from U.S. Department of Health and Human Services, Health Resources and Services Administration, Maternal and Child Health Bureau. (2007). *The national survey of children with special health care needs chartbook 2005–2006*. Rockville, MD: U.S. Department of Health and Human Services. Retrieved from http://mchb.hrsa.gov/cshcn05/MI/NSCSHCN.pdf

Commentary
Carly

Carly is a child with Fanconi anemia, a rare genetic disorder that affects many different organ systems. Carly averaged approximately three to four physician visits per month in her first 3 years of life. In addition, she had approximately 12 monthly visits with therapists and early intervention specialists. She saw professionals about her health and development almost every weekday. Below is a list of the medical specialists she saw in the first 3 years of her life and their role in her care. Following that is a list of the other health professionals and their roles.

Medical specialist	Role
Hematologist	Manages problems with blood
Immunologist	Monitors immune function
Infectious disease expert	Assists in choosing medication for infections
Orthopedist and hand surgeon	Plans and provides surgical correction of missing thumbs and boney abnormalities
Ear, nose, and throat specialist	Evaluates abnormal ears and hearing loss
Developmental-behavioral pediatrician	Evaluates nature and degree of developmental delays and recommends therapy and education
Endocrinologist	Evaluates short stature
Neurologist	Evaluates small head size

Other health care professionals	Role
Audiologist	Determines degree of hearing loss and fits hearing aids
Occupational therapist	Provides weekly treatment for fine motor skills
Physical therapist	Provides weekly treatment for gross motor skills
Speech-language pathologist	Creates goals and strategies to improve communication
Dietician	Adjusts caloric intake as child gains weight
Social worker	Assesses and treats parental emotional status

Table 2.5. Comparison of health care expenditures and utilization between children and youth with special health care needs and children without disabilities

Category	Children and youth with special health care needs	Children without disabilities	Comparison
Hospital days	464 days/1,000	55 days/1,000	8 times higher
Physician visits	4.6 visits/year	1.9 visits/year	2 times more
Nonphysician professional visits	3 visits/year	0.6 visits/year	5 times more
Prescriptions	6.2 medications/year	1.8 medications/year	3 times more
Home health provider days	3.8 days/year	0.04 days/year	95 times more
Health care expenditures	$2,669/year	$676/year	4 times higher
Out-of-pocket expenditures	$297/year	$189/year	1.5 times higher

From Newacheck, P.W., Inkelas, M., & Kim, S.E. (2004). Health services use and health care expenditures for children with disabilities. Pediatrics, 114(1), 79–85. doi:10.1542/peds.114.1.79. Reproduced with permission from Pediatrics, Vol. 114, Pages 79–85, Copyright © 2004 by the AAP.

Note. Secondary data analysis of the 1999 and 2000 Medical Expenditure Panel Survey, with total sample of 13,792 children younger than 18 years and overall response rate of 65.5. All comparisons are statistically significant.

Ironically, with the proliferation of subspecialists, children with disabilities and their families often cannot find general physicians or other professionals who are willing to provide routine care and play a coordinating role for them within the health care system. Without a coordinator, the care becomes even more fragmented and complex. In some cases, important issues can be missed; in others, care may be excessive. Families are often left to make sense of a vast array of conflicting information and coordinate care without any professional assistance.

Nonmedical Sources of Complexity

The sources of complexity go beyond the number of providers and services. Disabilities occur disproportionately among the poor and socially disadvantaged. Table 2.6 shows the rates of disability among racial/ethnic minorities in the adult U.S. population and demonstrates that they are highest among American Indians and Alaska Natives. Among adults with severe disability, 27.1% were living in poverty in the 2005 survey, compared with 12.1% of those with moderate disability and 9.1% of those with no apparent disability (Brault, 2008). Poverty rates are also higher among children with disabilities than among children with no disabilities (Fujiura & Yamaki, 2000). Food insecurity or hunger, public or subsistence housing,

Table 2.6. Disability among U.S. adults,[a] by race and ethnicity

Race/ethnicity	Percentage with disability
Non-Hispanic White	20.3
Non-Hispanic Black or African American	21.2
Hispanic	16.9
Asian	11.6
Native Hawaiian or other Pacific Islander	16.6
American Indian or Alaska Native	29.9

Reprinted from Centers for Disease Control and Prevention. (2008). *Racial and ethnic differences in self-related health status among adults with and without disabilities*. Atlanta, GA: Author. Retrieved from http://www.cdc.gov/features/dsdisabilityandhealthstatus/index.html

[a]Age 18 years or older.

increased exposure to violence and stress, and other adverse living conditions, often associated with poverty, compromise health status over and above the impact of disabilities. If efforts at combating even some of the ravages of poverty become part of comprehensive care for children with disabilities, then health care will include additional steps, providers, time, communication, and challenges.

COSTS

The cumulative cost of health care for individuals with disabilities is high. *Public Health Reports* found that disability-associated health care spending for U.S. adults totaled $397.8 billion in 2006, almost 27% of all such spending (Anderson, Armour, Finkelstein, & Wiener, 2010). Annual health care expenditures for children with special health care needs are three to four times higher than those for children without disabilities. Families experience higher out-of-pocket expenses as well (Newacheck & Kim, 2005).

Individuals with disabilities also use therapeutic and supportive services to a far greater extent than do individuals with no apparent disabilities (Maag, 2000). The following is a list of such services and examples of each.

- Family supports, such as social workers and respite care
- Developmental supports, including physical and occupational therapy
- Hearing and communication services, such as audiology and speech-language pathology
- Services to support everyday function, such as independent living services, transportation, or personal care attendants
- Additional medical services, such as home health services

Each unit of supportive service is not particularly expensive in itself, certainly in comparison to hospitalizations or operations. However, because these services are required on an ongoing basis, their expenses accumulate. Among children with disabilities, 40% use supportive services. Though this proportion is high, on average, another 5%–10% report unmet needs for these services (Maag, 2000).

Lifetime Financial Costs

A report prepared for the National Institute of Neurological Disorders and Strokes (NINDS; Honeycutt, Dunlap, Chen, al Homsi, Grosse, & Schendel, 2004) reported estimated lifetime costs in 2003 dollars for a child with a disability born in the year 2000, over and above lifetime costs for a child without a disability. The estimates were staggering (Table 2.7); however, these calculations are an exaggeration of out-of-pocket expenses based on several assumptions and procedures. The first major assumption in the report is that the "majority of persons with DDs (developmental disabilities) require long-term supportive care or services" (p. 57). This statement indicates that the authors focused only on those individuals with the most severe disabilities. The majority of individuals with intellectual disability are classified as having mild disability, and many live in the community without any specific supports other than informal help provided by their family and friends. Most individuals

Table 2.7. Estimated prevalence and lifetime economic costs[a] for intellectual disability, cerebral palsy, hearing loss, and vision impairment, by cost category—United States, 2003

Developmental disability	Rate[b]	Direct medical costs ($ millions)[c]	Indirect non-medical costs ($ millions)[d]	Total costs ($ millions)[e]	Average cost ($ millions)	Cost per person
Mental retardation	12.0	7,061	5,249	38,927	51,237	1,014,000
Cerebral palsy	3.0	1,175	1,054	9,241	11,470	921,000
Hearing loss	1.2	132	640	1,330	2,102	417,000
Vision impairment	1.1	159	409	1,915	2,484	566,000

Reprinted from Honeycutt A., Dunlap, L., Chen, H., al Homsi, G., Grosse, S., & Schendel, D. (2004). Economic costs associated with mental retardation, cerebral palsy, hearing loss, and vision impairment—United States, 2003. *Morbidity and Mortality Weekly Report, 53*(3), 57–59. Retrieved from http://www.cdc.gov/mmwr/preview/mmwrhtml/mm5303a4.htm#tab

[a]Present value estimates, in 2003 dollars, of lifetime costs for persons born in 2000, based on a 3% discount rate.

[b]Per 1,000 children age 5–10 years, on the basis of Metropolitan Atlanta Developmental Disabilities Surveillance Program data for 1991–1994.

[c]Includes physician visits, prescription medications, hospital inpatient stays, assistive devices, therapy and rehabilitation (for persons ages <18 years), and long-term care (for persons aged 18–76 years), adjusted for age-specific survival.

[d]Includes costs of home and vehicle modifications for persons aged ≤76 years and costs of special education for persons aged 3–17 years.

[e]Includes productivity losses from increased morbidity (i.e., inability to work or limitation in the amount or type of work performed) and premature mortality for persons aged ≤35 years with mental retardation, ages ≤25 years with cerebral palsy, and aged ≤17 years with hearing loss and vision impairment.

with cerebral palsy have milder variants that allow independent mobility. Thus, it is critical to establish exactly which children with disabilities were considered in the calculation of the estimate and the implications of those decisions on the results.

The high estimates of cost summed medical expenses, nonmedical costs, and indirect costs. It seems reasonable to add nonmedical costs because they include home modifications to accommodate wheelchairs or other assistive technology, vehicle modifications, special education programs or tutoring, and special accommodations for recreation and leisure. However, it may not be reasonable to include indirect costs in these calculations. Honeycutt et al. (2004) included estimates of "the value of productivity losses in workplaces and households that occur when persons with DDs (developmental disabilities) die prematurely, are unable to work, or are limited in the amount or type of work they can perform." It is noteworthy that indirect costs accounted for the largest percentage of total costs (range: 63%–81%). Moreover, among total direct costs, special education accounted for a substantial percentage (range: 42%–82%) for each developmental disability. Institutionalization also contributed substantially to the estimates, even though rates of institutionalization have dropped precipitously since the 1970s. These figures may therefore give a false impression of the actual health care expenditures for this population.

Paying for Health Care

The costs of health care for people with disabilities are borne largely by the public sector; in the United States, this payer is Medicaid. Approximately 68% of Medicaid spending is associated with disability. Approximately 38% of all Medicare spending is also associated with disability, as well as 12% of health care costs for those with either private insurance or no insurance (Kaiser Commission, 2011). Sadly, despite these high expenditures, studies find that people with disabilities do not receive the same level of preventive care as people without disabilities, even though preventive care tends to be less costly and may improve health outcomes for individuals with disabilities.

In the past, many children with disabilities were institutionalized shortly after the diagnosis was confirmed, and the costs of institutionalization were often borne by the public. However, as a result of deinstitutionalization, financial responsibilities have shifted to the family (Anderson, Dumont, Jacobs, & Azzaria, 2007). Surveys have found that 18% of parents reported that their child's condition caused financial problems for the family, 20% reported more than $1,000 in out-of-pocket expenditures per year, and 24% indicated that they had to reduce work hours or resign to provide care for the child or youth (U.S. Department of Health and Human Services, 2007). Although significant, these figures do not reflect the social and emotional costs of care.

SUMMARY

Individuals with disability represent a substantial proportion of the child and adult population of the United States and the world. It is important to focus on children with disabilities because of the high prevalence of disabilities, the high complexity of care with resulting potential for error, and the high costs of care. Health care costs are at least 3 to 4 times higher for children with disabilities than for children without disabilities. In the United States, medical costs are borne predominantly by the public health care insurers, Medicaid and Medicare. Medical and nonmedical costs are also borne by families. However, if health care delivery and health care systems can improve the outcomes for children with disabilities by investments when they are young, then there is a strong possibility of long-term savings in terms of human and financial costs.

Exercises

1. Examine Table 2.1. Generate possible explanations for the range of values for percentage of individuals in the different countries with disabilities.
2. Discuss how changing the questions in the U.S. Census from the 1990 Census to the 2000 Census may have influenced the results of the census.
3. What are other methods or questions to obtain estimates of the prevalence of disabilities in the United States? What are other methods to obtain estimates of health care costs for children with disabilities in the United States?
4. Discuss the following scenario: An advocacy group has been pressuring politicians in the area for a respite care program. This program will offer families the opportunity to have a trained caregiver for their child with disabilities so that they can have short-term breaks from the care. How would you decide whether to institute such a program in your region? How would you finance the program?
5. A research team has developed a promising new medication to improve cognitive function in individuals with fragile X syndrome. How do you think such advances will affect the prevalence and severity of disabilities within that group and in general?

3

What Are the Challenges in Delivering Health Care to Children with Disabilities?

Dinah

Dinah is a 4-year-old girl with a severe seizure disorder and global developmental delays. She first experienced a series of seizures at 13 months of age, at which time she was hospitalized for several days. The attending neurologists ordered extensive work-up, including an electroencephalogram to document the seizure type, blood and urine tests, and a magnetic resonance imaging (MRI) scan to determine the cause. No clear explanation for the seizures was ever found. Dinah was started on antiepileptic medications, but she continued to have intermittent seizures. After several days, she was discharged with the hope that as the medication levels in her bloodstream increased, seizure frequency would decrease. However, seizures continued at irregular intervals. The neurologists changed the medications many times and recommended changes to her diet. Nonetheless, on several occasions, Dinah was rushed to the hospital because the seizures occurred in rapid succession or lasted for more than a few minutes. Each hospital stay led to further manipulation of the care plan. Each hospital stay was also highly disruptive to her family's life. One parent remained with Dinah at all times to monitor her status and communicate with the health care team; the other tried to maintain a normal life for her two older siblings.

When she was 3 years old, Dinah's family became concerned because she had minimal verbal communication and delayed fine motor and play skills for her age. They convinced the medical team that the focus should shift from trying to control seizures to improving Dinah's developmental status and function through education. The family enrolled Dinah in a special education preschool program. In addition to active participation in the development of her individualized education program (IEP), the parents had long conversations with the teaching and therapeutic staff members about Dinah's condition. The staff took a cardiopulmonary resuscitation course. A representative of the medical team came to school to teach the teachers how to manage seizures. The parents and staff made contingency plans to be used if seizures were to persist.

Dinah did well for about 6 months. Her receptive language skills increased, and to her parents' delight, she began to communicate verbally. Then, without warning, she had a prolonged seizure at school while working one to one with a new speech-language pathologist. The frightened therapist directly called the paramedics without consulting the school principal, who knew Dinah's emergency plan. The ambulance took Dinah to a small local hospital emergency room rather than to the larger children's hospital where she usually received care. Because the emergency room doctors did not know her patient history, they administered medications and ordered procedures, most of which had proven ineffectual in the past. When the parents arrived and asked for her to be discharged, the staff ignored their requests. Repeat MRI scans and electroencephalograms were done. An expensive hospitalization ensued, on the third day of which the parents prevailed and arranged for Dinah's transfer back to her usual place of care, where she was immediately discharged as per parent request.

It took multiple attempts and many years to create a health care plan that sufficiently stabilized Dinah's condition and allowed her to attend school. She never achieved a complete remission of seizures. And yet even after all that planning, breakdowns in the carefully crafted plans took place. A new therapist was not informed about the emergency care plan, and after another seizure, Dinah was again taken to the wrong hospital. There, a new group of doctors, meeting her in the emergency room and unfamiliar with her case, treated her as a child with an acute problem. They probably felt a need to act quickly and did not ask whether there was a care plan before proceeding with their management. Rather, they set in place a plan that developed momentum and continued on even after her parents arrived. Dinah underwent tests that she really did not need, that had been done in the past, and that would not have been expected to change her condition. Her parents' efforts to stop this process were not heeded. Dinah's case demonstrates the challenges of creating and maintaining an appropriate and well-coordinated health care plan for a child with a long-term health condition and accompanying disabilities.

Although medical care for children with disabilities advanced dramatically in the second half of the 20th century, health care delivery systems have not progressed at the same pace (Institute of Medicine & Committee on Quality of Health Care in America, 2001). This chapter explores challenges in delivering effective and efficient health care to children with disabilities. Although there are many interacting issues leading to these challenges, three main features not well suited to the care of children with disabilities are discussed:

- The emphasis of clinical encounters is often on establishing the appropriate diagnosis (a diagnostic focus), whereas the emphasis should be on taking care of the children after diagnosis (a management focus).

- The main objective of health care is often improving clinical indicators, such as the frequency or duration of seizures, whereas for children with disabilities, the main objectives of their families are functional outcomes, such as improvements in learning, communicating, self-care, and interacting with others.
- Health care interventions are often directed solely at the individual with the condition, whereas effective interventions may include changes in the physical, social, or service environment.

Many children with disabilities have significant unmet health care needs, and the services and supports they receive may not be the most useful for helping them successfully manage disability. At the same time, as in the case of Dinah, children with disabilities may receive excessive care that increases risks and expenses. It is necessary, then, to change the nature of health care delivery to improve outcomes for children with disabilities and their families.

SHIFTING FROM A DIAGNOSTIC TO A MANAGEMENT FOCUS

The hallmark of Western, or allopathic, medicine is the attempt to connect symptoms and signs of illness to an underlying cause for the disorder. In many cases, such as acute infectious diseases, the underlying diagnosis dictates the treatment plan. When the most common bacteria associated with the infection are known, then simply diagnosing the infection, such as an ear infection, can lead to selection of the right antibiotic. When many possible bacteria might be the cause, the infection is cultured and the bacteria identified in order to make the best choice of antibiotics.

The Western medical model continues to put considerable focus on establishing an accurate diagnosis in order to choose the appropriate treatment. That approach is on display weekly in the *New York Times* Sunday magazine. There is often a challenging medical case in which the individual presents with unusual findings. A physician or series of doctors embark on a carefully choreographed set of procedures, from obtaining a comprehensive history to careful examination of the patient and review of diagnostic tests. In the newspaper, the process, even if protracted, is typically successful in determining the cause. Eventually, the disparate findings gel into a cohesive understanding of the underlying cause of disease findings, and the appropriate treatment is offered. In the idealized Western medical model, the appropriate treatment restores the individual to good health.

In cases of children with disabilities, diagnosis may be elusive. In the opening vignette, many tests for possible genetic, metabolic, or neurologic abnormalities failed to determine why Dinah developed seizures. Even when an underlying cause can be determined, it does not necessarily dictate the treatment approach. For example, the evaluation of a child with seizures may detect a genetic explanation for the disorder. However, there may be no medication currently available that can correct the genetic defect or the abnormal proteins it expresses that result in epilepsy. A magnetic resonance imaging (MRI) scan may show a scar from a prenatal neural injury, a cause for which there is no specific treatment other than what is used generally to manage seizures. So, as in Dinah's case, the treatment is often directed toward the clinical signs and symptoms—the seizures—and not the underlying condition.

Even if the diagnosis is clear, health care for children with disabilities and other long-term conditions must shift away from obsessive investigations of underlying causes to actively taking care of the whole child. This comprehensive care of a person fits under the rubric of management focus. Focusing on management is a challenge for the Western medical model (Institute of Medicine & Committee on Quality of Health Care in America, 2001) because comprehensive plans must consider many diverse issues beyond the cause of the condition. Management often requires understanding the natural course of a condition and where the individual is within that progression. If a condition is likely to improve over time, then management may be conservative. If the condition is likely to deteriorate over time, then management must anticipate adverse events. In the care of children, management plans require consideration of the child's age and the circumstances of the family. For example, management of seizures is different at different ages. If a young child experiences seizures, the treating professionals in consultation with the family may decide to postpone treatment because the child is almost always in the company of adults, and thus would be safe if another seizure unexpectedly occurred. If an older child or adolescent experiences seizures, the team may begin treatment to reduce the risk of recurrence because the child is frequently in the community, where safety may be compromised if another seizure unexpectedly occurred.

Creating a management plan for children with long-term illness or disability requires active collaboration among many members of the health care team, including the family, the child, and others in the community (Institute of Medicine & Committee on Quality of Health Care in America, 2001). A physician in isolation may be able to complete a diagnostic work-up and choose the appropriate treatment for an acute medical problem. However, given the complexity of issues surround disability, creating and implementing a management plan requires a team.

The introduction of practice guidelines has supported the creation of comprehensive management plans for many disabilities. *Practice guidelines*, as the name implies, are recommendations regarding the care of a patient, in our case, a child with a specific disability. They are also called *best practices* or *recommended practices*. The recommendations are typically generated from a systematic review of the literature or, when evidence is not available, from the prevailing opinions of a panel of experts. Thus, they are evidence based, or at least scientifically motivated. They include a list of assessments or procedures that should be performed at specific intervals, and they may indicate how to proceed if the tests prove positive. Importantly, practice guidelines consider the broad sweep of issues that may arise in treating children with disabilities, including aspects of their functional profile, such as learning abilities, communication abilities, and emotional characteristics. Practice guidelines are available from professional societies for several disabilities. Here are a few examples:

- ADHD (Subcommittee on Attention-Deficit/Hyperactivity Disorder, 2011)
- Down syndrome (Bull & the Committee on Genetics, 2011)
- Neurofibromatosis (Ferner et al., 2007)
- Williams syndrome (Committee on Genetics, 2001)

The major advantage of practice guidelines is that they standardize an approach to the comprehensive management of the disability. They also reduce the chances that important health care issues will be missed or that unnecessary procedures will be done. They have therefore been highlighted in models to improve the delivery of long-term care (Improving Chronic Illness Care, 2011). The major criticism of practice guidelines is that they force the health care team to treat all individuals in the same manner, regardless of individual differences in the health condition, the patient's environmental circumstances, or the patient or family preference. In principle, practice guidelines should be sufficiently clear about when they can be overridden by clinical judgment. For example, they are often limited to a specific patient category. The practice guidelines for children with ADHD published by the American Academy of Pediatrics (AAP; Subcommittee on Attention-Deficit/Hyperactivity Disorder, 2011) cover children 4–18 years of age and should not be applied to those children less than 4 years old. The same guidelines recommend monitoring treatment success by using behavior questionnaires completed by parents and teachers. The guidelines, by necessity, must be modified for children who are home-schooled. Ideally, practice guidelines should allow sufficient flexibility to accommodate individual circumstances and needs. In the ADHD guidelines, the clinician must choose target outcomes for treatment in collaboration with parents, teachers, and if possible the child him or herself. The guidelines do not dictate the goals of management, allowing flexibility and individuation. Finally, the health care team should be able to vary their procedures in individual cases as long as they can justify the decision.

SHIFTING FROM CLINICAL TO FUNCTIONAL IMPROVEMENT

Once a management plan is created, possibly using practice guidelines, how is progress monitored? The usual medical approach is to establish clinical indicators that can be assessed at appropriate intervals. For example, in the management of diabetes, blood studies serve as a clinical indicator of how well the patient was able to control his or her blood sugar over the preceding several weeks. In the practice guidelines for Down syndrome, regular measurement of height and weight serve as a clinical indicator of nutritional and endocrine status.

In the care of children with disabilities, clinical indicators are often inadequate to assess the success of the management plan. Because disability is defined in large part as the impact of a health condition on function, the most important indicators are often functional measures. In Dinah's case from the opening vignette, functional measures might include assessments of her speech and language skills, whereas clinical indicators might include seizure frequency. Both kinds of information are important in evaluating the management plan and should therefore be monitored on a regular basis. If a medication reduces seizure frequency and also slows the development of speech and language skills, then the team, including the parents, needs to make tough decisions about how to proceed.

Addressing function issues is often relegated to specific professionals on the health care team. Physicians and the medical system, on one hand, tend to monitor clinical measures, aiming for cure or symptom reduction. Therapists, educators, and social workers, on the other hand, are far more likely than physicians to assess function. Unfortunately, information about the child's functional status is often divorced from information about the child's clinical status. Physicians, who focus on clinical issues, may work in different settings than therapists and educators, who focus on functional outcomes. They each establish their own treatment objectives without necessarily coordinating their efforts with the rest of the team. In such cases, ongoing monitoring and revisions of clinical plans proceed with an incomplete and uncoordinated data set. For example, the clinical indicators might suggest improvement after addition of a new medication, such as a reduction in seizure frequency or duration, whereas the functional indicators suggest deterioration, such as increased fatigue and somnolence. A clinician looking at only one set of indicators or measures might choose a plan that is inappropriate. A team that looks at both sets of measures and tries to understand the discrepancy is likely to choose a better approach. Therefore, shifting the objectives of health care from a clinical to functional improvement may demand greater levels of coordination than does an exclusive focus on clinical improvement.

EXPANDING FROM CONVENTIONAL TO ENVIRONMENTAL INTERVENTIONS

Table 3.1 reviews the features of the medical model of disability. Because disability resides solely within the individual as a function of the health condition, the major interventions are clinical in nature and are delivered at the individual level, such as medications, surgery, and therapy. This table also reviews the rehabilitation model of disability that is similar to the medical model, with the exception of a focus on function rather than disorder.

The social model stands in sharp contrast to the medical model. In the social model, the limitations in function result from the interactions of the individual with the external world and/or society. The social model emphasizes that disability is due to barriers in the environment rather than defects within the individual. The barriers could be physical, such as a lack of ramps at the entrance to buildings; attitudinal, such as prejudices of employers; or policy based, such as explicit exclusion of individuals with disabilities from housing or employment. If the environment could be accessible with accommodations and supports, and if society could set aside negative stereotypes about people with disabilities, then, according to this view, individuals would not experience limitations. Therefore, the major interventions for disability in the social model are at the societal level. They may include policies to implement universal design in building construction so that all buildings are readily accessible, or community awareness campaigns to combat prejudice. Table 3.1 also includes features of the social model.

WHO offers a view of disability that integrates the medical and social models (WHO, 2011). In this integrated model, disability is a complex phenomenon, reflecting an interaction between features of a person's body and features of the society in which he or she lives. Individuals are not determined to have a disability solely on the basis of their medical condition but rather as a combination of health conditions, environmental factors, and personal factors. The integrated model is often more appropriate for the care of children with disabilities because it pulls together elements from the medical and social models as needed for specific issues at specific times (Table 3.1).

Adoption of the integrated model of disability diversifies the interventions that children with disabilities may receive. In some cases, the best course of action may

Table 3.1. Features of disability within the medical, social, and integrated models

Feature	Medical model	Social model	Integrated model
Cause of the disability	Medical conditions	Social and environmental barriers	The interaction of a person's body and the social conditions of the society in which the person lives
Focus	Deficits	Strengths and assets	Strengths and needs
Terminology	Impairment = long-term or permanent loss of sensory, physical, or mental function	Disablement = limitation of opportunities to take part in the normal life of the community due to physical and social barriers	Limitations of activity of daily living and restrictions in social participation
Target for change	Individual	Society	Individual, community, and society
Goal of treatment	Prevention or cure	Improved functioning; greater social, educational, or economic opportunities for participation	Inclusion within the community and society; contribution as appropriate to age, developmental level, and ability; health
Ultimate decision maker, those with power to effect change	Physician, medical care team, and other professionals	Individual or family plus community	Individual or the family, with active support and input from the interdisciplinary professional and community team
Nature of the interventions	Medication, surgery, or prescribed therapy	Voluntary supports, resources, laws, and regulations	Medication, surgery, or therapy; voluntary supports, services, and anything that works
Results	Dependency, low self-esteem	Independence or interdependence, high self-worth	Inclusion, contribution, interdependence, high self-worth

Sources: Rieser (2000); Camilleri (2003).

prove to be medication, surgery, or therapy, interventions directed at the individual with the condition. For example, in the management of seizures, medications are effective at reducing seizure frequency and long-term complications of uncontrolled seizures. However, in other cases, the best course of action may be changes to the environment. For example, in the management of seizures, adaptations to the physical environment may improve the child's safety when an unexpected seizure occurs. Other interventions may include supports and services that provide the child with opportunities for functional improvement or parents the opportunities for social support. For children with severe and/or long-standing disabilities, clinical management over time may require a spectrum of services, from intense long-term hospital treatment to intermittent service within community settings. In Dinah's case, the management plan included special education services with the goal of improving her communication and learning and environmental preparations to ensure her safety.

Depending on the needs of the child and family, management may also include recreational activities and social opportunities within the community. Health care and educational professionals need not deliver all of the interventions of a comprehensive management plan. Contributors to the plan may include neighbors, coaches, or religious leaders. There are many advantages to capitalizing on the natural environment of the child, or natural supports for the family, in designing the management plan. These resources may persist over time as the child's situation evolves, whereas doctors, therapists, and teachers may change over time. Natural supports may be close to home, relatively inexpensive, and important for the development of identity and self-concept, as well as for improving health or functional status.

In a comprehensive management plan, the target of intervention may not even be the child or patient but rather the environment. For example, consider a school-age boy with cerebral palsy who begins to show increasing difficulty with gait. What interventions would be appropriate to restore him back to his highest level of function? If an evaluation uncovers that an important factor in his regression is a growth spurt and increasing muscle stiffness, then an increase in therapy or surgery to release tight tendons may prove the best plan. However, if an assessment reveals that regression began after budget cuts led to a reduction in the number of hours of physical therapy he was receiving, then surgery may be ill advised, at least until after physical therapy hours are restored. If regression relates to his lack of access to physical exercise and activity, then the plan may include increasing his opportunities to move. Some examples are as follows:

- Encouraging him to go to the neighborhood park on a daily basis
- Providing him with an extra gym class
- Giving him the task at school of delivering mail to each of the classrooms
- Giving him the job at home of walking his dog with his neighbor
- Enrolling him in a sports team or gym

If his regression was associated with a lack of follow-through on recommendations for a home program because of the parents' work schedules, then the management plan might involve finding alternatives or identifying resources to substitute for parents in reinvigorating the home program. In creating a comprehensive management plan, multiple factors must be simultaneously considered, some of which are found within the child and some within the environment.

EXPANDING AND COORDINATING THE HEALTH CARE TEAM

As the goals of management expand from clinical indicators to functional status and as the interventions expand from patient focused to environmental, the health care team involved in the management of long-term illness and disability must expand accordingly. In addition to the person and/or family, the team might include professionals from nursing, psychology, physical therapy, occupational therapy, speech-language pathology, clinical dietetics, audiology, and social work. The team may also include representatives of community-based resources and services that work with the child and family. The team can also think creatively about the informal supports in the child and family's world— a neighbor with shared interests in dogs, the local scouts leader, the family's religious leader—who may be able to help the child to join in the social life of his peers and community. (See the commentary on p. 39.)

The child and family may also need a wide range of indirect services, such as transportation services and respite care. Of course, the family and the child are also members of the team.

With a broad and diverse set of professionals and nonprofessionals involved in the treatment of a child with disabilities, coordination of care becomes extremely difficult. Health care has not established a standard definition of care coordination or a theoretical foundation for how care coordination should be approached. These issues are covered in greater depth in Chapter 10. Here, suffice it to say that in the past, many programs for children with disabilities were carried out by interdisciplinary teams that met concurrently. They often had a planning meeting to discuss patients before the clinic session and a case conference at the end of the session. By the conclusion of the final meeting, the various perspectives were fused into a single, multifaceted understanding of the child and family, and a comprehensive set of recommendations could be offered. Since the mid-1990s, many of the interdisciplinary teams have been disbanded, and care conferences have been abandoned because of strong financial pressures. It has become almost impossible to call together a meeting with representatives of all of the services and supports that a child and family use, especially if those supports include education, community-based social service, and natural supports. Accordingly, there is no consensus about goals, strategies, or monitoring. It is often unclear which professional or organization is responsible for which part of the management plan, and the care is highly fragmented.

As a result of these challenges, families often find themselves in the role of care coordinator. Their success at the role is based on their understanding of the child's condition and its treatments, their organizational skills, their communication and advocacy skills, financial resources, and other factors that tend to exacerbate disparities across children and families. For example, an uncoordinated approach to the number and scheduling of required clinical visits and treatments often is extremely burdensome for families. Complexity compromises the family's ability to adhere to clinical recommendations and interferes with everyday family life.

Commentary
Informal Supports

The attention to function in the health care of children with disabilities is ultimately to foster their involvement in community and their potential for contribution. Opportunities to work and play within the community are often the best way to achieve the goal. Informal or natural support networks build on relationships, shared interests, and regular contact. Informal support may come from neighbors, friends, coaches, teammates, classmates, relatives, and coworkers. For individuals without apparent disabilities, the informal network is the main source of social support. It would be great if that were the case for children with disabilities as well. Informal supports can provide opportunities, advice, and resources within the context of nonhierarchical and mutually beneficial relationships. Health care professionals must be cautious not to co-opt and professionalize all of a child's informal supports. In the end, if all of a child's relationships represent formal supports, provided through agencies and service organizations, then health care has defeated its primary purpose.

UNMET NEEDS

The net result of all of these challenges is that children's health care needs are often not adequately met (Table 3.2). The high prevalence of unmet needs can be found in several interview studies. For example, using the 2001 National Survey of Children with Special Health Care Needs, researchers found that in Massachusetts, 17% of the children with extensive long-term needs and 37% of those more severely affected reported unmet needs. Sadly, children with either high levels of functional limitations and unstable health status were about 3 times more likely to experience unmet needs than children with mild functional limitations or stable health status (Hill, Freeman, Yucel, & Kuhlthau, 2008). Among children born preterm, families also report high levels of unmet needs, especially for occupational therapy, physical therapy, speech-language pathology services, and early intervention (Hintz et al., 2008). These data demonstrate the importance families place on therapeutic and educational services that are likely to improve their children's functional status.

Dental care remains the most frequently cited unmet health need for children with elevated health care needs. Although they find it difficult to access routine preventive dental care, they have even more difficulty obtaining dental surgeries and other required treatments. Even among children with elevated health care needs, there are significant disparities in who receives adequate dental care. Adolescents; those who are poor, uninsured, or had insurance lapses; and those severely affected by their condition were the most likely to have unmet dental care needs (Lewis, 2009).

Substantial numbers of children with special health care needs also have unmet needs for mental health care services (Ganz & Tendulkar, 2006). Similar to the needs for dental care, those children who were poor, uninsured, and were without a usual source of care were significantly more likely to report unmet mental health care needs than those with more financial resources. In addition to those most severely affected by their disability, children with emotional, developmental, or behavioral conditions were also statistically significantly more likely to have unmet mental health needs. Families of severely affected children and of children with emotional, developmental, or behavioral conditions were also significantly more likely to report that their own mental health care needs went unmet. Unmet mental health needs compromise the family's ability to provide adequate support and service to their child.

Table 3.2. Examples of unmet service needs among children with special health care needs or disabilities

Service needed	Source
Family planning and reproductive health	Kaiser Family Foundation (2013)
Health insurance coverage	DeVoe, Ray, Krois, & Carlson (2010)
Medical or subspecialty care	Newacheck et al. (2000); Mayer et al. (2004)
Medications or eyeglasses	Newacheck et al. (2000)
Neurodevelopmental and behavioral health	Hintz et al. (2008)
Oral health and dental care	Kaiser Family Foundation (2012)
Occupational therapy, physical therapy	Hintz et al. (2008)
Social worker	Hintz et al. (2008)
Speech-language pathology services	Hintz et al. (2008)
Visiting nurse	Hintz et al. (2008)

In addition to direct medical services, families report a high prevalence of unmet indirect medical services. In particular, almost one quarter of families reported unmet needs for respite care. Responsibility for the care of children with disabilities has shifted from state institutions to families with deinstitutionalization (Chapter 1). When the child's needs are high, parents may be on call virtually every moment the child is at home. The parents' ability to remain caring and vigilant may suffer if they cannot get a break. However, the rates of unmet needs for respite are highest among the families of the most medically unstable children (Nageswaran, 2009; see the commentary below).

As suggested in the previous descriptions, many financial and sociodemographic factors are associated with having unmet health care needs. In the United States, health care services are better for those children who have health insurance than those who do not. Those children who become uninsured at any time are many times more likely to experience an unmet need than those insured continuously. In the 2005–2006 National Survey of Children with Special Health Care Needs, 62% of children nationally had continuous health insurance, up modestly from 2001 (Honberg et al., 2009). This study found that children with special health care needs were more likely to be insured than children without elevated needs, but they were less likely to be adequately insured (Honberg et al., 2009). Children who did not have health insurance were more likely to have unmet needs than those who did, and their families were likely to experience financial problems (Honberg et al., 2009).

Sociodemographic factors are also associated with unmet medical needs. Among children with elevated health care needs, sociodemographic risk factors

Commentary
Health Insurance as an Unmet Need

As employer-based insurance coverage for children has declined, coverage from public forms of insurance has increased. However, despite the availability of public coverage via Medicaid and the Children's Health Insurance Plan (or CHIP), many children do not have adequate health insurance coverage (Newacheck, Halfon, & Inkelas, 2000).

The National Survey of Children with Special Health Care Needs assessed the type of insurance held by children with special needs: 59% had solely private insurance provided by an employer, union, or directly from an insurance company; 28% had solely public insurance; 7% had a combination of private and public insurance; 4% were uninsured; and 2% had various forms of comprehensive coverage (U.S. Department of Health and Human Services, 2007). A comparison of the study in 2005–2006 with a previous version in 2001 demonstrated the decrease in the proportion of children and youth with special health care needs who had private insurance. In addition, two thirds of parents of children and youth with special health care needs thought that their child's coverage was adequate, but one third thought coverage was usually or always inadequate (U.S. Department of Health and Human Services, 2007). The adequacy of insurance coverage varied by the type of insurance. Given the high cost of medical services (Chapter 13), inadequate health insurance is tantamount to inadequate medical care.

course together. Children from a home where English is not the primary language are significantly more likely to be Hispanic or non-European American, be poor, have less educated parents, and reside in larger households, but less likely to receive cash assistance from welfare. Logistic regression showed that children with elevated needs who are from non-English primary language families were twice as likely to lack access to a medical home, a usual source of care, and family-centered care. They were 4 times as likely to lack health insurance, and their family members were also more likely to lack adequate insurance. Family members of these children were almost twice as likely to have to stop employment as a result of their child's condition (Yu, Singh, Yu, & Singh, 2009).

REDUNDANT AND UNNECESSARY CARE

Ironically, at the same time that many children with disabilities and their families have unmet needs, they may also receive redundant or unnecessary care. Health care providers are often unaware of what others who are providing care have recommended. Children, like Dinah in the opening vignette, get repeat diagnostic workups because one group of physicians cannot access the information that another group of physicians ordered or do not trust results from another institution. Families often understandably seek a second opinion regarding their child's condition. However, some families also seek a third or fourth opinion. Although additional information or a different perspective may be warranted in many cases, families often receive limited guidance about how to integrate all of the information they

Commentary
Clinical Pearls for Obtaining History

Obtaining a history from the family of a child with disabilities can be very time consuming, particularly for children who have received considerable treatment for their condition. Developmental-behavioral pediatrics programs routinely request parents complete an intake questionnaire prior to their first visit. The questionnaire asks information about the child's past medical problems and previous health care visits. Review of the questionnaire allows the team to focus on the most relevant information.

In addition to factual information, professionals often need to know what families understood from other professionals and their impressions about previous health care. This information may be particularly pertinent when families seek a second opinion or shift care to a new provider. One straightforward strategy to gather this information is to ask the parent to recount the history of medical visits in order. For each previous evaluation or treatment, ask the following: 1) Who did you see? 2) What did they do? 3) What did you think about what they did?

It is important to receive the information without any judgment. Parents have told me that they did not trust the previous doctor's diagnosis because he or she did not examine the child carefully. They have confided that they did not believe the professional because the information conflicted with what a family member had said. The information allows the treating professional to avoid previous problem areas while serving the child and family.

gather or how to choose among competing perspectives. Their persistent seeking of additional opinions may indicate a general problem within the health care system, such as the lack of a trusted professional who can answer all of their questions, investigate the reasons that the family remains unsatisfied, or coordinate care across different systems. (See the commentary on p. 42.)

Unnecessary care also results from failure to establish clear treatment goals or a thoughtful plan to meet each of the goals. Health care and education goals are often completely separate. Occupational therapists in both settings may be working on the same treatment goals, resulting in redundancy but not necessarily improved outcomes. Even within the health care sector, the problem is exacerbated when members of the treatment team are in different organizations or agencies. There may be good communication among the professionals within one organization but limited communication across organizations.

As service and supports are added to a care plan, ensuring compatibility becomes a key issue. Specific combinations of medications cannot be administered at the same time because together they are either not safe or not effective. Pharmacists become the gatekeepers, using integrated databases to ensure that potentially dangerous combinations of medications are not prescribed. No equivalent professional reliably monitors other aspects of treatment to ensure compatibility and safety. A speech-language pathologist at school may be working toward very different goals using different strategies than the speech-language pathologist in the health care system. The parents are often unable to evaluate whether this situation is positive, allowing a wider range of issues to be addressed in therapy, or negative, diluting the effect of each approach. Though probably not as lethal as the wrong combinations of medications, conflicting recommendations for therapy or behavior management can arise and compromise the child's care.

SUMMARY

Challenges to delivering comprehensive health care to children with disabilities include the diagnostic focus, reliance on assessment of clinical indicators rather than functional status, and the use of a medical model when an integrated model would expand the range of interventions to include increased services and supports and changes to the environment. The challenges lead to both unmet needs and unnecessary duplication of services. In order to address these shortcomings, we need a new paradigm that includes focusing on function, integrating care plans, carefully coordinating care, and empowering families and children. However, the first step is establishing the broad priorities for health care for children with disabilities and their families. It is to these priorities that the discussion now turns.

Exercises

1. Interview the family of a child with disabilities. Identify unmet needs such as problems getting health promotion advice, dental care, or mental health services. Identify examples of care that the family may now think were excessive.
2. Discuss strategies for meeting the unmet needs of the family interviewed.

3. Investigate strategies for care coordination. Who could serve as the care coordinator for the family you interviewed?
4. Communication systems among health care professionals are often poorly developed or poorly implemented. How could you redesign your notes to facilitate communication with the family and across the health care team?
5. Many interventions in health care have possible adverse side effects. How do we discuss the complexity of these situations with families and children? How can open communication reduce complexity without increasing parental anxiety?

II

Goals of Health Care for Children with Disabilities

4

Inclusion

The Making of an Inclusion Advocate

Liz did not set out to champion inclusion. In fact, in the early days after Bevin was born, she was intently focused simply on keeping her daughter alive. As she put it, "Life was a big struggle for a long time." Then, at some point, she had the growing realization that there was "no point to living unless you have a life."

Bevin was a child with complex disabilities and medical needs. As an infant, she was able to receive what was then called infant stimulation services, even though she was born before federal legislation supported services for children from birth to age 3 years. It surprised Liz that, when Bevin got too old for early intervention, the same organizations that had served her as an infant and toddler rejected her for their preschool programs. The most painful reason they offered was, "We only admit children who have a strong rehabilitation potential."

Fortunately, by then federal law required that all children age 3–21 years receive a free appropriate public education in accordance with their needs. With few other options available, an education official agreed that Bevin, though still a preschooler, could attend the public program for school-age children with severe physical and medical disabilities. The school shared the parking lot with another elementary school for typically developing children. Buses arrived at the same location, and one group of children went left, the other right. Liz began to wonder whether the two populations of children could intermix at least some of the time, using the same classrooms, sharing the same cafeteria, or playing together on the playground. She realized that if she had to fight to get her child a spot in a school designed for children with disabilities, she might as well push for a spot in a regular elementary school. As these ideas began to coalesce into a cohesive philosophy, she got elected as the parent representative for the three segregated schools for children with disabilities within the district. She could use this platform to advocate for inclusion.

Several key contacts and experiences increased her confidence in her position. At the suggestion of a progressive teacher, she joined TASH, an organization that promotes inclusion of individuals with severe disabilities in all areas of community life. She became a parent representative to a federally funded project called the Developmental Support Project that devised ways to provide education and therapy to children requiring prolonged hospitalizations. She met like-minded professionals and parents whose work cross-fertilized her efforts. She became cleverer and more insistent about strategies to bring children of all abilities together.

Liz recognized that systems change comes slowly, yet even she was surprised by the intransigence of the education system. At one point, she devised a strategy to get the students from the segregated schools included in neighborhood programs. She pointed out to district officials that students in the special education program attended school throughout the summer. Their old segregated school building was not air-conditioned, and the windows could not be opened to let in fresh breezes. She argued that temperatures became dangerously high during the summer. But the school district remained so resistant to inclusion that they air-conditioned the building rather than support an integrated summer program.

Undaunted, Liz pushed to the next level. She ran for the school board and was elected for two terms. She won by linking the issues of children with disabilities to the issues of others in the community, including senior citizens. She became a fierce advocate for her beliefs. As a member of the school board, she managed to move inclusion further and further.

After two terms, it was time for a different approach. Liz now heads The Parent Education & Advocacy Leadership Center, established in October 2005, an organization of parents of children with disabilities that reaches out to assist professional providers as well as other parents of children with disabilities. The center serves 43 counties in central and western Pennsylvania, with a focus on education and community supports.

Bevin completed high school and attended some college classes. She continues to live with her parents. Because she uses a ventilator to support her breathing, she needs a constant companion. She has a nurse with her during the day while her parents work. Liz continues to avoid the segregated programs for her daughter. Rather than participate in a sheltered workshop or adult day care program, Bevin spends her days with her nurse in the community, visiting friends, frequenting museums, participating in a walking group, and attending concerts.

Our health care systems and society at large have reached a stage at which the paradigm for health care and disabilities requires explicit and radical reform. For many health care clinicians, the primary purpose of health care for children with disabilities is simply to improve their health status. These clinicians treat children in the hopes that they will achieve stable or even good health, often defined in terms of clinical indicators such as seizure frequency or oxygen saturation. If the children are healthy, then they can be afforded opportunities to participate in selected programs such as special education or, later in their lives, sheltered workshops. If the children with disabilities succeed in those special programs, then they earn the opportunity to be included in settings for children or adults with no apparent disabilities, such as regular education or competitive employment. This book proposes to turn this paradigm on its head.

The three pillars of the approach proposed here are inclusion, contribution, and health, in that order. Health care must function in the service of inclusion and contribution. The ultimate goal of health care is that individuals be able to participate actively and fully in their community of family, friends, neighbors, classmates, co-workers, and society at large. This chapter discusses inclusion and why it has primacy in the triad of goals; Chapters 5 and 6 turn to contribution and health, respectively.

THE MEANING OF INCLUSION

Inclusion is a word that often engenders strong feelings and intense debates among self-advocates, families, clinicians, educators, and policy makers. Many debates hinge on the particular definition of inclusion. For the purposes here, inclusion is defined very broadly: *Inclusion* is a fundamental guarantee that individuals with disabilities will receive all of the rights, privileges, and protections of the society at large. Inclusion is not the placement of a child in a particular setting such as a neighborhood school or regular education classroom; it does not refer to any particular type of activity such as competitive employment. It is definitely not a political tool. Inclusion covers many different elements of everyday life. It can be characterized as follows:

- The state of being welcome and included in the broad social network of family, friends, and fellow citizens
- Living life with full human dignity
- Enjoying equality of opportunity and possibility
- Maintaining the prospect of making meaningful contributions to society

This is the definition of inclusion that motivated Liz in the opening vignette.

THE HISTORICAL CONTEXT

Inclusion is the culmination of a long historical development that moved individuals with disabilities from invisibility to social presence and from neglect and abuse to full human rights. Prior to the Enlightenment of the late 1700s and early 1800s, disability was entirely a personal or family issue. In the best scenarios, children with disabilities lived with their families and were assigned roles and responsibilities in line with their capabilities. In the worst scenarios, maltreatment was rampant and social protections nonexistent. Infanticide was not uncommon; children were abandoned by families who understood that if the children survived, they might end up in slavery or prostitution; individuals with intellectual disability might be sold to the rich for amusement (Kanner, 1964). Even advocates for the poor and disadvantaged often ended up supporting institutionalization. For example, in many cultures disabilities have been interpreted from a religious or metaphysical perspective, for example, as divine retribution for sins in the immediate or ancestral past.

Within this belief system, children with disabilities became constant reminders of an unspecified transgression and sources of shame. These beliefs reinforced misunderstanding, isolation, and maltreatment.

During the Enlightenment, a new social philosophy reframed basic concepts of human experience and human worth. Humanism gave value to all individuals, including children and adults with disabilities. A dominant philosophical tenet was the redemptive power of work. During the Enlightenment, medical practitioners began to take on the challenge of treating individuals with disabilities. The famous physician, Jean Marc Gaspard Itard, was one of these pioneers; he attempted the rehabilitation of the Wild Boy of Aveyron, a child who, according to legend, was raised in the woods by animals but who was more likely a child with autism abandoned by his parents (Plucker, 2012). The goal of the Enlightenment physicians was normality, the cure of intellectual deficits, and a restored ability to contribute to society through work.

With limited understanding of the causes of intellectual deficits, these well-meaning physicians had few therapeutic options. They believed that intensive instruction could be enhanced through exposure to fresh air, natural beauty, and healthy diets. In this spirit, they oversaw the construction of spacious residential educational centers in beautiful mountain settings. Unfortunately, even ideal educational programs and serene natural environments could not counter the consequences of many medical conditions that limit intellectual function. For example, in the 1700s and 1800s, cretinism, untreated congenital deficiency of thyroid hormones, was endemic, particularly in inland communities. The physicians of the time recognized the telltale signs of short stature and intellectual disability but did not yet know that cretinism was caused by a lack of iodine that led to failure of the thyroid gland to produce the hormones that promote physical growth and cognitive development. Individuals with untreated congenital hypothyroidism were among those admitted to the institutions for intensive habilitation. They were not substantially changed. When the centers failed to deliver the promise of cured citizens, they quickly evolved from educational or rehabilitation programs to crowded, custodial institutions that promoted segregation and social control (Kanner, 1964). In the 1800s, Dorothea Dix was a tireless crusader for individuals who were poor and insane. She found widespread appalling abuse in U.S. state systems that had been devised to care for these individuals, and her solution was the creation of state hospitals or asylums.

In the second half of the 19th century, such residential institutions flourished throughout Western Europe and America. However, as social Darwinist beliefs spread, attitudes toward institutionalization began to shift. The prevailing belief became that individuals with disabilities were a negative influence on the human race—a menace—and should not procreate or participate in community life. Many physicians abandoned their role in habilitation and participated in euthanasia and sterilization.

In the early 20th century, even as institutions flourished, the public school movement emerged, proposing among its principles the education of children with disabilities in their home communities. Public policy initiatives in the United States began to recognize the importance of children to society and the presence of children with disabilities in society. Gradually, the government began to provide supports and protections. The U.S. Children's Bureau was established in 1912 during the presidency of Theodore Roosevelt; it evolved into the Maternal Child Health Bureau (MCHB) in 1935 and was codified as Title V in the Social Security Act. One of its first programs was Crippled Children Services. Given the extremely high number of families touched by polio, there was strong support for an agency aimed at improving the lives of the many children with polio and other disabling conditions. Eventually, the MCHB migrated to the Health Resources and Services Administration, reflecting a conceptual shift that considered child health issues in public health terms rather than social service terms. In 1930, President Herbert Hoover, a president not known for progressive policies, hosted the White House Conference on Child Health and Protection that concluded that all children, including children with disabilities, regardless of condition, should be educated in their home communities (Children's Charter, 1930; Hoover, 1930).

Though the philosophy and the policy of the early 20th century were moving toward greater supports and services for individuals with disabilities, counter forces limited the extent of change. The eugenics movement, which advocated for restrictive immigration, sterilization, and institutionalization, was influential throughout the first half of the 20th century until the end of World War II, when Nazism and eugenics together were discredited. Another impediment to change was the advent of the Great Depression, followed by World War II; universally dire fiscal and social conditions stalled progress toward reintegration of children and adults with disabilities into society. In fact, during the 1930s, the population in institutions increased because unemployed parents could not care for their children, including their children with disabilities, within their homes (Kanner, 1964). In their attempts to ensure their children's survival, parents sometimes lied, describing a typically developing child as incorrigible or having a seizure disorder, so that they too would be admitted to the institutions.

In the aftermath of World War II, people with disabilities and their families and supporters became the driving force in the further development of disability rights and policy. Organizations of persons with disabilities, their families, and advocates were formed and advocated for better conditions for persons with disabilities. One notable organization, The Arc, was founded in 1953 as the National Association for Retarded Children, with the modest goal of altering perceptions of children with intellectual and developmental disabilities (The Arc, 2012). However, The Arc's advocacy intensified, and by the 1970s the organization became a key player in the ultimate enactment of important federal legislation guaranteeing education to all children, regardless of their ability or disability. In the 1960s, the Disability Rights movement found a passionate champion in President John F. Kennedy, whose older sister had intellectual disability and mental health disorders. He and his family sparked change through eloquent rhetoric, public discussion, and, importantly, federal commitments to build training programs for professionals who could work with children and adults with disabilities (Association of University Centers on Disabilities, 2011). They also promoted the development of social programs, such as the Special Olympics, to improve the life experience of individuals with disabilities.

LEGAL FOUNDATIONS OF INCLUSION

Since the late 1960s, public policy initiatives have provided the legal foundation for inclusion of individuals with disabilities in community life. The Rehabilitation Act of 1973 (PL 93-112) prohibited discrimination on the basis of disability in federal institutions and those that received federal funding, and called for accommodations in schools and workplaces. The Education of All Handicapped Children Act of

1975 (PL 94-142), reauthorized as the Individuals with Disabilities Act (IDEA; PL 101-476) and then amended in the IDEA Improvement Act, guaranteed children with disabilities the right to a free appropriate public education in accordance with their needs in the least restrictive environment. The term *least restrictive environment* was plain talk for the position that children with disabilities needed to be included to the greatest extent possible in their neighborhood schools, alongside typically developing children. During this time, deinstitutionalization also emerged as a movement, allowing children and adults with disabilities to make the transition from institutions to community life.

The developments in inclusion of individuals with disabilities have not been limited to the United States. Perhaps the broadest efforts have been through the UN and WHO. These international organizations have taken up disability rights as part of their human rights agenda. The United Nations declared 1983–1992 as the Decade of Disabled Persons and, in 1993, adopted the Standard Rules on the Equalization of Opportunities for Persons with Disabilities to set the moral and political context of equalization of opportunities for people with disabilities in member countries (United Nations Department of Economic and Social Affairs, Division for Social Policy and Development, 2006). The rules serve both as a context for policymaking and as a basis for technical and economic cooperation among countries. More recently, the Convention on the Rights of Persons with Disabilities was created to "promote, protect and ensure the full and equal enjoyment of all human rights and fundamental freedoms by all persons with disabilities, and to promote respect for their inherent dignity" (United Nations Web Services Section, 2006).

IMPLEMENTING INCLUSION

This section discusses implementation of inclusion at four distinct levels: the family, school, workplace, and general community. Although inclusion is the fundamental goal of health care, achieving it is not easy, straightforward, or inexpensive. Ensuring inclusion at each of these levels requires preparation of the relevant social units, deployment of resources, and investment.

In the Family

Some reading this book may think it unnecessary to discuss inclusion within the family. Yet, until the late 1980s, it was not at all uncommon for physicians and other health care workers, such as social workers or nurses, to recommend lifelong institutionalization for a child born with disabilities (e.g., Down syndrome) or diagnosed during childhood with disabilities (e.g., autism). Well-meaning families often followed physician recommendations, burdened with grief and guilt. (See the commentary below.)

Commentary
Darryl's Curse

As a resident, I took care of a 2-year-old child, Darryl, who had a rare condition known as Ondine's curse, in the intensive care unit of the hospital. Although this child was perfectly fine while awake, he stopped breathing as soon as he fell asleep.

He underwent a tracheostomy, which creates an opening in the wind pipe to allow breathing, and was connected to a mechanical ventilator every afternoon for his nap and evening for sleep. He remained hospitalized for years on the assumption that his family would not be able to provide this level of care in their home. To make his life seem normal, the nurses provided toys and activities to keep him engaged. One of his favorite toys was a doll with a tracheostomy, and he suctioned it lovingly as part of his play.

In my residency, almost all children on ventilators lived in a respiratory care unit or intensive care unit the entire time they remained supported on a ventilator. However, during the mid- to late-1980s in Pennsylvania, the situation began to change. Most children on ventilators could be cared for at home. Their parents learned how to manage a ventilator and suction. The state provided home nursing services for a portion of every day to allow the parents to either sleep or work.

A large body of research has documented the physical and emotional ravages of institutional care. In 1945, Renee Spitz published his observations of children raised in foundling homes or orphanages (Spitz, 1945). In the absence of a family environment, with care provided by nurses working on shifts, approximately one third of the infants died, even those with no apparent disabilities other than institutionalization; survivors typically had physical, emotional, and social impairments. Children with disabilities, such as Down syndrome, had similarly high mortality within institutions. Those who survived made minimal progress toward academic or social goals. The placement of a child in an institution thus became a self-fulfilling prophecy that the child could not learn. The results were used to perpetuate an unjust and harmful situation. (See the commentary below.)

Commentary
The Historical Perspective of Living with Spina Bifida

A 2012 Perspectives article in the journal Pediatrics *reminded me about how recently the situation has changed for individuals with spina bifida (Pruitt, 2012). The scientific debate about the selective "nontreatment" (p. 182) of newborns with spina bifida raged into the 1970s and 1980s. Medical attitudes proved to be self-fulfilling prophesies. Physicians predicted that children with spina bifida would live without the functional capacity to make friends, have jobs, or establish intimate relationships. So, the physicians recommended nontreatment. Untreated children either succumbed to infection or had such severe disabilities from hydrocephalus that the predictions proved accurate.*

Tragically, the debate continued even after intermittent catheterization reduced the rates of renal failure, improved shunts reduced the problems associated with hydrocephalus, improved neonatal care reduced complications of neonatal health problems, and education and social services improved educational attainment and social competence. In fact, by 1984, most children with spina bifida were capable of independent ambulation, achieved continence, and had typical intelligence (Pruitt, 2012). However, the poor attitudes of medical professionals outlasted the dramatic improvements in outcomes.

The situation has changed dramatically in a very short period. Now it is generally assumed that families will raise a child with Down syndrome or autism in their home. Children with complex medical needs are discharged to their families once stability is assured, even if that stability requires high-level medical interventions such as tracheostomy and mechanical ventilation.

Successful inclusion of such children in family homes and family life requires planning, resources, services, and often sacrifice. Parents, other family members, and caregivers need information about the child's condition and training about providing all components of the child's care. (See the commentary below.) When neonates with Down syndrome have severe feeding difficulties, their parents must learn how to ensure that they get adequate nutrition. When children with autism have severe, unpredictable tantrums, their families must learn how to manage aggressive and destructive behavior. When children with tracheostomy tubes and mechanical ventilation live at home, their families must learn how to manage equipment and to identify early warning signs of complications. Anna's parents in the commentary needed to learn to administer medications and assist in therapy exercises.

In the era of inclusion, financial costs have shifted to families. As in Anna's case, care within the family and at home may come at great cost: the direct cost of medication and equipment and the indirect costs of home adaptations, specialized child care, and work lost in order to provide care and attend medical visits. As discussed in Chapter 2, disability falls disproportionately on the poor. The ability of poor families to support a child with disabilities within their home is limited, and the difficulty with the costs may compromise the child's care or restrict the family's social mobility.

Commentary
Anna Lopez

The Lopez family immigrated to the United States to obtain good health care for their daughter, Anna. At the time, she was about 8 years of age and had severe cerebral palsy. She seemed bright but was completely nonambulatory and spoke with difficulty. Her parents provided all of her care—feeding her, dressing her, and carrying her to use the toilet. Anna was enrolled in school, recognized as both a student with a disability and an English language learner. An appropriate individualized education program was constructed that involved English education and speech-language pathology services, as well as occupational and physical therapy. The family found a clinic with a Spanish-speaking physician who arranged for vision and hearing assessments, consultation with a neurologist, and a visit to a Shriner's Hospital that could provide care for children with cerebral palsy at no cost to the family. The neurologist prescribed medication to reduce spasticity. The therapists taught Anna and her mother daily exercises to stretch tight muscles and improve movement patterns. The Shriner's Hospital helped her obtain braces, a walker, and a motorized wheelchair. Her mother dutifully assisted Anna with the exercises and helped her with her English studies so that she too could master the new language. With financial assistance from their church, the parents bought a small ranch house. They literally moved walls to allow the walker and wheel chair to negotiate freely throughout. After about 18 months, Anna was speaking in short sentences in English, eating on her own, getting to the toilet independently, making new friends, and thoroughly enjoying school.

The goal of inclusion of children with disabilities within their families is not possible without supports and services for families, often from health care providers. Care plans must consider the family's strengths and their ability to care for a child with disabilities. Education and training for the caregivers is essential. Families may need support for many aspects of family life, such as figuring out how to talk to siblings about their brother or sister's condition, how to modify the home environment for greatest ease in providing care, and how to find social opportunities that would be enjoyable for the entire family. Systems for ongoing support must be developed and implemented and certainly may include parent-to-parent support. Financial issues must be faced squarely, and implicit compromises about who supports what aspects of care must be made explicit. Although the costs in terms of health care dollars are higher for these children than for children in the general population, in most cases, children benefit enormously from staying at home with their families; ultimately, those raised in loving families have greater independence and less need for social supports. Providing financial and social supports can be conceptualized as investments in these children at young ages, likely to yield financial—and, more important, social—benefits over time.

In Schools

The topic of inclusion in education remains highly controversial. Among parents of children with disabilities are those who argue passionately that their child must be in a regular classroom in the neighborhood school. At the same time, some parents advocate for their child to be in a special educational program exclusively focused on their child's disability because that is the only way to find teachers who understand how to educate the child with a specific condition. There is disagreement among educators and administrators about placing children with disabilities in regular classrooms because of the alleged positive and negative effects on those children and on those typically developing students, and because of financial considerations.

The Education of All Handicapped Children Act (PL 94-142) set the standards for special education in the United States:

> To the maximum extent appropriate, children with disabilities, including children in public or private institutions or other care facilities, are to be educated with children who are not disabled, and that special classes, separate schooling, or other removal of children with disabilities from the regular educational environment occur only when the nature or severity of the disability is such that education in the regular classes with the use of supplementary aids and services cannot be achieved satisfactorily. (U.S. Department of Education, 2007)

The conditions within education in the early 1970s formed the backdrop of the legislation. Of the 8 million children with disabilities in the United States at that time, half were not receiving any educational services (Douvanis & Hulsey, 2002). Students were evaluated for suspected disabilities without notice to their parents and without any opportunity for recourse if their parents disagreed with the assessment. At the same time, parents were able to exclude their children from compulsory attendance regulations without oversight or consequence. Even among those children with disabilities who attended school, many were systematically excluded from meaningful educational experiences (Douvanis & Hulsey, 2002).

Today, worldwide, the United Nations estimates that school enrollment rates for children with severe disabilities in developing countries may be as low as

1%–3%. The result is that many children with disabilities remain unable to read and write (United Nations Department of Economic and Social Affairs, the Office of the United Nations High Commissioner for Human Rights, & Inter-Parliamentary Union, n.d.). The underlying belief that motivated the legal language of PL 94-142 was that success in special schools or special classes, even those offering outstanding educational opportunities, would not adequately prepare students for full participation in an integrated society. If the goal of education is preparation of children for adult life and roles, then children with disabilities must have opportunities to interact with children with no apparent disabilities.

Inclusion is similar to but distinct from mainstreaming. Inclusion implies a commitment to educate children, to the maximum extent appropriate, in the school and classroom they would have attended had they not had the disability (Wisconsin Education Association Council, 2007). If children need specialized instruction, the first choice is for those supports and services to come to them within their classroom rather than for them to leave the class or school to receive the supports and services. Mainstreaming generally implies limited and selective placement of students in regular education classes only when professionals deem such a placement to be feasible and appropriate. Mainstreaming assumes that students earn placement in regular education by demonstrating the ability to keep up with the work assigned to the other students in that classroom (Wisconsin Education Association Council, 2007). In this model, supports and services are generally restricted to the specialized classrooms or schools.

U.S. educational law does not use the terms *inclusion* or *mainstreaming*. It states only that children should be educated in the least restrictive environment. The law has been interpreted to require school districts to have a continuum of placements available, extending from regular education classrooms with minimal supports or services to intense residential programs. With this wide array of options, the law envisions that an interdisciplinary team, including school professionals and family members, would collaborate to determine the appropriate educational setting as part of designing the individualized education program. The placement and the time spent in different settings or receiving different services should be based on the student's strengths and needs, not on parental or educator philosophy or on financial factors.

Because of the ambiguity in the law, the courts have had to interpret the law through specific cases. In general, decisions have supported inclusion over mainstreaming (Douvanis & Hulsey, 2002). In other words, when in doubt, the default action should be placement of a child with his or her typically developing peers. In its programs, the United Nations clearly supports inclusion in education as part of its human rights agenda (United Nations Department of Economic and Social Affairs, the Office of the United Nations High Commissioner for Human Rights, & Inter-Parliamentary Union, n.d.)

The law calls for supplementary aids and services to support children in the least restrictive environment. These aids and supports include specialized instruction methods and adaptations to the usual curriculum. Adaptations may include accommodations, alterations in the formats to increase accessibility, and alteration in the content. For example, specialized instruction for children with reading disabilities includes explicit instruction to increase the students' awareness of the sounds of the language and to master sound–symbol correspondences, skills typically acquired in preschool by good readers. Adaptations for children with reading disabilities include presenting material in visual as well as auditory formats, providing extra time to complete class assignments, modifying expectations about what students should achieve in fixed time frames, and offering different homework assignments.

Many different models of inclusive education are available: special education teachers can serve as consultants, team members, or co-teachers. The choice among models is a function of many factors, including the number of children in the class, the nature of their learning needs, and the extent of behavioral and emotional needs. Collaboration among the teachers is a key to success regardless of model. The commitment to educating children in the least restrictive environment requires, among other adaptations, appropriate preservice preparation of teachers for the diversity of student learning abilities, in-service reinforcement of the principles and practices that work, technical assistance for schools and teachers to accommodate the students with disabilities in their classes, and teacher performance evaluations that include student learning profiles as part of the evaluation.

The great fear among parents and teachers is that either the children with disabilities or their typically developing peers will not learn well in inclusive settings.

Commentary
Lawrence Crosby

Mr. and Mrs. Crosby sought consultation for their son, Lawrence, an 11-year-old with a speech-language disorder and reading disability, about which middle school he should attend in the coming academic year. His disabilities were diagnosed while he was in preschool, where he received appropriate interventions but made slow progress. He attended kindergarten and first grade in a public school with special education supports. However, his parents became very concerned that he was not receiving adequate intervention to improve his speech and language skills. Lawrence was also teased by one of his first-grade classmates with sufficient negativity that it bordered on bullying. The parents then enrolled him, at great financial expense to the family, in a private school specializing in the education of children with communication disorders. Over the next few years, he made good friends there, and he participated in the Special Olympics. His parents were reconsidering academic placement because middle and high school would require a greater financial commitment at a time when Mr. Crosby had reduced to part-time work to be available to his son for support in school and transportation to after-school programs.

At the consultation, the psychologist asked Mr. and Mrs. Crosby what their long-term goals were for Lawrence. They hoped that he would be able to do some post-secondary training, either college or technical school, in order to get a decent job. The psychologist reiterated the question to Lawrence. The parents realized that they had not engaged their son in this discussion. Lawrence talked about his interest in mechanics and cars. The psychologist then asked the parents what skills and experiences would allow their son to achieve those goals. The parents came to realize that practicing social interactions with potential customers and bosses would be extremely valuable for their son. Lawrence talked about an elective after-school class he had heard about at the public middle school that taught the students about car mechanics. Together they created a plan for investigating all of the options for the following year and for sharing in the final decision making.

Many parents are also concerned about the social and emotional consequences of attending the regular classroom, as expressed in the commentary on p. 57. Teachers worry about their ability to meet the demands of students with a wide range of abilities. Ideally, to address these concerns, consultants would have available comprehensive data on indicators of academic success as a function of the educational model. Families and professionals would be able to review academic progress, graduation rates, postsecondary schooling, employment, adult inclusion in the community, and psychosocial or emotional health based on randomized placement in inclusive versus noninclusive settings.

Public policy has advanced faster than research in education; thus, experiments using randomized clinical trials or other careful scientific methodology have never been completed. The data that do exist make several major points:

- Placing children with disabilities in regular classrooms gives them access to the general curriculum that they may not have otherwise encountered.
- Early studies of the academic performance of mainstreamed and segregated students with mild conditions found that the integrated group outperformed the segregated students (Wisconsin Education Association Council, 2007).
- Meta-analyses confirm a small to moderate beneficial effect of inclusion education on the academic and social outcomes of students with disabilities (Wisconsin Education Association Council, 2007).
- Advantages of inclusion for children with disabilities include greater social skills and language abilities, the domains of function most correlated with later occupational success. Attendance rates are also better in inclusive schools, indicative of the preferences of students and their families (Wisconsin Education Association Council, 2007).
- Worldwide research shows that children, including those with significant disabilities, who are included in regular education are more likely to finish school, go on to postsecondary education and training, get jobs, earn good incomes, and become active members of their communities (United Nations Department of Economic and Social Affairs, the Office of the United Nations High Commissioner for Human Rights, & Inter-Parliamentary Union, n.d.).
- Among the students with no apparent disabilities, there are several advantages to participation in inclusive programs. In surveys, parents and teachers have reported that they experience increased comfort with disabilities and improvements in self-concept (Peck, Carlson, & Helmstetter, 1992). They also develop warm and caring friendships with the students with disabilities (Bogdan & Taylor, 1989). These friendships develop when the student with no apparent disability attributes thinking to the student with disabilities, sees that person's individuality, views the other as a reciprocal partner, and defines a social place for that partner (Bogdan & Taylor, 1989).

Parents often favor segregated settings, in which their children with disabilities receive one-to-one attention, or small group instruction, where they get individualized education in a supportive, low-distraction setting. (See the commentary on p. 57.)

They choose segregated education for conditions such as blindness because they think that the instruction offers specialized approaches to concept formation, mobility, and social interactions, issues that may be challenging to children with visual impairment. These factors may be beneficial for some children and, if so, should be considered in designing their educational program. However, children must also be able to generalize their education from the specific lesson to other situations and other settings. An exclusively segregated placement limits the children's abilities to apply their knowledge in real-world situations and everyday social environments.

Another fear of adults, including the parents introduced in the vignette, is that children with disabilities will have negative social experiences in regular classrooms, resulting in poor self-esteem, limited willingness to participate in education, and poor chances for decent employment. Fueling this fear is the increased attention to bullying that has occurred in part because of increases in school violence. Approximately 3.7 million U.S. schoolchildren have bullied and 3.2 million children have been bullied (Hoover & Stenhjem, 2003). Physical weakness is a consistent predictor of being bullied (Hoover & Stenhjem, 2003), placing students with disabilities at risk for maltreatment. However, educational placement does not cause or prevent aggression toward children with disabilities. Placement in a large class with typical learners may increase exposure to potential bullies. However, separation of students on the basis of academic abilities may exacerbate their perceived weakness and imply that they are not similarly valued in the community. Bullying prevention requires a school culture that values all students, offers adult modeling of respectful interactions, provides opportunities for all students to participate in social and academic interactions, monitors the social and academic experiences of the learners, and implements fair and meaningful consequences for bullying. These precautions can be implemented in inclusive settings. At the same time, students with disabilities must be prepared for social interactions with children and adults with no apparent disabilities regardless of their placement in school. There is no better defense against bullying than an individual's strong social skills, self-confidence, integration with others, and ability to get adult help when necessary.

Another fear regarding inclusion is that children with disabilities will have difficulty making friends in school. Here again, the ability to make friends is independent of classroom placement. The ability to make and keep friends should be part of a children's educational program for typical learners and for children with disabilities. Marsha Forest and Jack Pearpoint created programs to facilitate social interactions for children in inclusive education (Forest & Pearpoint, 2001). One, Making Action Plans (MAPS), is a collaborative action planning process that brings together the key actors in a child's life. In the spirit of cooperation, this team creates a plan of action to be implemented in a regular classroom setting. Another, Circle of Friends, prepares schools and students for inclusion by making explicit social contacts for each child. Four circles of contacts are the circles of intimacy, friendship, participation, and exchange. As the students construct circles for themselves and for other students, their willingness to engage with children with disabilities often increases. These simple, straightforward strategies can be used regardless of where children spend most of their time and are particularly important for children in inclusive settings.

Critics of both inclusion and segregated programs each point to financial issues in the decision to promote whatever position they favor or to denigrate the ideas of their opponents. Inclusion is often conceived as an expensive and therefore unsustainable policy. Inclusion is also criticized as driven by an unrealistic expectation that money will be saved (Wisconsin Education Association Council, 2007). As discussed in the United Nations Enable program, inclusive educational settings are generally less expensive than segregated systems simply because one single, integrated educational system tends to be cheaper than two separate systems (United Nations Department of Economic and Social Affairs, Division for Social and Policy Development, 2006.). However, most important is the recognition that the costs of special education are generally higher than regular education in either scenario. According to the U.S. Special Education Expenditures Program, the average cost per pupil for a regular education in 2005 was $6,556. The average cost per student in special education in the same year ranged from $10,558 for students with learning disabilities to $20,095 for students with multiple disabilities. The differential expense for inclusive versus segregated education is small in relation to the difference between special and regular education. Again, these costs are an investment in the children's and society's futures.

The goal of inclusion of children with disabilities within their neighborhood school in classes with typically developing children requires a commitment of the educational, medical, and social service systems. Education plans must consider the child's strengths and needs in terms of academics, social functioning, behavior regulation, and motivation. Consultation, technical assistance, and support for teachers are essential. That preparation of teachers should begin in preservice training and continue as in-service training once teachers experience real-world situations. Inclusive education requires a team effort. (See the commentary on p. 61.) Health care providers play a fundamental role in assisting schools in promoting inclusion. Special educators, therapists, psychologists, and social workers must share their perspectives to help the students succeed. Opportunities for team collaboration must be implemented. Financial issues must be faced squarely. Inclusive education is not an inexpensive option but does not need to bankrupt a school district. Ideally, a middle ground in the intense debate between promoters and opponents can be reached by focusing on the strengths and needs of individual learners in educational planning. The vast majority of children benefit enormously from opportunities to attend the same school as their neighbors and siblings. Ultimately, interactions with typically developing peers prepare them for social participation in a broad social context, encourage independence, and ideally lead to reduced needs for later social supports. As with inclusion in the family, inclusion in schools is a social investment in children with disabilities at a young age.

In the Workplace

As more individuals with disabilities are reaching adulthood with the benefits of living with their families and receiving a strong educational foundation, especially inclusive education, their goal can then become securing employment with good wages and benefits in workplaces along with individuals of all abilities. For individuals with disabilities, the term *competitive employment* is often used. Recognizing that work can be considered from the vantage of inclusion, I discuss employment in the next chapter on contribution.

In Community Life

Inclusion in the community remains a very substantial challenge. Successful inclusion depends on the beliefs, attitudes, and practices of many different individuals, organizations, and institutions. As described previously in the sections on inclusion in families and schools, successful community inclusion also relies on the availability of supports and services. Because this book focuses on children with disabilities, I discuss these issues only briefly.

One important element of community life is where people choose, or are able, to live. Individuals with disabilities often choose to live in their own homes over

Commentary
Barbara Minzenberg, Ph.D.

Who are the children who are the most challenging to include in regular educational programs? To seek to answer this question, I interviewed Barbara Minzenberg about her experiences creating systems change for inclusion of preschoolers in Allegheny County, Pennsylvania.

Barbara Minzenberg is an educator who became sensitized to the issues of inclusion after the passage of federal legislation regarding early intervention. In 1989, she and a colleague successfully competed for a U.S. federal grant to institute an innovative model program of inclusion for preschoolers within the Pittsburgh public schools. They reasoned that the biggest impact would come from including the most seriously affected children into regular programs in the first wave of the MOSAIC program.

As Dr. Minzenberg recalls, the most challenging group to include with typically developing learners was children with severe behavioral and emotional problems. In the past, school districts often met the legal requirements to serve such children in the least restrictive environment by engaging a consultant who made rare appearances in the classroom, offered cursory recommendations, and then suggested alternative placements at the first breakdown in the plan. Their program replaced the consultant with the positive support team, an interdisciplinary team of psychologists, educators, and mental health professionals. The team consulted with schools and teachers even prior to the introduction of the child with behavioral difficulties to the school or class and remained actively engaged over time. They conceptualized their consultation as a dialogue with the teacher, inquiring about what has worked for other students in that class and how the new student was doing. Their consultations might suggest changing the physical features of the classroom, the schedule of activities, or the number of distracters. Teachers met monthly to discuss the issues among themselves, sharing their successes and ongoing issues.

Another group that was challenging to include in the MOSAIC program was children with complex medical problems because of the lack of on-site nursing in neighborhood preschools. A similar team concept brought health professionals to the schools and classrooms to assist with preparation and ongoing support of the student and to serve as a liaison with the medical specialists involved in the child's care.

Dr. Minzenberg conjectures that the intense preparation that went into introducing inclusion into the classrooms was the key to success. Empowering the teachers within the system and garnering support of the administrative leaders changed attitudes and expectations. All of these elements were fundamental to the long-term success of the program.

other residential options. For this reason, the availability of domestic supports is very important. The beginning of Chapter 2 described the intensity with which individuals with disabilities lobbied for in-home supportive services. Without these services, many of those protesters might have not been able to live in a community setting.

Another important area of community life is social relationships. Many social systems, such as athletic teams, book clubs, and churches, are made up of homogeneous groups. It is difficult for other people to break in, particularly when they have a disability. Moreover, legal protections may not typically cover clubs and teams, particularly those that do not receive government financing. Supports and services are less available in social institutions than they are in schools and workplaces.

Inclusion is easier for those individuals and families who have built strong relationships with others in the community at school and/or work; they have the foundation of a social network. After all, networking is how most people find friends, dates, jobs, and satisfying recreation. When these connections are positive, the results can be extremely satisfying to the individual with disabilities and the rest of the community. Some communities are designing and creating venues where individuals of all abilities can readily come together to enjoy common interests. However, as of this writing, this area is still a frontier to be explored and developed.

SUMMARY AND CLINICAL IMPLICATIONS

Health care providers may not always think explicitly about inclusion as the ultimate goal of the treatments they provide to children with disabilities. They may implicitly see their main purpose as improving health status, such as decreasing seizure frequency or reducing spasticity. However, improving the health status of a child should ultimately allow that child to enjoy integration within the family, school, workplace, and community to experience a typical everyday life. Treatments that result in segregation must be carefully evaluated.

It is important to determine whether health plans and treatments ultimately allow children with disabilities to be a part of family, school, work, and community; thus, they should be reviewed with regard to their commitment to inclusion. If an intervention does not meet this criterion, directly or indirectly, then it may not be necessary or wise. When multiple alternative approaches are possible to treat a health condition, an approach that promotes inclusion should be preferable to one that leads to isolation. When periods of isolation or institutionalization seem inevitable because of the nature or severity of a health care condition, then plans for transitions back into family, school, work, and community should be constructed at the initiation of the intervention. These plans may focus on changing the environment more than treating the individual and are appropriate targets in a health care system that embraces the integrated model discussed in Chapter 3. When inclusion requires supports and services to succeed, then those supports and services should be arranged as part of the health care plan. Inclusion should be viewed not as an option but rather as a fundamental human right.

Exercises

1. Enlightenment physicians were highly enthusiastic about the possibilities of remediating individuals with disabilities. Modern day genetics researchers are also excited about remediation of disabilities on the basis of understanding the genetics of disorders. Compare and contrast these two groups of physicians in terms of their goals, strategies, promises, and risks in the care of children with disabilities.
2. A church builds a ramp to allow individuals with disabilities to participate in services. However, it does not immediately see an increase in the number of congregants with disabilities. How would you advise the church to increase participation of individuals with disabilities?
3. Imagine you are at a social event and you hear someone making derogatory jokes about individuals with disabilities. How would you handle the situation? What if you heard that person complaining about social expenditures for special education or workplace accommodations for individuals with disabilities?
4. What personal actions could you take to increase the inclusion of individuals with disabilities in your community?
5. A child care center in your area asks for consultation to diversify the students in the program by including children with disabilities. What initial steps would you take to evaluate their readiness for diversification? What would you want to see in place prior to acceptance of a child with disabilities? Who might be available in the community to assist the center in its exciting new endeavor?

5

Contribution

Evan

Evan was 3 years old and could not feed by mouth. He had food pumped directly and continuously into his stomach through a gastrostomy feeding tube. He also had delays in language and cognitive abilities that his parents hoped could be remedied once he started preschool. However, his feeding pump was connected to a tall, heavy stand that the child could not move. When he entered school, tethered in this way, Evan was unable to move through the classroom and participate in activities. So his parents called an urgent meeting with his health care team, and together they fashioned a backpack-feeding pump. They also bought a toy cart that he could put it in and still move around if he got tired. These accommodations allowed Evan to interact with his classmates at school.

Josie

Josie had a severe neuromuscular disorder. She was unable to walk independently and had severe limitations in self-care. Throughout her public school years, she used a power wheelchair for mobility. Her parents provided her personal care at home; an aide at school provided personal assistance during the school day. Josie was an outstanding student. As she approached the end of high school, she decided that she wanted to attend a college away from her family. In addition to the usual considerations in choosing a college, she had to assess the accessibility of classrooms and the attitudes of teachers and administrators. She also had to learn how to assess, hire, and train personal aides who would come to her dormitory room early in the morning and late at night to assist with personal care. She graduated college with honors.

Scott

Scott was a 29-year-old with Down syndrome whose test scores indicated that his functioning was in the mild range of intellectual disability. After he completed high school, he worked part time at a restaurant, first with the support of a job coach and then independently. He was selected to sit on the advisory board for a nonprofit organization as a community member. Initially, he attended the meetings with a mentor, but after four meetings, he participated independently. He was very active in the community, taking public transportation to meet up with friends for social activities, including monthly dances and bowling on Saturday afternoon.

Inclusion is fundamental for children and adults with disabilities to counter the isolation, neglect, and abuse that can occur with segregation. Inclusion reflects the integration of individuals of all abilities into the same physical locations and same social structures. However, society could accept individuals with disabilities into community life as passive observers. If such were the situation, despite their physical presence, children and adults with disabilities might continue to experience limitations and lost possibilities. Moreover, in spite of good intentions, many social efforts have created only token roles for children with disabilities or opportunities that maintain their primary identities as patient, client, or person with a disability. Barriers to participation persist in our communities and society. It is vitally important that social systems afford children and adults with disabilities the opportunities to be fully engaged and make meaningful contributions to their families, schools, workplaces, and communities. The children and young adults described in the opening vignettes each contributed to their social groups, as appropriate to their age, developmental level, interests, and strengths.

Contribution is the second pillar in the health care goals of people with disabilities. Health care supports contribution by focusing on the individual's functioning in his or her everyday life and in the community. Health care interventions should be designed to enhance function and thereby to allow the individual, whether child or adult, to contribute to his or her social context.

Contribution implies that the children are involved within their social structures, play meaningful roles, engage in activities, or assume responsibilities. In many cases, contribution reflects actions on the part of the children. However, contribution can occur without deliberate action because the individuals have a positive impact on others around them. Contribution does not mean that all individuals with disabilities can or should eventually earn high wages, although Josie in the opening vignette indeed did. Children, like Evan, contribute in many ways though they are not yet wage earners. Like all children, depending on age, they interact lovingly with their parents and siblings, learn to their best ability at school, make friends with neighbors and classmates, join clubs or teams, or participate in worship and service projects at their religious institutions. Contribution does not require that children with disabilities perform at the same level as others in their social settings. They may not have the same chores as their siblings, earn the same grades as other children in the regular classroom, or earn comparably high salaries at the workplace, although all of these are real possibilities. Each individual has unique strengths and talents that, when combined with those of others, create social groups and communities that work well.

Contribution reflects the interdependence that we all experience, each of us contributing what we have and receiving what we need. What is essential is that like all children, children with disabilities have equality of opportunity to contribute, free of any preconceptions that limit what they can do or how far they can go. Health care should further the child's abilities to contribute in meaningful ways.

This chapter first considers the benefits of contribution and then provides a framework for incorporating a focus on contribution or function into health care delivery.

REASONS TO FOCUS ON CONTRIBUTION

The most compelling reason to promote contribution is that it, like inclusion, is a human right, and its importance is fundamental for the child or adult with disabilities. All individuals want to feel wanted, needed, and appreciated. The opportunity to contribute brings with it a feeling of self-worth and positive self-concept, with downstream positive impacts on health and well-being. Moreover, the opposite—feelings of uselessness, for example—creates stress, loneliness, and depression. Over time, the inability to have an impact on the physical and social environment can generate feelings of hopelessness. Stress and hopelessness are associated with adverse effects on physical and mental health that can accumulate over the life span (Middlebrooks & Audage, 2008)

From the standpoint of the social group and society, helping the individual with disabilities to contribute also brings positive benefits. Individuals who are contributing are likely to be seen as a person first and more likely to make friends and develop their own social lives. They are less likely to depend on their families, siblings, or government programs for all of their social activities. They are more likely to earn wages and pay taxes as they become adults. Society gains more productive citizens than it would otherwise have. The financial and social benefits are not the primary motivation for the focus on contribution. Indeed, some children and adults with disabilities may continue to live with their families and use government assistance all their lives. They still can contribute to their neighborhood, places of worship, community organizations, and family. However, ensuring opportunities for contribution, supporting children to seize and shape the possibilities around them, and advocating for removal of barriers that block contribution are likely to bring societal as well as personal advantages.

CURRENT CLINICAL PRACTICE

To enhance an individual's ability to contribute, health care for children with disabilities must focus on the child's functioning for success in everyday life. (See the commentary below.) Rehabilitation specialists, including physical therapists, occupational therapists, and speech-language pathologists, typically create goals, objectives, and strategies for care that are based on the child's function. For example, in

Commentary
Clinical Pearls

A child's functioning, present and future, is highly salient to his or her family. Often at the time of diagnosis of a disability, parents ask, "Will my child go to college?"

or "Will my child ever marry and have a family?" The disability label wrecks their dreams for their child's future. Of course, health care professionals cannot provide any honest reassurance for the parents of a child with disabilities any more than they could promise college and marriage to the parents of a child without disabilities. What parents seem to be asking is, "Will my child be functional?" or "Will my child be able to contribute to society?" The health care team shares the family's commitment to supporting the child's ability to contribute.

Thus, it is often better to speak to the anxiety rather than answer the question directly. One option would be, "I see how worried you are about your child and your child's future. I want to assure you that the health care team will work diligently with you to allow your child to make meaningful contributions. How does that sound to you?" Offering positive models of contribution may be helpful after the anxiety is acknowledged.

the care of a child with a neuromotor disorder, such as Josie in the opening vignette, the initial goals of the physical therapist are often to improve the child's mobility so she can participate more easily at home and school, and not simply to build strength or reduce muscle spasticity. Specific objectives under the goal might include assisting the child in building motor patterns that ultimately lead to standing and walking. Specific objectives might also include increasing strength or reducing spasticity, but it is particularly important that these objectives be conceptualized as intermediary steps that ultimately promote mobility. Spasticity may lead to hip dislocation, pain, and further immobility; therefore, reducing spasticity is also an appropriate goal when it serves to maintain function over time. If a child's condition is sufficiently severe that independent walking is unlikely, the goal for that child remains improving mobility. In such circumstances, the therapist may shift strategies and provide the child with a walker or with a wheelchair.

To broaden to a focus on function is challenging for medical care, because physicians are trained to focus on symptom management or cure. They often pay more attention to the signs and symptoms of illness than to the whole person, and they sometimes focus on the immediate issues without taking a longitudinal perspective. Those physicians who are committed to a broader orientation find it challenging to focus on function because of insufficient time and resources to craft care plans in collaboration with families and community resources and services. Among physicians, three different subspecialists who pay particular attention to function include developmental-behavioral pediatricians, physical medicine and rehabilitation specialists, and geriatricians. The conditions that these professionals treat, such as autism, spinal cord injury, or dementia, respectively, share the feature that they usually cannot be cured. Without the possibility of cure, improving or maintaining function becomes the central clinical focus. Interestingly, although the populations these three subspecialists serve are very different, the modes of operation are similar: the professionals often work on teams alongside psychologists and rehabilitation specialists such as physical and occupational therapists and speech-language pathologists. Their work also involves collaborating with community-based resources and services to improve the environmental factors that affect function.

It is important in the care of children with disabilities that all treating clinicians share a commitment to enhancing the child's functioning. (See the commentary on p. 69.)

Although their primary work may not be directly involved in improving functioning, they should appreciate how their clinical focus contributes to a larger plan. In Section III of this book, I present tools designed to facilitate a broad and inclusive approach that integrates clinical and functional goals.

INTERNATIONAL CLASSIFICATION OF FUNCTIONING, DISABILITY, AND HEALTH

Function is multifaceted and difficult to define. What should be included within this broad concept? The functional consequences of retinitis pigmentosa include blindness, whereas the functional consequences of bacterial meningitis include deafness. Is it necessary to consider the functional consequences of each health condition individually, or would it be possible to find a unifying framework and a systematic approach for defining and classifying function that would be appropriate for many different health conditions? The functioning of an infant is very different than that of a late adolescent. Is it necessary to consider function differently for different ages

Commentary
Seamus

Seamus was adopted at 18 months of age and diagnosed with a bilateral moderate-to-severe sensorineural hearing loss at 3 years. He was then fitted with hearing aids and finally learned language. When he got to school age, he was found to have low average intelligence and a language-based learning disability. He struggled but succeeded at learning to read. As he entered adolescence, he developed an anxiety disorder that limited his interest in going out with other kids or even leaving home. When he was 14, a treating psychiatrist told his parents that he might have autism and that they should expect him to require institutional care as an adult. The parents were devastated. His mother eventually decided to seek a second opinion when he was 15.

The consulting developmental-behavioral pediatrician concurred that Seamus had a learning disability and anxiety but put more importance on the hearing loss and anxiety as explanations for shyness and social withdrawal. The pediatrician thought it extremely premature and unnecessary to plan for institutional care before an aggressive treatment plan for all of the issues Seamus faced had been tried. Instead, the recommendation was to focus on his functioning at home, at school, and in the community.

Armed with this new approach, the parents found a new psychiatrist to treat the anxiety disorder with both medication and cognitive behavior therapy. They returned to the audiologist, who realized that Seamus might benefit from new hearing aids, especially because in high school the FM system he had used in elementary school to improve his hearing was impractical in the setting of many class changes. The parents returned to the school and asked for a new individualized education program. Seamus was consulted to gauge his goals and aspirations. New social and vocational goals were added to the previous academic goals. The parents found several strategies to increase Seamus's sense of maturity and independence at home, including giving him an allowance and allowing him greater input into family outings and activities. Seamus responded with improved mood, greater social engagement, and better academic performance.

or developmental stages, or would it be possible to find a unifying framework that would serve across the age span?

The International Classification of Functioning, Disability, and Health (ICF) offers a common framework for describing function across all health conditions and across ages. The World Health Organization (WHO) developed the ICF to understand, codify, and evaluate the impact of disease and disability on individuals and on populations (WHO, 2002). The framework is applicable to individuals regardless of age, social circumstance, culture, or clinical condition. Developed by an international group, the language is descriptive, simple, and easily translated into multiple languages. The overall framework is designed to have universal cultural applicability rather than to favor a particular philosophical or national approach.

Brief History

WHO has been at the forefront of efforts to standardize health-related information on a worldwide basis through its WHO Family of International Classifications. These manuals standardize terminology, which enables improved communication. They facilitate collecting, evaluating, and interpreting public health statistics, particularly if a goal of the statistics is to compare across countries or states or eras. Physicians and other health professionals in the United States are very familiar with one manual: the *International Classification of Disease* (10th ed.; ICD-10; World Health Organization, 2011) used to classify diseases and injuries. After every health care encounter, the clinician is obligated to choose the appropriate ICD codes that indicate the reason for the encounter. ICD development dates back to 1853, when an internationally applicable classification system for causes of death was commissioned. The resulting lists of conditions went through several revisions and were mainly used to calculate mortality statistics. In 1948, the First World Health Assembly endorsed an international classification of diseases that expanded to include diseases, injuries, and causes of death. Revisions in the classification continued approximately every 10 years, expanding the previous listings. The ICD-10 was adopted by WHO member states in 1994.

WHO began discussions of a system to address the consequences of disease in 1972 and, in 1980, published the first version of a classification system designed to relate physical function to health conditions. Originally, the manual was called the *International Classification of Impairments, Disability, and Handicaps* (Grimby & Smedby, 2001). It was based on a very linear underlying model that assumed that impairments at the level of the body affected activities at the intellectual/emotional level, which then influenced the individual's relation to the social group. Early versions of the ICF were field tested in 61 countries between 1994 and 2001, involving 1,800 experts who evaluated its feasibility, reliability, and validity (Simeonsson, 2003). In 2001, the name was changed to the International Classification of Function, Disability, and Health. This version broadened the perspective, abandoned the biomedical orientation, and offered a highly interactive model in which function is the result of health conditions as well as environmental and personal factors.

Core Concepts

The ICF perspective on child health and disability has informed many of the core constructs of this book. Its fundamental tenets include the following (WHO, 2011):

- Disability is a universal experience, rather than an experience isolated to a minority within the population.
- It is more important to focus on human function than on disability.
- Common experiences can follow different etiologies or diseases. For example, limitations in mobility might arise from amputation, severe arthritis, cerebral palsy, or congenital heart disease. Therefore, the language is neutral in reference to diseases or etiologies.
- A single approach is appropriate across the life span and not only at distinct developmental stages.
- The conceptual model is interactive and integrative; medical and environmental factors both impact function. It is important to address the *context* in which an individual must function as well as the person whose function is under consideration.

The current ICF model conceptualizes that health conditions affect function at three levels: body functions, body structures, and activities and participation (Figure 5.1). *Body functions* are defined as physiological functions of body systems, including psychological functions. *Body structures* are anatomical parts of the body such as organs, limbs, and their components. *Activity* is defined as the execution of a task or action by an individual. *Participation* is involvement in a life situation (WHO, 2002). These levels are mutually interacting. Body functions may affect participation; conversely, participation might impact body functions. Contextual factors also affect function at all three levels. Contextual factors consist of both environmental factors and personal factors. *Environmental factors* make up the physical, social, and attitudinal environment in which people live and conduct their lives. Environmental factors can serve as barriers or as facilitators. *Personal factors* have not yet been codified.

The ICF also uses specific terminology for issues or challenges that arise within any of the domains of function. *Impairments* are problems in body function or structure such as a significant deviation or loss. *Activity limitations*, or simply

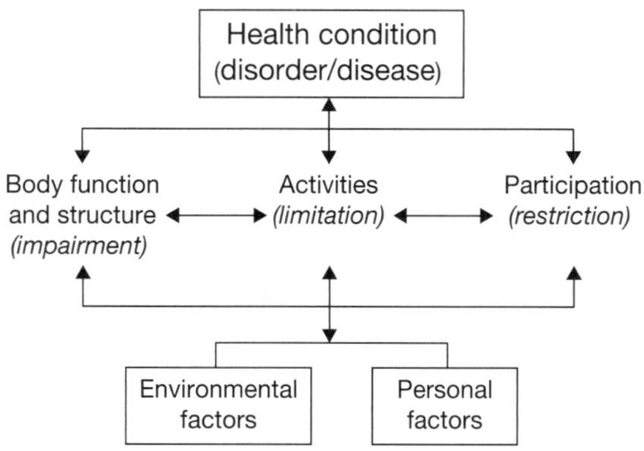

Figure 5.1. Basic model of the *International Classification of Functioning, Disability, and Health*. (From World Health Organization. [2002]. *Towards a common language for functioning, disability and health: ICF* [p. 9]. Geneva, Switzerland: Author. Retrieved from http://www.who.int/classifications/icf/training/icfbeginnersguide.pdf; adapted by permission.)

limitations, indicate difficulties an individual may have in any of the activity categories. *Participation restrictions*, or simply *restrictions*, are defined as problems an individual may experience in involvement in life situations.

It is important to emphasize that the focus of the ICF is function. For instance, one category of activity is mobility. Mobility is distinct from walking, although most people achieve independent mobility through walking. A child with paraplegia who cannot walk may or may not have a limitation in mobility. If she has available to her a wheelchair, and if she attends a fully accessible school, she may not have any limitations in mobility. Thus, on ICF Item d4601, "Moving around within buildings other than home," no functional problems would be indicated.

Coding System

Within the ICF coding system, letters indicate which of the three levels of function are indicated: body functions (*b*), structures (*s*), and activities and participation (*d*). Each of these levels of function has been subdivided into domains that provide increasingly finer levels of description. The subdivisions are organized as chapters, indicated as a single digit (e.g., b1, s2, d3) after the letter code. These chapters are further divided into specific functions, represented by three to four digits. Environmental factors impacting health and function are indicated by the letter "e" and are similarly divided into chapters, indicated by a single digit, and subdivisions, indicated by three or four digits. Personal factors have not yet been organized into chapters or subdivisions. Table 5.1 lists the major sections, chapters, and a few subsections within each chapter.

In 2007, WHO released a modification of the ICF called the *ICF Child and Youth Version* or *ICF-CY* (WHO Workgroup for Developmental of Version of ICF for Children & Youth, 2007). This revision was designed to capture unique aspects of child functioning. Body functions and body structures are very similar in the two versions. Activities in the ICF-CY that are not in the original version include learning through symbolic play (d1313), pretend play (d1314), and engagement in play as a major life area (d880).

Uses

The ICF provides a systematic and universal framework that can be used at the individual, institutional, or social level. At the individual level, it can be used to describe the individual's level of function across the wide range of human functioning that can be impacted by disease and disability. Perhaps even more important, at the individual level, the ICF can be used to plan interventions for the individual (Reed et al., 2005). It allows health care to consider which treatments or interventions can be put in place specifically to maximize specific aspects of functioning. Once the interventions have been tried, it provides a framework for evaluating the outcomes in terms of function in order to determine whether the intervention has been useful. The ICF can promote communication across the health care team by using a shared language. Because it uses plain language, it avoids the jargon that leads to breakdown in communication. The ICF also can be used at the institutional level by describing the population cared for by that organization.

The ultimate goals of health care for children with disabilities, particularly as they transition into adulthood, should be full social participation and contribution.

Table 5.1. Domains, chapters, and representative subdivisions of function and structure within the *International Classification of Functioning, Disability and Health for Children and Youth*

Domain	Chapter	Subdivision
b Body function	b1 Mental functions	b110–139 Global mental functions b140–189 Specific mental functions, including attention, memory, and psychomotor function
	b2 Sensory functions and pain	b210–229 Seeing and related functions b230–249 Hearing and vestibular functions
	b3 Voice and speech functions	b310 Voice functions b320 Articulation functions b330 Fluency and rhythm of speech
	b4 Functions of the cardiovascular, hematological, immunological, and respiratory systems	b410–429 Functions of the cardiovascular system b430–439 Functions of the hematological and immunological systems
	b5 Functions of the digestive, metabolic, and endocrine systems	b510–539 Functions related to the digestive system b540–559 Functions related to metabolism and endocrine systems
	b6 Genitourinary and reproductive functions	b610–639 Urinary functions b6330–679 Genital and reproductive functions
	b7 Neuro/musculo/skeletal and movement-related functions	b710–729 Functions of the joints and bones b730–749 Muscle functions b750–789 Movement functions
	b8 Functions of the skin and related structures	b810–849 Functions of the skin b850–869 Functions of the hair and nails
s Body structures	s1 Structures of the nervous system	s110 Structure of the brain s120 Spinal cord and related structures
	s2 The eye, ear, and related structures	s210 Structure of the eye socket s220 Structure of the eyeball s240 Structure of the external ear
	s3 Structures involved in voice and speech	s320 Structure of the mouth s330 Structure of the larynx
	s4 Structures of the cardiovascular, immunological, and respiratory systems	s410 Structure of the cardiovascular system s420 Structure of the immune system s430 Structure of the respiratory system
	s5 Structures related to the digestive, metabolic, and endocrine systems	s510 Structure of the salivary glands s520 Structure of the esophagus s530 Structure of the stomach
	s6 Structures related to the genitourinary and reproductive systems	s610 Structure of the urinary system s620 Structure of the pelvic floor s630 Structure of the reproductive system
	s7 Structures related to movement	s710 Structure of the head and neck region s720 Structure of the shoulder region s730 Structure of the upper extremity
	s8 Skin and related structures	s810 Structure of areas of skin s830 Structure of the nails
d Activities	d1 Learning and applying knowledge	d110–129 Purposeful sensory experiences d130–159 Basic learning, including acquiring language, learning to read, and learning to write d160–179 Applying knowledge, including thinking, reading, and solving problems

(continued)

Table 5.1. *(continued)*

Domain	Chapter	Subdivision
	d2 General tasks and demands	d210 Undertaking a single task d220 Undertaking multiple tasks d230 Carrying out daily routine d240 Handling stress and psychological demands d250 Managing one's own behavior
	d3 Communication	d310–329 Communicating—receiving d330–349 Communicating—producing d350–369 Use of communication devices and techniques
	d4 Mobility	d 410–429 Changing and maintaining body position d430–489 Carrying, moving, and handling objects d450–469 Walking and moving
	d5 Self-care	d510 Washing oneself d530 Toileting d540 Dressing d550 Eating d560 Drinking d570 Looking after one's health
	d6 Domestic life	d610–629 Acquisition of necessities d630–649 Household tasks
d Participation	d7 Interpersonal interactions and relationships	d710–729 General interpersonal interactions d730–779 Particular interpersonal relationships, including unfamiliar, formal, informal, familial, and intimate relationships
	d8 Major life areas	d810–839 Education d840–879 Work and employment d860–879 Economic life, including economic transactions and economic self-sufficiency d880 Engagement in play
	d9 Community social and civic life	d910 Community life d920 Recreation and leisure 9930 Religion and spirituality d940 Human rights d950 Political life and citizenship

Source: World Health Organization Workgroup for Developmental of Version of ICF for Children and Youth (2007).

The focus on social participation characterizes the goals for children with no apparent disabilities as well. When children are preschoolers, the focus of their parents and teachers is their learning to communicate. However, as they age, the focus shifts to applying communication skills to completing school, obtaining employment, and building meaningful social relationships. Similarly, when children are school age, their parents and teachers focus on their learning mathematics. However, as the children approach adulthood, particularly for those who have difficulty learning math, the focus becomes more practical, including whether they can succeed at domestic tasks, such as managing their bank account or making change, as well as use math as needed for employment and participation in the community.

The ICF combines activities and social participation under the same letter in the coding scheme (*d*). The highest level tasks that emphasize social participation are as follows:

- *Domestic life*: Acquisition of necessities, household tasks, caring for household objects, and assisting others

- *Social relationships*: Intimate, close, informal, formal, distant
- *Major life areas*: Education, employment, financial resources
- *Other community engagement*: Recreation and leisure, religion or spirituality, political life and citizenship

If the child has impairments of body functions or structures that negatively impact activities, then the impairment should be addressed. Within the ICF framework, impairments in body functions and structures can be addressed either by treatment in the health care system or by changes in the environment. For example, if a child has difficulty with speech production, then he or she may be a candidate for an augmentative and alternative communication device that bypasses the use of the vocal system.

Limitations

The ICF is not an assessment tool but rather a system for analyzing function (Reed et al., 2005). Practical methods for operationalizing the ICF in health care, rehabilitation, and education are being developed at the time of this writing and are discussed in greater detail in Chapter 8. However, current functional assessment tools can be used to map on to the ICF categories (Ogonowski, Kronk, Rice, & Feldman, 2004). The ICF also has an interview schedule that addresses major domains and can be used for clinical care, research, or public health surveys. Finally, because the ICF is an omnibus framework, it is very lengthy. It is not readily apparent how many and which functional areas should focus on health care planning for any particular individual or group. Researchers have attempted to develop core sets of items for specific clinical conditions so that the entire ICF does not have to be addressed at each visit. Nonetheless, when to expand beyond the core sets is not clear.

Employment

One of the most obvious indications that an individual is making a contribution as he approaches adulthood is his ability to work. Though work may seem a distant goal to families of children with disabilities or the clinicians who treat them, planning for the eventuality of work should begin early in life. Unfortunately, for individuals with disabilities in the United States, obtaining competitive or inclusive employment is a significant challenge. Table 5.2 shows data from the U.S. Department of Labor, Bureau of Labor Statistics (US Bureau of Labor Statistics, 2012), in which a person

Table 5.2. Employment status (in thousands) of the U.S. civilian population over 16 years of age for July 2012

Category	People with disability	People with no disability
Civilian population	28,007	215,346
Civilian labor force	5,791	150,735
Participation rate	20.7	70.0
Employed	5,004	138,112
Unemployed	787	12,613
Unemployment rate	13.6	8.4
Not in labor force	22,216	64,611

Source: U.S. Bureau of Labor Statistics, Division of Current Employment Statistics (2012).

with a disability was defined as having at least one of the following conditions: is deaf or has serious difficulty hearing; is blind or has serious difficulty seeing even when wearing glasses; has serious difficulty concentrating, remembering, or making decisions because of a physical, mental, or emotional condition; has serious difficulty walking or climbing stairs; has difficulty dressing or bathing; or has difficulty doing errands alone, such as visiting a doctor's office or shopping, because of a physical, mental, or emotional condition. The proportion of individuals with disabilities who met this definition was 11.2%. The table documents that among the population of adults older than 16 years, the vast majority were not participating in the labor force. Even in the slow recovery from recession, the vast majority of individuals with no apparent disabilities were employed. Moreover, the data indicate that among those adults participating in the labor market, the unemployment rate was higher for those with disabilities than for those without disabilities. In the United States, public policy often includes disincentives to work; for example, if an individual who is disabled uses public health care insurance, then the individual may decide not to accept a job if it means that he may lose his health insurance. A Developmental Disabilities Assistance and Bill of Rights Act of 2000 (PL 106-402) listed 10 "Areas of Emphasis" that would have a strong impact on the lives of individuals with developmental disabilities; employment was on the list because unemployment rates are unacceptably high among this population.

The lack of work opportunities for individuals with disabilities is a problem worldwide. The United Nations Enable (United Nations Department of Economic and Social Affairs, Division for Social Policy and Development, 2006) program states:

> In every society, persons with disabilities have not been fully integrated into the labour market. Most are either unemployed or have been dissuaded from actively seeking work. Among those who are working, many are underemployed, paid below minimum wage, and work below their capabilities. This lack of economic participation has a

Commentary
Abilities United

Abilities United, in Palo Alto, California, includes employment services among its programs for adults with physical and intellectual disabilities. Several features of this program allow it to stand out from others in the same community. First, when an employer considers whether or not to employ individuals with disabilities, the executive director Lynda Steele and her capable staff ensure that the addition of the client is based on a business plan for the company and not simply on the company's interest in doing a good deed. "Our experience shows," explains Ms. Steele, "that the situation remains far more stable if the company has a sound business rationale for the hire." In addition, the agency made a bold move to eliminate "subminimum wage" options in 2008, explained Sheraden Nicholau and Jeff Weber, leaders in adult employment services. Clients sign individual contracts with the hiring company, even as they are supported by Abilities United. This shift has allowed the agency to put into action their philosophy of supporting individuals with disabilities in living the lives they choose. The agency succeeds in this mission by providing related services and support, including independent living and volunteer work opportunities. Their staff is cross-trained so they can provide multiple supports to the same individual.

significant impact on the lives of persons with disabilities, as they are then unable to earn an adequate standard of living (article 28) and to live independently in the community (article 19).

The issue of employment for individuals with developmental disabilities that were acquired prior to the age of 21 has grown in importance as more children with disabilities survive to adulthood and more adults with disabilities live in the community. In the 1950s and 1960s and continuing to some extent to the present, the solution for providing work opportunities for adults with physical or intellectual disabilities was the sheltered workshop, a protected and segregated environment in which individuals work under supervision. Income to the workshop usually comes from a combination of contracted work and government subsidy. The work is typically highly repetitive, including packaging, simple assembly, or stuffing envelopes.

Many features make these sheltered programs an unacceptable or inadequate solution to the issue of employment. Wages are very low, below minimum wage. A 1998 national report indicated that sheltered workshop clients earned an average of $65 per week, whereas rehabilitation clients working in the competitive labor market earned an average of $272 (Taylor, 2002). Even for people with severe intellectual disability, earnings are significantly higher in competitive employment. Workshop clients earned a weekly average of $37, and workers in competitive employment made $110 (Taylor, 2002). Work is often sporadic; employees may show up at work only to learn that they are not needed that day because of a lack of contracts. Another major problem is that opportunities for advancement are very limited. Only 3.5% of people in sheltered workshops move into competitive employment in a given year, even though the stated aim of the workshops is preparation for other employment opportunities (Taylor, 2002).

Competitive employment is a term used to imply inclusion in employment; it means working in positions alongside individuals with no apparent disabilities and being paid a decent wage, including benefits. (See the commentary below.)

Commentary
Two Workers at Abilities United

I interviewed two adults with Down syndrome who had used employment or independent living skill programs at Abilities United about their work and life experiences. Jane lives on her own and works in a volunteer program within the community that is designed to help participants get work experience. In this program, several adults with disabilities regularly participate in maintenance activities in local parks and animal care at nearby farms. I couldn't help but notice that she was wearing a shiny red jacket and glittery gloves for the interview. I gently inquired about her outfit. It turns out that immediately after the interview she was heading to a Halloween party, dressed as Michael Jackson.

Jillian lives with her mother in a nearby town. She works 20 hours per week at a supermarket. Jillian is particularly proud that she had personally landed a volunteer position at the office of a local politician, doing office work. She anticipates that this placement will lead to a good job if she does well. She is also working on independent living skills in order to obtain her own apartment in the near future.

Commentary
Bender Consulting Services

"Hiring people with disabilities should not be thought of as a charitable act; it is a business solution for your corporation or organization. Your hiring managers will be making a good business decision that will pay off in dividends, and will also be the right thing to do."

Joyce Bender, CEO, Bender Consulting Services (Bender, 2012)

Most people get their jobs through networking, including social contacts in the community, opportunities to show their work to potential employers, or excellent reputations in their field. Some individuals with disabilities require assistance to secure and maintain competitive employment. To this end, employment specialists, known as job coaches, may assist, particularly in the early phases when training takes place and establishing accommodations is the most critical. Job coaches are typically supported by state and federal programs and sometimes by employers. They may provide training for coworkers to support the new employee. The job coach may be reintroduced if work requirements change, if new training is necessary, or if changes in the individual's status require adjustments to the accommodations (see the vignette about Scott and the commentaries about Abilities United and two workers in the program). Individuals with disabilities can learn many job skills and requirements; the onus is on the teachers to figure out how to teach (Wolfensberger & Thomas, 1998).

If the individual with disabilities requires more assistance in finding a position, learning the job requirements, and adjusting to work life, a transitional step toward competitive employment, called *supported employment*, may be an option. Supported employment uses an employment specialist to assist in establishing goals and making plans with the worker; the coach may assist in the job search and through initial training phases. Follow-up support systems may remain available until the individual no longer wants assistance. The important features of supported and competitive employment are that the work occurs in the community among coworkers with no apparent disabilities, compensation is fair and steady, benefits are available, and the options regarding desired work are centered on the individual's preferences and skills.

Legal protections for competitive employment are included in the ADA, which protects individuals with disabilities from historical discrimination in all employment practices, including job application procedures, hiring, firing, training, pay, promotion, benefits, and leave. Individuals with disabilities also have the right to be free from harassment resulting from the disability. Most importantly, individuals with disabilities have the right to request a reasonable accommodation in the hiring process and on the job. *A reasonable accommodation* is any change or adjustment to a job, the work environment, or the usual procedures that would allow one to apply for a job, perform job functions, or enjoy equal access to benefits available to other individuals in the workplace. Some of the most common types of accommodations include the following:

- Environmental changes such as installing a ramp or modifying a work space or restroom

- Sign language interpreters for people who are deaf or readers for people who are blind
- A quiet work space or changes to reduce noisy distractions for someone with a mental disability
- The provision of written materials in an accessible format such as braille, audio tape, or computer disk
- Telecommunication devices for use with telephones by people who are deaf, and hardware and software that make computers accessible to people with vision impairments or who have difficulty using their hands
- Time off to receive treatment for a disability

As in the case of inclusion of children with disabilities in their families and in schools, employment of adults with disabilities requires commitment, support, incentives to employers, and changing social beliefs and expectations. Preparation of the workplace and support for the worker may both be required for a successful match.

SUMMARY AND CLINICAL IMPLICATIONS

The second major priority for health care for children with disabilities is that they have meaningful opportunities to contribute within the social world (e.g., school, clubs, neighborhood, place of worship, work). To achieve this, health care for children with disabilities needs to expand from a focus on diseases, symptoms, and clinical indicators to include a focus on function. Health care plans must include strategies to enhance function, particularly at the level of social participation. The ICF provides a conceptual framework and a coding system to categorize function. Within the ICF, the ultimate goal for an individual is social participation. Changes to the physical or social environment can often compensate for restrictions in activities or impairments in function, as can medical procedures. The importance of supporting contribution remains unchanged; even after many advances promoting inclusion, employment statistics for individuals with disabilities are poor, and far below the levels of their peers without disabilities, even when work abilities may be the same.

Exercises

1. What formal assessment measures or other methods could be used to allow reliable and valid coding using the ICF or ICF-CY?
2. What characteristics would you put into the personal factors in the ICF? How would you suggest that they be assessed?
3. Use the ICF Functional Interview with a child with disabilities or his or her family. How well does it work to assess function in this individual? What additional information would be important to obtain? How might you obtain it?
4. Consider your work or school situation. How welcoming is your setting to individuals with sensory, motor, cognitive, or social disabilities? What kind of

accommodations might make your work or school situation more accessible for individuals with disabilities?

5. Identify the agencies and organizations in your community that provide vocational counseling and job training for individuals with disabilities. How are these organizations funded? What kind of data do they keep on their success rate? What kinds of positions do their clients get?

6

Health

William

William had trisomy 21 and a serious heart condition that left him with oxygen levels in his blood stream that were far lower than normal. When he was about 10 months of age, he had major surgery to correct the heart defect but suffered many complications following surgery. His oxygen levels did not immediately improve to normal, and he required prolonged mechanical ventilation in the intensive care unit (ICU). When his heart and lungs began to improve, he developed pneumonia, prolonging his stay in the ICU. This pattern of moderate improvement and severe complication persisted for months. He moved from the ICU to the hospital floor and then required readmission to the ICU. His parents took turns staying at the hospital every night to ensure that changes in his fragile status could be detected as soon as possible and relayed to the health care team.

After hospital discharge 5 months later, the erratic swings in health status continued for almost 2 years. During that time, Will had multiple hospitalizations for adjustment of heart medication or treatment of breathing difficulties, which for convenience were called asthma attacks. At age 3, he finally began to stabilize. His parents threw a family party when he had gone 6 months without a hospital visit.

At 3½, William was very delayed in his development. He did not walk or talk. His parents consulted the general pediatrician about enrolling him in a preschool program for children with developmental delays. The pediatrician deferred to the cardiologist and pulmonologist, who both advised against enrollment, fearful that Will would catch a cold or other infection that could send him back to the hospital. His parents tried to support his development with private therapies, but the doctors were also not in favor of his going into waiting rooms within the hospital.

At age 4, Will was slipping farther behind his peers in terms of functional abilities. His parents decided that they should not wait any longer to enroll him in school. They requested an evaluation for special education services, and Will was found eligible. They enrolled him in a community preschool, and he received special education supports within his classroom. His parents consulted with the program to establish a safety plan in case he became ill. Will loved the ability to be with other 3- and 4-year-old children and began to make developmental progress. He never required another hospitalization for heart or lung conditions.

Improved health is the third pillar of the triad of goals for health care for children with disabilities. However, a philosophical shift needs to take place that moves health care from a primary emphasis on the care and protection of the body to one of support of children's functioning, as illustrated in the opening vignette. Health care for children with disabilities should be designed to support their participation fully in everyday life, through both inclusion (Chapter 4) and contribution (Chapter 5). When health care is planned and provided in line with these priorities, children with disabilities can enjoy lives of personal satisfaction and well-being. In Will's case, the corrective cardiac surgery was necessary for him to survive, let alone participate in his family, school, and community. However, in the aftermath of that surgery, his physicians resisted any attempt to provide him with education, social experiences, and other activities that would allow inclusion and support contribution. His parents had to push against well-meaning and overly protective professionals for him to enjoy the activities that are part of everyday experience for children his age.

In contrast to a strictly medical focus, a broad definition of health is needed to cover the many issues that compromise function in children with disabilities. Health care that meets this definition supports not only physical health but also social and emotional functioning, and it requires the coordinated efforts of treating clinicians, the health care system, and the community. The Chronic Care Model (Improving Chronic Illness Care, 2011), as it is called by its developers, is an underlying model for comprehensive long-term clinical care. In order to allow health care to support inclusion and contribution, clinicians, collaborating with parents, must make explicit the functional outcomes and specific target objectives of the health care interventions for children. At the broader systems level practice guidelines should be created that include interventions to address the child's and family's function. Quality improvement activities at the office, clinic, hospital, or organizational level should emphasize the importance of functional outcomes in the assessment of care. Professional organizations, health insurance companies, and public health officials at local, state, or national levels should consider how to ensure that health care supports social participation.

A BROAD DEFINITION OF HEALTH

Health can be defined narrowly as being free from illness, injury, or pain. Almost everyone desires to be healthy according to this definition. However, if we use this definition to determine the scope of health care for children with disabilities, then health care is limited to preventing or curing illness, mending injuries, and/or reducing pain. Such a narrow scope of health care would not serve even those of us without apparent disabilities. Under this definition, it is difficult to justify providing services we have come to expect from the health care system, such as reproductive health services, glasses for individuals with near- or far-sightedness, or hearing aids for people with hearing loss.

The World Health Organization (WHO) formulated an alternative, expansive definition of health as "a state of complete physical, mental, and social well-being and not merely the absence of disease or infirmity" (WHO, 1946, p. 100). Under this definition, health care encompasses approaches and strategies that seek to improve the physical, mental, emotional, and social conditions of individuals. Though the broad definition can be criticized as vague and overly inclusive, it also has many advantages, especially with regard to the care of children with disabilities.

Children or adults with disabilities typically do not consider themselves ill or injured. Fortunately, most are not in pain (Chapter 1). They require health services to improve or maintain their functional capacities and to address their individual physical, mental, emotional, and social conditions. They look to health care for a broad range of services that derive from the WHO definition that would be considered unnecessary, even frivolous, according to a narrow definition of health. The following are some examples of clinical scenarios that would fall under the umbrella of health care according to an expansive definition:

- A toddler who has been exclusively tube fed after hypoxic-ischemic brain injury at birth is evaluated by an interdisciplinary feeding team composed of occupational therapy, dietetics and nutrition, and psychology professionals to develop a plan to transition the child to oral feedings. The plan includes direct interventions with the child and frequent educational sessions with the family.
- A child whose cleft lip and palate were successfully repaired obtains the services of a speech-language pathologist because of a persistent communication disorder after corrective surgery.
- The treatment plan for a preschooler with ADHD includes behavior management training for her parents and consultation with the early care and education team at the local school.
- A toddler with autism who is uninterested in the environment and nonverbal receives 3 hours of applied behavioral analysis in his home every weekday.
- The mother of a child with severe disabilities acknowledges that she is sad, unable to sleep, and withdrawn from her friends and family; she receives psychotherapy for adjustment reaction with depressive features.
- The family of a child with a rare genetic disorder receives the services of a social worker to assist them in finding parent-to-parent support with similar families. They also receive counseling from a geneticist and genetics counselor about the probability that another child might have the same disorder.

What these diverse examples have in common is that the treatments serve to allow the children and/or their family members to function more successfully in everyday life than would have likely occurred without the treatment.

After accepting the broad definition of health, a corollary is that health care does not need to be delivered only in clinical offices and hospitals, and not even exclusively by clinicians in the medical system. Health care can be conceptualized as encompassing various community resources and services that seek to improve physical, mental, emotional, and social well-being. For children, health care and education become inextricably intertwined. Children with learning problems, communication disorders, and social skill deficits may benefit from services that are offered in both the health care and educational systems. Health care also encompasses informal supports: families, friends, schools, religious institutions, neighborhood groups, and others. Though these social networks usually do not have a primary mission to improve a child's health, they foster caring interactions and provide instrumental support that inherently enhances and reinforces wellness.

HEALTH CARE DELIVERY SYSTEMS

The Chronic Care Model (Improving Chronic Illness Care, 2011) offers a conceptual framework for health care delivery under the broad construct of health. Figure 6.1 depicts the model, showing the basic elements of the health care system at the community, organization, practice, and patient levels. In the classic version of the model, informed patients take an active role in their own care. Health care providers form prepared and proactive interdisciplinary practice teams with adequate resources and expertise to anticipate and meet the needs of their patients. Their bidirectional interactions with health system and community support lead to improved outcomes. The Chronic Care Model, as adapted for children, is depicted in Figure 6.2. The two main differences are that 1) in this model, a supportive and integrated community interacts with a prepared and proactive practice team as well as with the informed

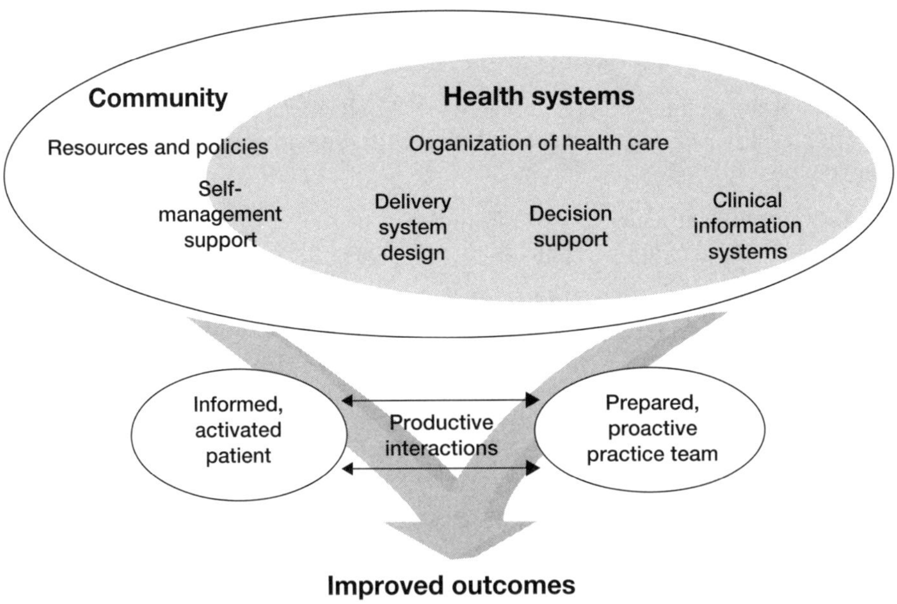

Figure 6.1. The Chronic Care Model for adult health care. (From Wagner, E.H. [1998]. Chronic disease management: What will it take to improve care for chronic illness? *Effective Clinical Practice [1]*1, 2–4; reprinted by permission.)

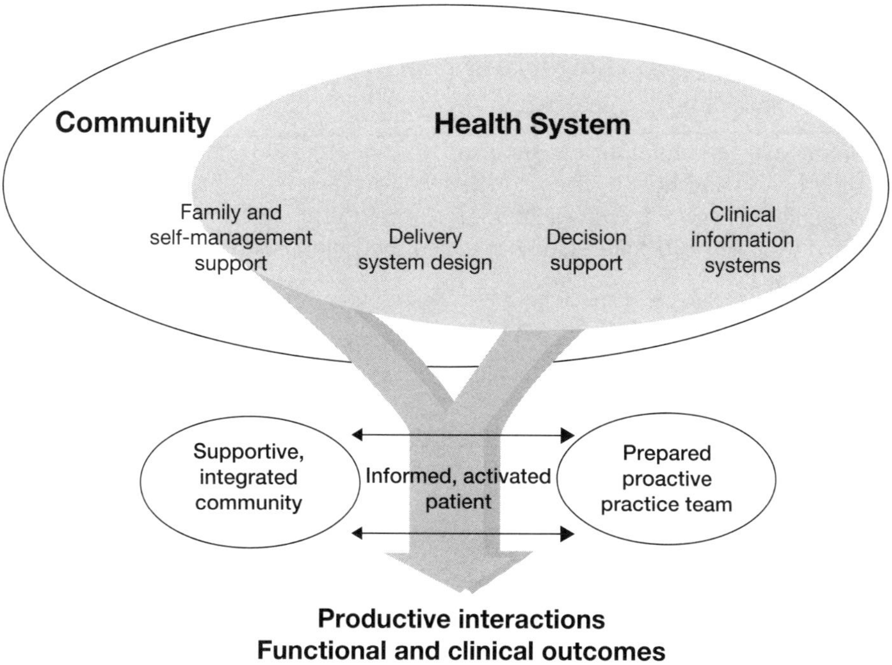

Figure 6.2. The Chronic Care Model for child health. Note that the informed and activated patient interacts with the prepared and proactive practice team and with the supportive and integrated community. (From Wagner, E.H. [1998]. Chronic disease management: What will it take to improve care for chronic illness? *Effective Clinical Practice [1]*1, 2–4. As adapted by the National Initiative for Children's Healthcare Quality; http://www.nichq.org/how_we_work/care_model_for_child_health.html; adapted by permission.)

and activated patient (and, I would add, family) and 2) the result is improved clinical and functional outcomes.

In both models, the interactions of patient and health care team are supported by four innovations in the health care system:

1. Clinical information systems organize patient and population data to facilitate efficient and effective care. Among the opportunities with improved information systems are sharing information between families and providers and among providers, creating interdisciplinary care plans (Chapter 8), and monitoring outcomes of the plan.

2. Decision support promotes clinical care that is consistent with scientific evidence and patient preferences. Research documents that quality of care can be improved when treatment decisions are based on clinical research and practice guidelines, though pitfalls and harms are also possible. Decision support allows guidelines to become readily available in daily practice, shared with families, and used to design educational interventions for providers as information changes with new research (Woolf, Grol, Hutchinson, Eccles, & Grimshaw, 1999).

3. Delivery system design ensures the delivery of effective, efficient clinical care and self-management support. Because of the complexity of care, delivery system design spells out the roles, responsibilities, tasks, and accountabilities for

members of the health care team and ensures that children get planned follow-up as appropriate to their conditions. In the modern information age, delivery system design can specify modes of interaction other than the traditional office visit to accomplish clinical care.

4. Self-management empowers and prepares children and their families to manage their health and health care. Effective self-management support acknowledges the family's central role in their child's care, fosters a sense of responsibility, and provides basic information, emotional support, and strategies for living with the condition.

The improving Chronic Care Model also emphasizes that community resources and services must be mobilized to meet needs of patients and their families. (See the

Commentary
Ashley

Remember Ashley, the child we met in the opening of Chapter 1? She was the child who was born very prematurely and developed respiratory difficulties, cerebral palsy, learning difficulties, and mental health problems. Ashley's after-hospitalization care was overwhelming for her parents. They ricocheted from one subspecialty group to another trying to meet all of their daughter's needs. They decided that her mother would quit work in order to focus on obtaining Ashley's health care.

When Ashley reached 10 months of age (6 months of age adjusted for the degree of prematurity), she made her first visit to the high risk infant follow-up clinic at the hospital of her birth and neonatal hospitalization. The interdisciplinary team at the clinic—a pediatrician, nurse coordinator, physical therapist, dietician, and social worker—was available at that visit. Partnering with the family, they assessed many different aspects of Ashley's health and integrated the findings into a single coordinated plan. The team noted high muscle tone and delayed motor development and referred the child for publicly funded early intervention services in the community. When Ashley turned 2, the team made the diagnosis of cerebral palsy. Though the parents were sad to get this news, at least they felt prepared and grateful that Ashley had been receiving weekly physical and occupational therapy for 18 months. They always credited those services for Ashley's ultimate ability to walk and to write.

When Ashley turned 3 years old, she graduated from the follow-up program. It was established for children from the neonatal ICU only until they reached age 3. Ashley and her family faced another challenge, as her graduation left them without the needed therapeutic support. The parents turned to her pediatrician for advice about her progress and the services appropriate for her ongoing delays. Though the pediatrician was kind and attentive, her knowledge about community resources was limited. As in the early days after Ashley's hospital discharge, the family was on its own to find community-based resources for their daughter. They eventually connected with a parent-to-parent support group for children born preterm. Other parents of children with disabilities became their guides through the health care system, sharing tips about what was available and who was the best clinician or service to provide the care.

commentary on p. 86.) Within this category are community programs that support or expand care. Also within the category are formal and informal social networks that encourage participation and social well-being. Partnerships among community services and linkages between community organizations and the health care system support children and families and develop interventions to fill gaps in needed services. For example, health care teams can form partnerships with schools or early intervention programs to ensure that children receive prescribed treatments and appropriate physical activity. Local and state departments of health and other agencies often have information regarding health conditions and their care. National disease-centered organizations link families with similar life experiences, provide valuable information, encourage self-help strategies, and advocate for pertinent policy change. The community is also essential for advocating for policies to improve patient care. Unfortunately, the health care system often misses opportunities to make the most of such resources.

PURPOSES OF HEALTH CARE INTERVENTIONS

If health care is defined broadly as a state of general well-being, and if health care systems incorporate community resources and services, then what constitutes appropriate health interventions? Health care incorporates more than the services and supplies required for diagnosis and treatment; interventions should include services that improve, maintain, or restore functional ability. However, the interventions should be clearly and specifically targeted to the clinical or function goal. Consider two contrasting cases. (See the commentaries below and on p. 88, respectively.)

In the first case, Des had orthopedic surgery specifically in order to restore his walking to a previous level of gross motor function. The interdisciplinary team became engaged at an early phase in the change of his gait patterns. When the child, family, and team concurred that the desired improvements were not occurring, they sought objective information from a gait analysis. Data from the gait laboratory

Commentary
Des

Des is a 15-year-old with cerebral palsy. He had achieved independent ambulation as a preschooler, though his gait remained unsteady and slow. However, as a teenager, when he began a growth spurt, his posture began to deteriorate, and his gait became less efficient. His doctors and therapists explained that although cerebral palsy is a nonprogressive condition, its manifestations change over time. Many problems arise when an adolescent's bones grow more quickly than the muscles lengthen. Des increased the frequency of physical therapy and physical activity for several months, but his gait did not improve. He then underwent an analysis of gait in a specialized laboratory. The interdisciplinary team determined that orthopedic surgery was likely to improve his gait, at least back to his baseline condition, so he and his family agreed to the procedure. They planned for the recommended operation in the summer between 10th and 11th grade, when he would be able to dedicate time to postoperative rehabilitation without the conflicts of homework and clubs. The plan resulted in noticeable improvements in his walking and made it easier for him to hang out with his friends and participate in his many extracurricular activities.

documented the problems and provided direction to the orthopedic surgeons. The final decision about whether to proceed with surgery was the result of an active collaboration among many professionals involved in Des's care, his parents, and Des himself. The success of the operation could be evaluated on the basis of specific target objectives, and the result was very positive.

In the second case (see the commentary below), Maria had a similar orthopedic procedure. In her case, the desired outcomes were not clearly articulated. The decision to do the operation was made without the collaboration of the health care team, and her physical and occupational therapists were not contacted or consulted. Her operation appeared to the therapists to be designed to treat the decreased mobility at the ankle, the symptom of cerebral palsy, and possibly to avoid the development of contractures, but they were not sure. Moreover, they noted that conservative management had not been adequately tried. The reason for release of hip muscles was not clear to the therapists who were treating her. Performing the operation at such a young age often necessitates future operations because linear growth may lead to increased spasticity or decreased range of motion. The operation neither improved Maria's level of function at the time it was done nor substantially improved her parents' ability to care for her. It actually led to a significant decrement in her mother's ability to leave the house and take her into the community and may contribute to future difficulties for her and her family.

The first step in providing care for children with disabilities that supports inclusion and contribution is to establish explicitly the desired results or target outcomes of treatment, with a long-term view of improving function. These objectives should drive the decision making about specific health care interventions. In acute health care, desired results or target outcomes are often implicit, and treatment does not need the involvement of an interdisciplinary team. For example, if a child suddenly

Commentary
Maria

Maria was a 3-year-old child born prematurely who developed cerebral palsy. Her trunk was hypotonic, but her legs were extremely hypertonic. She could not sit, stand, or walk. Physical and occupational therapy began a bit late, at age 2 years, after she received a definitive diagnosis. After a brief trial of therapy, her physical and occupational therapists recommended that she wear orthotic braces to stretch the muscles and tendons at the ankle joints and to allow her feet to be flat on the floor. They then recommended the use a passive standing frame to support her in an upright position. The stander allows the child to enjoy a different position and to learn about the world from that new vantage point. The therapists also ordered a special stroller for the child. Before these plans were fully in place, before the stander and stroller were even delivered, Maria's mother canceled several therapy visits. When the therapists called to ask why, Maria's mother reported that an orthopedist she had consulted decided to do an operation on Maria to relax her hip and ankle muscles. In the aftermath of surgery, Maria wore a cast from her waist to her feet. This meant that whenever her mother needed to go somewhere with her, she had to carry her wearing these heavy casts. Her mother experienced back problems after the surgery, and it was 3 months before therapy resumed.

develops a fever and ear pain, the family takes the child to the pediatrician to find a treatment that reduces the fever and pain and returns the child to her usual state of health. Though the objective is never stated, the treating physician and the family share the same objective. The choice of treatment is predicated on an accurate diagnosis of the problem. Similarly, in the opening vignette of this chapter, William had a serious, life-threatening congenital heart condition, and the cardiac operation was designed to correct his physiological function.

In long-term care, several benefits ensue from making target outcomes explicit. First, the choice of target outcomes may influence or even dictate the appropriate intervention. For children with cerebral palsy, the choice of target outcomes often suggests what intervention makes the most sense. Second, differences in the objectives across different members of the team or between the family and the treating clinician can be discussed. Because issues of disability are complex, and because approximately half of individuals with disabilities have more than one long-term condition, many target objectives for treatment are possible. The objectives of the individual, family, and clinicians may differ. The clinical process involves coming to consensus about the most important issues so as to focus efforts and avoid exhausting the child and family physically, emotionally, or financially. The consensus may help in staging the treatment plan so that the prerequisites have been accomplished before the main treatments are begun. Failure to negotiate about differences and to come to consensus lead to high dissatisfaction with health care. Third, knowing the target outcomes is essential for evaluating the success of interventions. If the child fails to meet the objectives, then the treatment team, including the family, can problem solve to determine the barriers to success. The problem may have been that the plan was overly ambitious or that it was not fully implemented. In Des's case, he first chose increased physical therapy and physical activity, and he gave therapy an adequate trial. When he did not meet his objectives, he and his family and interdisciplinary team turned to orthopedic surgery. In the second case, the desired results of the surgery were not made explicit, at least not with the family or the therapists. The results of the surgery could not be fully evaluated because there were no pre-established standards by which to evaluate it. Whether the treatment was in fact warranted remains an open issue.

This principle of establishing clear objectives has been a core feature of education law since passage of the original federal legislation making education for all children an entitlement (Wright & Wright, 2011). According to IDEA, once a child is determined to be eligible for special education services by documentation of a disability as defined in legislation, an individualized education plan (IEP) is developed. The IEP includes a description of the child's present level of performance and the unique needs based on the child's disability. The IEP is a written statement of the objectives for the child and the educational program designed to meet all of the child's individual needs. In short, it says what the child should accomplish in a year. Every child who receives special education services must have an IEP. In the current iteration of IDEA, the IEP is fully reassessed every 3 years. Establishing objectives that are measurable allows an evaluation of whether the plan is working and a reconsideration of the plan if it is not.

The American Academy of Pediatrics (AAP) recognized the value of articulating target objectives when it first published practice guidelines for the management of ADHD (AAP, 2003; Subcommittee on Attention-Deficit/Hyperactivity Disorder

Committee on Quality Improvement, 2001). The first step in the recommended management of ADHD is to recognize that ADHD is a long-term condition. Manifestations are generally apparent during the preschool years, although they may not come to medical attention until school age or even adolescence. The traits tend to persist into adulthood, even though some individuals no longer meet diagnostic criteria for ADHD as they get older. The next step in the recommended progression is to establish the target outcomes of treatment. Several tools for assisting pediatricians, other clinicians, and family members in arriving at the targets are included in a toolkit developed as a companion to the guidelines. The central issue here is that the treatment plan may vary as a function of the target outcomes agreed upon by clinicians, families, and children.

The establishment of target objectives is typically an iterative process. As the child progresses, often as a result of an intervention, the objectives shift, and the plan must be modified accordingly. Interventions bring along desired effects and adverse effects; the plan may need adjustment because of the severity of the adverse effects. For example, a child with persistent pain that limits concentration and social interaction may need medications to reduce the pain. However, the medication may blunt the child's cognitive abilities and reduce learning. It may also be challenging to balance short- and long-term objectives. For example, if a child is developing scoliosis, surgical intervention may temporarily cause a setback in mobility and community participation. However, early treatment may be more effective than waiting to prevent respiratory compromise from scoliosis.

All of these factors demonstrate that articulating target outcomes is a challenging step in the clinical process. Nonetheless, what is most important is that the target outcomes for intervention be made explicit. If they are stated, they can be discussed and if necessary debated among the team of health care professionals, the family, and the child, when appropriate. If they are stated, then it is easier to determine if the chosen treatments have a reasonable chance of leading to the desired results. If they are explicit, then the treatments can ultimately be evaluated.

AT THE SYSTEMS LEVEL

Health and medical care has expanded dramatically in the last 100 years. At the beginning of the 20th century, medical science was just learning that microorganisms were the cause of many diseases. The only available vaccinations were for smallpox and rabies. The use of x-rays to see within the body was quite new. No chemotherapy had been developed for cancer. Physical therapy had been recently recognized as a profession, occupational therapy was just conceived, and audiology and speech-language pathology had not yet emerged. At the beginning of the 21st century, we have learned about many viruses and bacteria that cause illness. We use MRI scans to see within the brain and the body. Many effective treatments are available for once-fatal illnesses, and interdisciplinary teams are in place for the care of children with disabilities and their families.

As opposed to a century ago, the challenge of this era is to choose effective and cost-effective approaches for the treatment or management of long-term conditions. The possibilities for intervention are vast. It is easy to overtreat some children while undertreating others. This problem is exacerbated in the current U.S. health care system because care is fragmented, delivered by many different professionals without systematic mechanisms for communication and coordination across the health care team (Institute of Medicine, 2001). New tools are needed to ensure that health care clinicians know about the availability of different treatments or strategies and how they can be applied appropriately and effectively.

Practice Guidelines

Practice guidelines have become one modern approach to guide the health care team in delivering appropriate interventions. They provide systematic recommendations for prevention, treatment, or management of specific conditions and include concise instructions on steps to take and interventions that work. They are designed to improve health care quality by disseminating information to treating clinicians and by reducing unnecessary or unwarranted variability in clinical processes. To be useful, the practice guidelines must be general enough to address the care of many different individuals who nonetheless share a diagnosis or clinical circumstance. At the same time, they must be specific enough to provide detailed guidance for the clinicians, in particular about when they are applicable and when they can be overridden. They often involve a step-by-step approach to diagnosis or treatment.

Practice guidelines are often qualified with the term *evidence-based.* This designation indicates that paths and decisions have been validated through rigorous scientific study. It encourages clinicians to base their decisions on scientific findings rather than on personal experience. Practice guidelines are often informed by systematic reviews of medical and health care literatures. When such scientific evidence is not available, then the guidelines may be created through a process of expert consensus.

Practice guidelines advantage children with disabilities, their practice teams, and health care systems. When guidelines promote effective interventions and discourage ineffective treatments, the net result is an improvement in clinical or functional outcomes. They are designed to reduce variations in health care that are based on what should be irrelevant variables, such as the specific clinician evaluating the child or the region of the country in which the care is taking place, variables unrelated to the clinical condition or the personal experience of the child and family (Woolf et al., 1999). Guidelines can thus reduce disparities and promote social justice. They are very useful to practitioners with limited experience and improve clinical decision making. Practice guidelines for children with disabilities can improve care by identifying nonmedical interventions, including therapy, education, parent support, and community education, elements of an effective plan that might otherwise be overlooked in treatment planning.

A potential harm of practice guidelines arises if they are flawed, poorly prepared, or based on inaccurate information (Woolf et al., 1999). Sometimes, particularly in the care of children with disabilities, the scientific foundation for decision making is highly underdeveloped because many pediatric conditions are relatively rare. It is difficult to amass a large group to evaluate or compare treatments. Entities that can identify an adequate sample and fund large studies include pharmaceutical companies or medical equipment manufacturers. These commercial units may have conflicts of interest and yet unduly influence the recommendations of the studies. Of course, these same issues arise when treatment proceeds without the benefit of practice guidelines. Another potential harm is that they might be applied to the wrong individual or clinical circumstance. When the guidelines include recommendations not to use specific interventions, that may lead to reduced access to that service or to a lack of insurance coverage for services. Recommendations for expensive interventions on the basis of flimsy evidence may displace limited resources that would be better spent on other services of greater value (Woolf et al., 1999).

The trend in health care is for increased reliance on practice guidelines. Governments and insurance carriers favor this development as an approach to controlling health care costs. However, clinicians and families often interpret the guidelines as an affront to personal autonomy. The development of clinical practice guidelines can be very helpful in managing long-term disability as long as the guidelines remain flexible and can be modified or ignored when clinical factors dictate a lack of supporting evidence for that condition or circumstance.

Quality Improvement

Another approach to improving health care delivery is quality improvement. Quality improvement has been an important focus in business and industry for many years; in that setting, it was designed to improve efficiency and reduce error. When it became clear that these issues were also important to patients and families, health insurance plans, and employers who contribute to health insurance, then the approach migrated into health care. The Institute of Medicine highlighted the need for quality improvement in health care in two important published reports (Institute of Medicine, 2001; Kohn, Corrigan, & Donaldson, 1999). The introduction of quality improvement methods has generally been associated with improvements in health care outcomes (Institute of Medicine, 2001; Kohn et al., 1999).

The process of quality improvement usually begins with evidence of a problem. Then data are collected to understand the cause of the problem and its impact. Changes in the system are made, and the data are reassessed. Quality improvement in hospitals is often focused on reducing waste, improving safety, reducing errors, identifying efficiencies, and reducing costs.

Quality improvement could be a strategy for improving clinical and functional outcomes of children with disabilities in the health care system. In this variant of quality improvement, an analysis of clinician fidelity to practice guidelines or other measure of clinical effectiveness would be obtained and associated with measures of children's functional status. Strategies for encouraging adherence to the guidelines would need to be created. The American Board of Pediatrics requires pediatricians to participate in quality improvement activities as part of the maintenance of their board certification. The impact of closer adherence to guidelines on child and family outcomes would be an interesting and important research project.

Practice guidelines and quality improvement are but two ways to focus on transforming health care to support inclusion and contribution. In the next chapter, I consider in more depth how to get health care aligned with functional outcomes.

SUMMARY

In the care of children with disabilities, at least in the present era, curing the condition is rarely a possibility. Health care for these children must be predicated on a broad and inclusive definition of health that is consistent with the overarching goals of inclusion and contribution. To that end, health care interventions should be designed to explicitly improve specific issues. The improvements in functioning should be the target outcomes of the intervention. Achieving improvements in function requires a team that is prepared to care for the child and a family that is well informed about the choices and considerations. This kind of coordinated health care system would fully utilize information technology capabilities to identify the children with high levels of need and to provide data-driven or scientifically motivated treatments. Community resources and services and informal supports are also actively engaged in supporting the child and family. It is also important to articulate explicit and measurable health care goals for individual children and their families and to evaluate whether those goals are met. Although good health is a fundamental goal, considerations about how to achieve clinical improvement should not trump interventions to improve functional outcomes. Functional outcomes can be conceptualized broadly from the individual level to participation in the greater society. Practice guidelines provide direction for health care for some specific populations or clinical problems and can be modified to include interventions that improve function. Quality improvement efforts may be useful to evaluate whether care processes are achieving desired functional outcomes within systems of care.

Exercises

1. Review critiques of the WHO definition of health. In what ways are these criticisms valid? How could you modify the definition to address these criticisms?
2. Consider the care of the children in the vignettes in this chapter. What community resources might they have used as toddlers, preschoolers, school-age children, and adolescents?
3. Investigate an electronic medical record. Does it have the capacities outlined for clinical information systems in the Chronic Care Model?
4. Evaluate a practice guideline in your clinical field. What is the clinical problem that the guideline addresses? Which groups are covered under the guideline, and which groups are excluded? How is the impact of this guideline on clinical care evaluated?
5. Investigate quality improvement programs at an institution where you work or in your field of study. What is the clinical problem that the program addresses? What are the measures that the program will follow to ensure that quality is improving? Evaluate this program from your point of view. In what ways might this program improve the care that you deliver? In what ways may it impede what you consider good care?
6. Design an alternative to the individual clinical visit for monitoring progress of a child with a learning disability.

III

Strategies and Tools to Achieve Goals

7

Focusing Health Care on Function

Anthony

At age 7 Anthony was diagnosed with attention-deficit hyperactivity disorder (ADHD). His parents and teachers concurred that he had many symptoms of inattention, hyperactivity, and impulsivity that had been present since he was a preschooler. The symptoms led to academic difficulties, including poor grades and weak performance on group-administered standardized tests. He also had significant difficulties in making and keeping friends. His pediatrician carefully followed the practice guidelines of the American Academy of Pediatrics (Subcommittee on Attention-Deficit/Hyperactivity Disorder, 2011) to make the diagnosis. She recommended a trial of stimulant medication, and the parents agreed. It took about 4 weeks and minor adjustments to the dose and schedule of medication for Anthony to achieve a maximum reduction of symptoms with minimal adverse side effects. His parents were very pleased that the daily notes and calls from school decreased substantially.

At age 8, at a planned follow-up visit, the parents expressed their surprise that although disruptive behaviors had seemed to subside, Anthony's grades and performance on standardized tests had not changed all that much since the medication was started the previous school year. Even more disappointing to them and to Anthony was that he had not been able to make new friends. The pediatrician recommended changes in the medication dose and schedule. After several modifications, the parents concluded that Anthony's residual academic and social issues would not be effectively managed with medication alone.

At the parents' insistence, the pediatrician referred the family to a highly respected child psychologist. He guided the parents in developing a behavior management program that initially rewarded Anthony for focus and persistence. Over time, working collaboratively, the parents shifted the targets of behavior management to rewards for accuracy and high quality of work. Anthony's school performance improved perceptibly, though not dramatically. The parents also wanted to address his social problems but could not afford social skills training while also paying for behavior management treatment. At the recommendation of other parents, they discontinued Anthony's participation in Little League and instead enrolled him in a Saturday martial arts class with an experienced master teacher who had an excellent reputation for teaching children of all abilities. Anthony loved the structured program. His mother invited a couple of the other students and their mothers out for lunch after the third class; the outing was so successful that lunch became part of the Saturday routine. Anthony and his classmates began to get together at other times of the week as well.

To achieve the vision of inclusion, contribution, and health for children with disabilities, major changes are required at multiple levels of the health care system. Some of these changes may take, well, an act of Congress. Other changes can begin without much funding or fanfare, however, as individual health care professionals work with children and their families. I will begin at the level of the individual practitioner, where change is readily attainable, and gradually work in subsequent chapters to the policy level (Chapter 13).

At the present time, physicians and many on the health care team who treat children with disabilities prioritize clinical goals. Surprisingly, achieving clinical goals does not necessarily result in improving functional outcomes. As Anthony's story demonstrates, the reduction in the number and severity of symptoms of inattention and hyperactivity, an indication of clinical improvement, does not necessarily lead to better grades at school or to meaningful friendships in the neighborhood. In order to achieve better grades, satisfying friendships, and improvements in his functional status, functional goals had to be made explicit and had to be addressed in a comprehensive treatment plan.

This chapter will define function and review functional assessment tools currently available. Members of the interdisciplinary team who treat children with disabilities already focus on function in their work but use different measures for different purposes. Even when function is assessed and used to inform treatment, the team is poorly informed about the broad functional perspective and how their individual work can contribute to an integrated plan of care. I make several recommendations to create integrated plans, using the International Classification of Functioning, Disability and Health (IFC) as the organizing framework.

DEFINITIONS AND FOCUS OF FUNCTION IN HEALTH CARE

Functional status can be defined as how an individual engages in and interacts with the world. Functional status encompasses the roles that people play and the purposes and meaning of those roles for the individual. Another term used to describe functional status is *adaptive behavior*. Functional status is highly influenced by health and may be the consequence of an individual's health status, but it is an independent construct (World Health Organization, 2002).

Focus of Function within the Medical Model

In the traditional medical model, the focus on function is secondary (Chapter 3); the physician's primary goal of treatment is to prevent or cure the patient's condition. If prevention and cure are beyond medical reach, then treatment is designed to alleviate the condition by reducing its signs and symptoms. For example, in cerebral palsy, treatment should reduce spasticity or dystonia, and in ADHD (as in the opening vignette), treatment should eliminate or at least minimize distractibility and fidgetiness. (See also the commentary below.)

In the medical model, the focus on function is typically relegated to nurses and to therapists, including physical and occupational therapists, speech-language pathologists, audiologists, rehabilitation counselors, and behavioral therapists. The services of these therapists typically require the referral of the physician. The physician determines the need for treatment, the amount, and the frequency. In the

Commentary
Personal Reflections

I came to understand the narrow focus of the medical model when my aging father developed glaucoma. Glaucoma is an eye disease characterized by increased fluid pressure in an anterior chamber of the eye. Untreated, the pressure injures the optic nerve and ultimately limits the individual's visual acuity and visual fields. My father's glaucoma was detected late in this process. His ophthalmologist treated the glaucoma first with medication and then, when the pressures remained high, with surgery. The doctor was delighted with the success of the surgery because the fluid pressure within the eye dropped to ideal levels.

Despite this apparent success, my father's vision did not improve. Rather, it continued to decline and began restricting his occupation and his recreation. By chance, I had met the director of a rehabilitation center for individuals with blindness and visual impairment. Sharing my father's frustrations with his medical care, I contacted the director to take him up on his kind invitation to visit his facility with my dad.

There, the entire program was designed to maximize each client's residual visual capacity. When visual impairment limited daily activities, the counselors and clients worked together to identify creative solutions to the problems. The staff immediately interviewed my father about his activities and interests. Because he needed to read, they showed him magnifying glasses with various lighting designs that would allow him to see small print. Because he loved to play bridge, they introduced him to playing cards with large numbers and to variations in the rules, such as having players name their cards as they play them. They helped him with eyeglass filters for glare so he could continue to enjoy walks on bright and sunny days, and they taught him how to increase the font size on his computer. At the end of this 2-hour visit, my father had a renewed sense of hope that he could cope with visual loss.

Clearly, the ophthalmologist was necessary to the care of my father's glaucoma. The surgery probably halted the progression of injury to the optic nerve. However, the ophthalmologist was not sufficient for a comprehensive plan; the rehabilitation counselor provided the keys to stabilizing function. My disappointment was that the ophthalmologist did not know to make the referral to a low-vision expert.

care of a child with ADHD, a family may directly contract with a psychologist or behavior therapist for treatment. However, the health insurance company often reimburses only care that is prescribed by physicians. Unfortunately, the clinical and functional perspectives often operate in parallel, with minimal communication and coordination.

Status of Function within the Social Model

In the social model of disability, the focus on function is primary (Chapter 3), and the goal is the individual's independence and participation within the community. The social model attributes disadvantages experienced by children and adults with disabilities primarily to environmental and social factors; thus, the interventions are aimed at the environmental and social level. From the perspective of the social model, a child with cerebral palsy who requires a wheelchair for mobility has functional limitations if she cannot afford the wheelchair or if her neighborhood is not wheelchair accessible. In addition, poor attitudes on the part of adults in the child's life might result in her reluctance to use the wheelchair, limiting her mobility and contributing to poor self-esteem, depression, and reduced social interaction. Similarly, a child with ADHD has functional limitations because of characteristics of the classroom or instructional approaches that do not accommodate the child's learning style.

The social model, like the medical model, is also limited in its pure form. It does not recognize that health and individual characteristics also contribute to functional status. For example, if the child with cerebral palsy has spasticity that causes pain or a growth spurt that compromises mobility, then the limitations may not be based on social and environmental features but rather on factors inherent to the individual. For this child to maintain function, physical therapy to relax muscles or surgery to correct painful hip dislocations may become central to the care. Similarly, the child with ADHD may have sufficient difficulties with attending and learning that he cannot achieve grade-level skills or output, even with classroom accommodations.

Function-Focused Care: Assisted Living as an Example

The term *function-focused care* has been proposed in the literature on assisted living. It is defined in that context as the implementation of a philosophy of care in which nurses and direct care workers help older adults to participate in self-care, as well as physical and recreational activities (Resnick, Galik, Gruber-Baldini, & Zimmerman, 2010, 2011). Adults move into care facilities when their function has declined and they lack sufficient supports to maintain independent living. Historically, in nursing homes and institutions for individuals with disabilities, the individuals' interests, needs, and individuality were subjugated to professional dominance and efficiency. Their mealtimes were set, their meals chosen for them, and their daily activities determined exclusively by staff. In function-focused assisted living, by contrast, the older adults assume as much personal responsibility as possible. They make personal choices such as when to eat, what to eat, and how to spend their time. The model encourages activity, such as physical exercise, over a sedentary lifestyle. Function-focused assisted living is not only respectful of the clients but also conducive to good health. Older adults who remain active and in control of aspects of their lives may use less nursing and direct worker time and attention without a reduction in safety (Resnick et al., 2011). It is important to note that even in function-focused assisted living, however, the medical model dominates. Function-focused care is relegated to nurses and the workers they supervise. The model does not specify whether or how these clinicians provide feedback to the physicians and other therapists to maximize the function of the adult residents. Thus, function-focused assisted living fails to integrate the functional focus across the interdisciplinary team. It is an isolated component of the total health care plan.

Function Focused: Expanding to Care for Children with Disabilities

An expanded variant of function-focused care would be particularly beneficial for the health care of children with disabilities. In children, functional expectations and capacity evolve over time. Developmental progress usually occurs even in the presence of disability, although disability may alter the rate or direction of developmental change. In the care of children, even those with severe disabilities, developmental change will propel increased functional capacity. Treatments geared toward improving function can capitalize on developmental changes in children's abilities. With appropriate interventions, recovery, at least to some degree, may also be possible. (See also the commentary below.)

This form of expanded function-focused care signals the primacy of functional improvement as the goal for the entire interdisciplinary team that treats children with disabilities, regardless of the child's setting. The child and family identify their primary goals, with support from the interdisciplinary team; the team shares responsibility for implementing the interventions that lead to improvement. All possible means can be deployed to this end: medical care, therapy, education, family training, adaptive equipment, formal or informal support, and ultimately self-care.

FUNCTIONAL ASSESSMENT

A prerequisite for the implementation of function-focused care is assessing how children function in their everyday life. Assessments of function provide an understanding of the child at baseline, prior to treatment, and an index of the type and

Commentary
Anthony as a Teenager

Anthony, the child in this chapter's vignette, remained on stimulant medication for about 5 years. By age 13 he had developed a passion for computer programming. He recognized that he needed strong math skills in order to accomplish what he wanted with the computer, and with this sense of purpose (as well as a stable group of friends), he had come to enjoy school as he grew older. At the beginning of the eighth grade, he decided that he did not like how the medication made him feel. He pleaded with his parents and with his pediatrician for a medication holiday. Reluctantly, they deferred to his wishes.

His parents noticed that off medication, he was sometimes too talkative and often easily distracted, but he had clearly progressed substantially since he was an early elementary school student. The family returned to the psychologist for a refresher course in behavior management, this time bringing Anthony to the sessions. He never went back on stimulant medication.

degree of change. Functional assessment may include formal measures, such as tests, surveys, or questionnaires, or informal strategies, such as observing the child at school or collecting work samples in a portfolio.

Functional assessment is fundamental in many disciplines working with children with disabilities. It is particularly pertinent in physical and occupational therapy, in which it encompasses evaluations of mobility and manipulation. However, even in physical and occupational therapy, functional assessment competes with clinical evaluations of tone, balance, spasticity, and sensory processing.

Unlike the standardized, norm-referenced tests (e.g., intelligence testing) that are typically used for evaluating children for disabilities and involve testing in controlled, decontextualized environments, functional assessment approaches describe the child's performance in the real world. Thus, assessment can be more meaningful but also more challenging, because functional competence within any domain is likely to vary across settings and situations. For example, a preschooler with a communication disorder may use more advanced syntactic structures with his mother at home than he does with his teacher at school or with an unfamiliar speech-language pathologist completing an evaluation. A child's decontextualized function in the office or the clinic offers only one perspective on that child's abilities and may not be representative of her behavior in other comfortable and familiar settings. Clinicians may therefore not be able observe the child's actual functional status as it appears within the child's natural environments. The problem is particularly acute for young children, who have not yet been to school and who, developmentally, do not understand the demands of the testing situation (Neisworth & Bagnato, 2004).

Methods of Functional Assessment

In order to obtain an accurate or authentic (Neisworth & Bagnato, 2004) evaluation of the child in his or her real world, functional or adaptive behavior measures often ask informants who know the child well to provide the information. Such measures may come in the form of questionnaires, surveys, or interviews. The usual informants are parents and teachers, and the measures rate the child's abilities in the home or at school, respectively. One well-known functional measure is the Vineland Adaptive Behavior Scales, now in the second edition (Sparrow, Cicchetti, & Balla, 2005). It assesses four functional domains: socialization; communication; daily living skills; and, in young children, mobility. Parents or teachers may be interviewed or asked to complete a survey form. Older children, adolescents, and adults may report on their own functional status. On the basis of response patterns, the

Commentary
Other Uses of the Term Functional Assessment

The terms functional assessment *or* functional behavioral assessment *may be used in a specific way for children with behavioral issues. In those cases, the terms denote a process focused on a problem behavior and seeking to determine the triggers, the function or purpose of the behavior for the child, and factors that maintain the behavior in the child's repertoire. Here, we are using* functional assessment *in a more general way.*

measure generates a standard score and an age equivalent. Assessments such as this one are evaluated according to the same psychometric properties used in the evaluation of standardized measures, including reliability and validity. However, because they use parents or teachers as respondents, they are more subjective than standardized measures. Functional assessment measures vary in the number of domains they assess, the specific domains included, and the items used to assess those domains. Table 7.1 lists several formal functional assessment tools currently available. Functional assessment may also use informal measures, such as a portfolio of work products.

Functional Assessment versus Standardized Testing

Assessment serves several functions: determination of eligibility for services, treatment planning and progress monitoring, and program evaluation. Standardized measures remain the gold standard for determining eligibility for services such as special education or early intervention. The criteria for eligibility are based on the degree to which a child's performance varies from the norms of typical development. Cutoff scores are established to make administrative decisions about which children meet eligibility criteria and, by implication, need services. However, using standardized measures as the sole criterion for establishing eligibility may prove problematic. For example, children with significant functional difficulties in school may be able to perform well in the highly structured and controlled environment of a standardized test.

Standardized tests do a poor job of determining the child's individual plan for therapy or education. The items that make up the standardized test are those that have proven useful in discriminating among age groups and also among diagnostic groups. For example, a good test item might be one that is answered correctly by only a few 4-year-olds, more 6-year-olds, and almost all 10-year-olds. However, the items that succeed at this discrimination function may or may not be important

Table 7.1. Selected set of functional assessment measures

Assessment measure	Age range	Domains assessed	Publisher
Adaptive Behavior Assessment System–Second Edition	0–89 years	Ten skill areas, three adaptive domains, and General Adaptive Component	Western Psychological Services (Torrance, CA)
Child and Adolescent Functional Assessment Scale (and related measures)	5–19 years	Eight areas of function for youth, two for caregiver	MHS (North Tonawanda, NY)
Functional Independence Measure for Children	6 months to 7 years or older for children with disabilities	Six areas	Systems for Medical Rehabilitation (Buffalo, NY)
Pediatric Evaluation of Disability Inventory	6 months to 7 years or older for children with disabilities	Three scales	Pearson (San Antonio, TX)
Vineland Adaptive Behavior Scales, Second Edition	0–90	Four domains and Adaptive Behavior Composite	Pearson (San Antonio, TX)

in the life of a child and may be irrelevant to the child's treatment plan. To plan a child's treatment program, additional measures, such as those based on developmental trajectories or academic curricula, need to be added to the standardized test at some point in the assessment process.

Standardized measures are also poor indicators for program evaluation. A child's score on the standardized measure is, by design, relatively stable over time. However, the measures that are most useful for program evaluation are those that document how a child has changed and grown through program participation (Neisworth & Bagnato, 2004).

Functional assessment has come to play an increasingly prominent role in the diagnosis of intellectual disability. In the past, scores on an IQ test were the major factor in deciding if a child functioned in the range of intellectual disability. The current definitions require limitation in both intellectual abilities, including reasoning and problem solving, and in adaptive behavior, including learning, social skills, and activities of daily living (American Association on Intellectual and Developmental Disabilties, 2010). The centrality of adaptive function in the definition prevents the application of the label to children who are shy, primary speakers of a language other than English, impaired in expressive communication, or unfamiliar with the rigors of formal testing, all of whom might do poorly on standardized measures of intelligence. Emphasizing the assessment of adaptive behavior acknowledges that some individuals may perform poorly on tests without experiencing equivalent difficulties in real-world activities. The integration of standardized and functional assessment improves the choice of therapies and supports for individuals who experience difficulties in everyday life. (See the commentaries on pp. 102 and 104, respectively, for examples.)

Commentary
Ellen

Ellen, age 3 years, 4 months, returned to the interdisciplinary team at the clinic with her distressed mother. The child had been diagnosed with autism approximately 4 months previously. Her mother followed the team recommendations and requested an evaluation for special education services at the local school. To her mother's surprise, Ellen was denied special education services on the basis of the school's evaluation. On the Preschool Language Scale, Fourth Edition (Zimmerman, Steiner, & Pond, 2002), the child scored an 84, based in large part on her ability to label pictures. On the Goldman-Fristoe Test of Articulation 2 (Goldman & Fristoe, 2000), she scored at the 96th percentile, based on clear articulation during labeling and imitating. No other assessments were conducted before she was declared ineligible for educational services.

The team deployed its speech-language pathologist to the school with data on the child's functional communication skills. Ellen could not answer simple questions such as, "What is your name?" or "How old are you?" She could not initiate a conversation. She did not follow two-step commands. She did not even use her vocabulary to make requests. Rather, she would stand before the desired item and throw a tantrum while the parents frantically tried to figure out what she wanted. On the basis of this functional description and as a result of the strong team advocacy, the school reversed course and found her eligible for services.

Commentary
Stanton

After having been diagnosed with childhood apraxia of speech at age 3, Stanton was brought back to the interdisciplinary team at the clinic 4 months later by his distressed mother. His mother had followed the team recommendations and requested an evaluation for special education services at the local school. He was tested with the Wechsler Preschool and Primary Scale of Intelligence, Third Edition (Wechsler, 2002) and the Goldman-Fristoe Test of Articulation (Goldman & Fristoe, 2000). His Full-Scale IQ was 67. He had a similar score on the articulation measure, during which all of his productions were imitative. The school recommended a segregated class for children with intellectual disability and 30 minutes per week of speech-language pathology services in a group setting.

The interdisciplinary team reviewed the results of the school's assessment and realized that the decision making was based on the Full-Scale IQ, despite a significant difference between low average nonverbal skills and impaired verbal skills. In addition, Stanton's unintelligibility had not been factored into the poor performance on the Verbal scale. The team deployed its speech-language pathologist to the school with data on his clinical and functional communication skills. Stanton had variable errors in vowels and consonants and struggled with pronunciation, especially as sentence length increased or creative uses of language were required. As a result of this functional description and the strong team advocacy, the school reversed course and found Stanton eligible for services on the basis of speech-language impairment. More important, the frequency and nature of speech therapy services were changed.

Functional Assessment versus Health-Related Quality of Life Measures

Health-related quality of life measures are designed to generate a profile of the respondents' function and well-being in relation to their health status. These measures assess the burden of disease on individuals and on populations and may be useful for tracking the benefits of medical treatments. Respondents are asked to evaluate changes in their functional status in relation to what they attribute to their health condition. One frequently used quality of life measure is the Short Form 36 (Version 2; Medical Outcomes Trust, n.d.). This measure asks whether health has resulted in recent changes in vigorous activities, climbing stairs, walking, or dressing. It also assesses whether physical health has resulted in a reduction in the time a person works, the amount accomplished, or the kind of work the person was able to do.

For children with disabilities, functional assessment measures are more useful than health-related quality of life measures at the clinical level. Health-related quality of life measures are designed to provide an evaluation of the perceived health burden of a condition and the relief offered by various treatments. However, the measures are not sufficiently detailed to guide treatment planning, as they do not take into account the individual's developmental or functional status. Individuals with disabilities may already have limitations in mobility or self-care, and the measures have limited sensitivity to changes in status. Importantly, they do not assess the influence of social and environmental factors on domains of function, even though these external factors may be highly relevant to the maintenance of functional capacity.

Health-related quality of life measures may be appropriate at the clinical level under specified conditions. They can be used as follows:

- To detect changes in functional status
- In adults who were previously in good health and highly functional
- In adults who can report on their status

For children, in whom assessment should be intimately tied to intervention because the possibility of change is so high, these measures are less generally useful.

FUNCTIONAL CLASSIFICATION

Different members of the interdisciplinary teams that treat children with disabilities address different domains in their assessments and treatments. Many of these disciplines have well-established protocols and assessment tools to evaluate the child's functioning within their domain or domains of interest. However, they lack a shared overarching framework, common language, and a standard method of classification; they are thus prone to fall back on discipline-specific terminology or diagnosis. It becomes difficult to share results across health care disciplines and even harder to share results with educators, public health officials, and policy makers. A single taxonomy that could be used across settings and professionals would be highly valuable and should have applicability to all members of the team.

The ICF, developed by WHO, provides a universal framework for describing a comprehensive view of children's function abilities (Chapter 5). Classification on the basis of functional characteristics as opposed to diagnostic category facilitates a holistic and nonstigmatizing approach to disability (Simeonsson et al., 2006). The framework not only describes the abilities of the individual but also captures environmental support and barriers that influence the individual's capacity to perform within his environment. As a comprehensive classification system, the ICF can serve to integrate the results of different measures within a single overarching system. (See the commentary on p. 105.) The ICF-CY facilitates the use of this model in the care of children with disabilities (WHO Workgroup for Developmental of Version of ICF for Children & Youth, 2007). The ICF-CY includes domains and codes that specifically apply to young children, whose body functions include heightened imagination and whose primary activities include play. ICF-CY contributes to interdisciplinary clinical practice in several important ways (Simeonsson et al., 2006, p. 4):

1. Provides a unifying framework for interdisciplinary practice (see the commentary on p. 107)
2. Yields profiles of child functioning across a wide range of domains at the level of the body, the individual, and the individual in a social setting
3. Clarifies clinical diagnoses and coexisting conditions
4. Provides the basis for planning individualized treatments and interventions
5. Allows tracking of the outcomes of the interventions and documentation of the changes within and across domains
6. Standardizes documentation of variables in research

The underlying conceptual framework of the ICF-CY can be found in Chapter 5. Recall from that chapter that functioning is an umbrella term, encompassing three levels: body functions and structures, activities of daily living, and social participation. Body functions and structures include mental and sensory functions as well as digestive and musculoskeletal functions. Activities of daily living include learning, communication, mobility, and self-care. Social participation includes interpersonal interactions and community and civic life. The model posits a dynamic interaction among the health conditions and these components of functioning, thereby capturing the complexity of long-term health care problems; the health conditions may be simultaneously the cause of functional limitations and the effect of functional factors. The ICF model also posits that environmental and personal factors interact at all levels of the system, directly and indirectly, in a bidirectional manner.

The ICF provides specific alphanumeric codes (see Table 5.1) for each functional domain: the integrity of body structures and functions, the ability of the individual to perform activities of daily life, and the scope of the individual's social participation. Alphanumeric codes are also included for environmental factors. The basic structure of the ICF is described in Chapter 5. The International Classification of Diseases (ICD), which provides numeric codes for clinical conditions rather than function, is well known in the United States because it is used for billing purposes. For example, cerebral palsy carries the code 343.2. Children with cerebral palsy may have mild problems with mobility over distances or may have severe difficulties

Commentary
The Importance of Functional Classification in the Absence of Team Meetings

In the 1980s and 1990s, premier programs that evaluated children with disabilities, such as those at the Leadership Education in Neurodevelopmental Disabilities Programs, relied on a large interdisciplinary team of medical, therapeutic, and other professionals, working contemporaneously to assess children and their families. After the data gathering, the team would meet to share findings and observations. At this team meeting, they forged a common understanding of the child and prioritized the issues within a treatment plan. The plan included a mix of medical, rehabilitation, environmental, and social interventions, organized around common objectives.

In the late-1990s through the present, many such teams have been dismantled for financial reasons. Though billing codes exist for team meetings, insurance companies recognize only face-to-face clinical time. Agencies and organizations have disbanded the teams even though their contributions were invaluable. Thus, it is very common for individual clinicians to work in isolation with children and families.

The net result is a problematic fragmentation; goals and strategies for treatment are not necessarily integrated.

In this era, the need for a common system and language such as the International Classification of Functioning, Disability and Health–Children and Youth Version has become even more important than in the past. Moreover, because the International Classification of Functioning, Disability and Health focuses on function, uses common vernacular, and is independent of the underlying condition, it may be highly useful for coordinating the health care team with the education team.

Table 7.2. *International Classification of Functioning, Disability and Health–Children and Youth Version* codes indicate areas of functional difficulty for two school-age children with the diagnosis of cerebral palsy (ICD Code 343.2) and similar motor function

Child 1: Gross Motor Function Classification System 3		Child 2: Gross Motor Function Classification System 3	
b1400	Sustaining attention	b117	Intellectual functions
b1254	Persistence	b1342	Maintenance of sleep
d345	Writing messages	B1671	Expression of language
D420	Transferring oneself	B3302	Speed of speech
D450	Walking	D132	Acquiring information
D540	Dressing	D240	Handling stress and demands
		D330	Speaking
		D420	Transferring oneself
		D450	Walking
		D465	Moving around using equipment
		D540	Dressing
		D750	Informal social relationships

walking. They may have other challenges as well, including speaking, toileting, dressing, and participating in social relationships. The set of codes and qualifiers from the ICF enriches the ICD coding and serves as the child's comprehensive functional profile, differentiating these poles of function (Table 7.2).

The codes and the overall profiles derived from the ICF have a direct and practical implication in the development of treatment plans (Simeonsson et al., 2006). Identified difficulties become target objectives for the treatment team. In addition, children's strengths and assets can be coded, as can their weaknesses and needs. In this way, care plans can capitalize on strengths and promote assets as well as address weaknesses and needs. In addition, the ICF environmental codes identify contextual factors that may facilitate change and environmental barriers that may impede function. These environmental codes suggest strategies directed toward the physical and social environment that might prove useful in allowing the child greater functional

Commentary

Introducing the World Health Organization Disability Assessment Scale

The World Health Organization has created a functional assessment tool called the WHO Disability Assessment Scale (WHODAS II; WHO, 2010), now in a second iteration. It has been created to interface easily with the International Classification of Functioning, Disability and Health and International Classification of Functioning, Disability and Health–Children and Youth Version. Advantages of the WHODAS II are that it was developed with attention to cultural issues, has strong psychometric properties, and uses a hierarchical structure that can generate a general disability factor that is useful regardless of the individual's underlying health conditions. The WHODAS II assesses six domains and generates a general disability score. As with the other functional assessment measures, the WHODAS II can be used to identify individual or group needs; define the interventions appropriate for an individual or group; track functioning over time; and measure outcomes, particularly in relation to treatments.

capacity. In some cases, direct individual therapy might be ideal. In other cases, changing social attitudes and modifying the built environment might be appropriate. Changes in the codes over time indicate changes as a result of development and therapy. (See the commentary on p. 108.)

Although this chapter emphasizes the use of functional assessment and classification for individual children, the ICF codes can be useful for public health planning. For example, it is possible to track the changes in functional status for all children with a specific degenerative condition to know the likely needs for the population as it ages and the likely expenses associated with the condition. It is also possible to evaluate the degree of improvement after specific treatments for children with comparable levels of function prior to the onset of therapy.

RECOMMENDATIONS FOR CLINICAL PRACTICE

What would a shift to function-focused care look like in clinical practice? It would change the practices of medical specialists on the health care team, as in the following examples:

- Neurologists diagnosing children with cerebral palsy would reliably note the child's status on the Gross Motor Function Classification System (Palisano et al., 1997). They would categorize the child in a five-level system, reflective of the child's status as a function of age. Although the diagnosis of cerebral palsy is shocking for many families, if it is qualified as Level 1, 2, or 3, then the parents can expect that the child will develop effective systems of mobility. Improving a child's functioning is almost universally possible, although the degree of improvement varies greatly across conditions and individuals.
- Otolaryngologists (ear-nose-throat specialists) would work closely with audiologists and speech-language pathologists. Decisions about surgery would be informed in part by practice guidelines and recommended practices and also by understanding how conditions affect the child's functioning. A child with fluid in the middle ear but no hearing loss, delays in the development of speech or language, or pain may not need tympanostomy tubes, especially because early placement of the tubes does not improve developmental outcomes (Paradise et al., 2001, 2007).
- Orthopedic surgeons would study a child's gait closely, in consultation with physical and occupational therapists, experts in durable medical equipment such as walkers, and the child's family, before deciding on corrective surgery.
- Pediatricians of all types would reliably gather information from teachers, school counselors, and coaches when evaluating a child for ADHD or any other neurodevelopmental or neurobehavioral disorder. On the basis of that information, they would work with the child, parents, and school to fashion a treatment plan that capitalizes on strengths and minimizes the negative consequences of weaknesses.

The shift to function-focused care would also change the approach of other professional members of the interdisciplinary team. For example,

- Psychologists would launch an evaluation of a child with an assessment of function and use the intelligence test only when it helps to explain pervasive problems in function. They would emphasize the capabilities of individuals with intellectual disabilities and investigate vigorously if children are not able to meet those expectations. For example, a child who functions in the range of mild intellectual disability should be able to read. If a patient scores in the range of intellectual disability and cannot read by mid-elementary school, that child gets the same thorough workup as a child of average intellectual ability who does not learn to read.

- Speech-language pathologists would emphasize a child's ability to carry on conversation, describe his day, and answer questions after listening to a story over scores on standardized measures of language. They would emphasize intelligibility in everyday conversation over scores on tests of articulation.
- Physical therapists would use neurodevelopmental training procedures only if they lead to documentable changes in mobility or related functions.
- Occupational therapists would evaluate sensory integration and other process-oriented treatments in relation to specific functional goals. If the child did not meet those goals they would discontinue that form of therapy.

The next step, once the interdisciplinary team is reliably integrating functional assessment into their routines, would be to integrate the results into a functional classification. The ICF and ICF-CY are available for this integration and have been used for these purposes in isolated settings. To create and maintain a functional classification system for individual children will require increased levels of communication and collaboration across the interdisciplinary team. Teams are often no longer located within a single institution and may never meet face to face. Functional classification results need to be integrated with the medical records, which are also often fragmented in many different locations. It is highly likely that to achieve this integration will require creative information technology approaches. The importance of an integrated assessment and plan is the topic of the next chapter.

SUMMARY

A major transformation in the health care for children with disabilities can begin without fanfare or major infusions of funding. It can begin through the deliberate and consistent use of functional assessment and functional classification for children with disabilities. Functional assessment should play the pivotal role in determining eligibility and treatment planning for children with disabilities. The need for assessment typically arises because a child is having functional difficulties in the world; for example, he or she may not learn as quickly as other children his or her age, cannot communicate effectively, or cannot build reciprocal social relationships. When the evaluation is stimulated by the presence of such difficulties, then the initial efforts to understand the child and his or her circumstances should begin with an analysis of the functional difficulties that brought the child to clinical attention. All members of the interdisciplinary team that serve children with disabilities and their families need to adopt this perspective, adjust their clinical practices, and communicate frequently and effectively across the team.

Exercises

1. Discuss the following situations in terms of the school policy and evaluations:
   a. Jacqueline's teacher referred her for evaluation for the gifted and talented education program in her school district because of her consistently outstanding academic achievement in the classroom across several years. The program requires that children score at least 2 standard deviations above the mean on an IQ test. Jacqueline was rejected for the program because she scored a 122, below the cutoff of 130.
   b. Evan's parents insisted that he be tested for the gifted and talented education program because his older brother was in the program. Evan earned As, Bs, and Cs on his report card because of strong math abilities, weak writing skills, and poor persistence for sustained academic activity, such as reading novels and preparing reports. He earned an IQ score of 131 and was accepted into the program.
2. Children with autism who learn to understand and use language may show persistent difficulties in initiating and sustaining conversation, creating narrative discourse, and understanding the nuances of language. What standardized measures are available to assess a child with these difficulties? What functional approaches are available to assess a child with these difficulties?
3. Evaluate the functional assessment tools used in your discipline. What are their psychometric properties? How do experienced practitioners perceive them? Under what circumstances are they usually used?
4. Use the ICF-CY to create a functional profile for two children with the same disability. Notice in which domains the two children have similar codes and in which domains the children have different codes.
5. Compare and contrast the profile from a functional classification system like the ICF-CY with an IEP based on IDEA. In what ways are these two documents similar? How do they differ? What strategies might be available to allow easy reconciliation of the two approaches?

8

Comprehensive Integrated Care Plans

Devi

I participate on a countywide collaborative of health, rehabilitation, education, and legal agencies that meets monthly to discuss children with complex health conditions, disabilities, or family circumstances who use the services of many of the participating agencies. This team tries to integrate care for the individual children discussed and to uncover systems issues that create barriers to optimal care or outcomes. Parents provide informed consent for the discussions, and the professional who brings the case to the collaborative has the responsibility to provide feedback to the family about the interdisciplinary recommendations.

On one particular occasion, one of the agencies wanted to discuss whether to file a child abuse report on the parents of a 3-year-old girl, Devi, with severe feeding difficulties. Devi had been fed by feeding gastrostomy, a tube directly into her stomach, throughout her first year and a half of life because of complex congenital conditions and repeated operations that together precluded her ability to feed by mouth. Oral feeding was first attempted when she was over 18 months of age. Initially, Devi seemed indifferent about eating, and over time, she developed an aversion to oral feeding. Her committed parents tried to give her food by mouth but frequently resorted to tube feedings because they were very worried that otherwise she would not receive adequate nutrition.

The public agency bringing the case to the collaborative had recently assigned an occupational therapist to work with Devi and her family on feeding issues. The occupational therapist began with exercises to desensitize the child to tastes and smells, and experimented with strategies to encourage the child to finger-feed the few salty items she was willing to put in her mouth. However, when the occupational therapist did a home visit to evaluate the setting for eating at home, she was shocked to see these same caring parents tying the child into a high chair and forcing spoonfuls of cereal into her mouth. The feeding was so harsh and so counter to the goals of therapy that the occupational therapist thought it bordered on abuse. Several clinicians at the meeting agreed.

A developmental specialist who knew the family well remembered that their pediatrician had also referred them to a local feeding clinic that was known to promote force-feeding in children who refused oral feeding. The specialist conjectured that the parents might be following the clinic's recommendations. So, rather than sending a report to child protective services, the collaborative created a plan in which the occupational therapist and public health nurse would jointly speak to the family to obtain a thorough history on how the parents came to use the force-feeding procedures and, if the hypothesis that it came from the clinic proved correct, would explain their concerns about force-feeding.

The plan was very successful. The parents acknowledged that they had been taught the techniques at the feeding clinic. They did not like to use them because they made their daughter so upset. They decided they preferred to stick with the occupational therapist's gradual approach. On follow-up several months later, the occupational therapist reported back to the collaborative that Devi was making slow but steady progress toward oral intake.

The care of children with disabilities is highly complex (Chapter 3). Multiple clinicians are required in many cases to assess and treat the many issues that the child and family face. It is quite easy for confusion to arise. As illustrated in the opening vignette, the advice from different professionals may be contradictory. This young child and her family saw two different programs for the same feeding problem, oral aversion. The two programs had very different approaches, and Devi's parents did not realize that the two approaches could not be sensibly undertaken simultaneously. This case demonstrates that overtreatment and conflicting approaches can readily arise in the care of children with disabilities.

This chapter recommends integrated health care plans for children with disabilities and their families. The chapter begins with a description of the current situation, the fragmented and uncoordinated assessment and planning process that most children with disabilities and their parents in the United States currently experience. It then presents a strategy, multiaxial assessment, to reduce this fragmentation. Multiaxial assessment replaces the use of a single diagnostic category with the use of a structured multidomain method for delineating health issues, functional consequences, and environmental conditions.

Two multiaxial assessment systems have been established within psychiatry to allow for a comprehensive assessment of individuals with mental health disorders. These systems can serve as the models for an integrated assessment of children with disabilities within their social and physical environment. The multiaxial assessment forms the frame of an integrated health care plan that includes all the pertinent clinical conditions and target outcomes for each condition. Additional information appropriate for the plan includes strategies, coordinators, and time lines for each condition. A successful integrated care plan joins treatment approaches aimed at functional objectives (Chapter 7) with those aimed at improving clinical conditions.

THE CURRENT SITUATION: FRAGMENTATION

In the U.S. health care system, children with disabilities visit or are supported by many specialists and subspecialists, including physicians, therapists, counselors, and educators. Each professional tends to focus on a slice of a child and family's issues. They do their own assessments and create their own plans, primarily or exclusively for those problems that fall narrowly within their scope of practice. These assessments and plans remain separate and are housed in a variety of different places, such as hospital medical records, therapy clinic records, and school-based reports. No centralized, cohesive plan integrates all of a child's health care issues and the plans associated with them. It is not uncommon for each of the professionals involved with a child and family to have only a partial accounting of who else is involved in the care, what their assessments show, what treatments are in place, and the future plans for the child or family.

Families try their best to maintain comprehensive records. They sometimes come to health care visits with multiple thick binders of information from the various professionals involved in their child's care. Some organized families have multiple tabs and cross-references to help them find information. Other families put the information into chronological order and then need to remember which professional they saw and when they saw them. Despite these valiant efforts, many families still have an incomplete understanding of how the pieces of their child's treatment fit together. It is hard for the families to step back and look at the whole. Like Devi's parents, they may be confused about what treatments work well together and what treatments contradict others. Wanting the very best for their child, they seek out as many services as are available, hoping that more outcomes equal better outcomes.

Consequences of Fragmentation

Multiple problems may arise from this fragmentation of care and record keeping. First and foremost, fragmentation threatens patient safety (Institute of Medicine, 2001). For example, two different physicians treating a young child with disabilities might inadvertently order different medications, each of which would be appropriate for the child's condition in isolation but become dangerous when taken together. Fortunately, pharmacists often have access to integrated medication databases to provide a vital safeguard. Warnings about dangerous drug combinations are typically programmed into the database, alerting the pharmacist, who in turn alerts the prescribing physician or the patient. Many electronic medical records also detect incompatible medication combinations before the prescription is signed, establishing an even earlier warning system.

When the treatments do not consist of medication, incompatibility may be more difficult to detect. The above vignette is a case in point. Regardless of whether you agree or disagree with force-feeding a child with oral aversion, what is clear is that if the force-feeding and gradual desensitization strategies are used simultaneously, then each approach is likely to cancel any potential gains from the other. In such cases, the family is often the only safeguard for avoiding initiation of incompatible treatments. However, if they do not recognize that recommendations are contradictory, if they are uncomfortable discussing the differences in approach with one or both professionals, or if the professionals refuse to acknowledge the potential problems when the family points them out, then incompatible treatments may proceed unchanged, and patient progress may be limited. When the family is not able to detect the contradictions, a trained care coordinator—a primary care physician, a nurse, or another family advocate—may also serve as a safeguard (Chapter 10).

Fragmentation also may lead to both unacceptable gaps in service and excessive treatment. For example, when there are two different treating therapists working in isolation, one at school and one in a private office, then each may assume that the other is providing a necessary treatment for the primary problem. Each may move to a secondary issue, deferring to their colleague for the other treatment. In this case, the child fails to receive any intervention for the primary problem. Alternatively, two therapists involved with a child and family may be working on the same goals. In some situations, more therapy may be better. In other situations, more therapy may lead to unnecessary expenses and to child and family exhaustion. To avoid such problems, families need a system that systematically creates a comprehensive picture of the child, his or her health conditions, and the treatments in place or planned.

A third negative effect of fragmentation is that it leaves families feeling confused, overwhelmed, and lacking control. They often get mixed messages about parenting or caring for their child, and they do not know who to turn to, who to ask, or who to trust. As in the vignette, their attempts at coping with this stress may be misinterpreted and may compromise the support that the family receives.

Imagine traveling by car from New York City to San Francisco and departing without a map or GPS. It would be quite easy to end up completely lost, going around in circles or backtracking over already-covered territory. You then might ask different people for directions and have to decide which to follow. Similarly, in navigating the uncertain road of providing longitudinal health care for children with disabilities, a map—an overarching organizational tool—would be very useful. A map in this case would begin with a comprehensive assessment and would then link treatments and plans to that assessment.

MODELS FOR INTEGRATION: MULTIAXIAL ASSESSMENTS

When I was in medical school, we were taught to create a problem list as a strategy for integrating health care information. At an initial encounter, outpatient or inpatient, a clinician was expected to start this master list, which would include subjective and objective data that defined each problem, an assessment, and a plan. At each subsequent encounter, the clinician ideally would review the list and, if necessary, add any additional items on the basis of incoming information. The idea of tracking all the child's problems makes excellent sense during a hospital stay to ensure that all of the health problems have been addressed, observed data have been accounted for, and each component of the plan has been duly executed.

A severe limitation of the problem list, particularly for longitudinal care, is the lack of any internal organization or prioritization. The list is usually generated chronologically. Major long-term conditions may be embedded within a long list of less serious or acute problems. I remember once reviewing the problem list of a child with Down syndrome. It looked something like this:

- Down syndrome
- Eczema

- Acute otitis media
- Normal thyroid function
- Acute otitis media
- Leukemia
- Eczema
- Acute otitis media

On the basis of this format, the problem list gave apparently equal weight to eczema, an annoying but rarely life-threatening skin condition, and leukemia, a serious cancer of the blood. This failure to prioritize among the issues limits the utility of the problem list. I admit that I rarely checked or updated the list in my outpatient clinics because I found that they grew longer and longer, failed to prioritize the issues, and led to a confusing and unhelpful view of the child.

An alternative to the disorganization of the problem list is the *multiaxial assessment*, a "contextual and standardized description of the clinical condition through a number of highly informative, therapeutically significant and systematically assessed axes or domains" (International Guidelines for Diagnostic Assessment [IGDA] Workgroup & World Psychiatric Association, 2003a, p. s52). This dimensional diagnostic approach was introduced into psychiatry in 1980 with the publication of the *Diagnostic and Statistical Manual for Mental and Emotional Disorders, Third Edition* (*DSM-III*; American Psychiatric Association, 1980). Until that time, psychiatric diagnoses, like medical diagnoses, were usually coded as a single entity; in the case of psychiatry, it was the primary mental or emotional disorder, such as schizophrenia or depression. The multiaxial assessment system expanded from the primary diagnosis to provide systematic and clinically relevant information for care of the patient with schizophrenia or depression. Like psychiatric disorders, disabilities are long-term and complex conditions. In fact, psychiatric disorders are likely to qualify as disabilities because they limit routine functioning in everyday life. Therefore, this approach from psychiatry serves as a useful model for comprehensive diagnostic formulation for disabilities other than mental health disorders.

DSM-IV and *DSM-5* Models

DSM-IV (American Psychiatric Association, 1980) recommended a five-axis system (Tables 8.1 and 8.2). Axis I included all of the psychiatric disorders that would be the major focus of attention or treatment in the mental health system. Axis I might include schizophrenia or depression. Axes II–IV were factors that, if present, would moderate the severity of the major conditions or modify the approach to treatment. Axis II included personality disorders and intellectual disability because these factors were likely to change the presentation or treatment of the primary psychiatric disorder. For example, adolescents with intellectual disability and depression may not be good candidates for certain forms of cognitive behavior therapy. Axis III included any medical conditions that might be related to the cause of the psychiatric condition or a complication increasing the severity of the condition. For example, the presence of cancer might have caused depression or might exacerbate depression in an individual with the emotional disorder. Medical conditions

Table 8.1. Five-axis multiaxial assessment based on the *Diagnostic and Statistical Manual for Mental and Emotional Disorders, Fourth Edition (DSM-IV)*

Axis	Definition	Examples
I	Clinical disorders	Attention-deficit hyperactivity disorder, obsessive-compulsive disorder, generalized anxiety disorder
II	Personality disorders/mental retardation	Borderline intellectual functioning, narcissistic personality disorder
III	General medical conditions	Obesity, failure to thrive
IV	Psychosocial/environmental problems	Inadequate housing, inadequate parental supervision
V	General assessment of function	Scores 0–100

might also affect treatment. The presence of liver disease might change the types of medications that can be safely administered to the person with a psychiatric condition. Axis IV listed environmental and psychosocial problems that may affect the diagnosis, treatment, and prognosis of the main conditions. Parental divorce, interpersonal violence, substance abuse, and mental health disorders in the parents all might exacerbate the condition in the child. Clinicians, recognizing the presence of multiple psychosocial stressors, might put less importance on parental behavior management approaches in treatment of the child's condition. The presence of parental substance abuse might change the clinician's choice of medications for a child with a behavioral condition.

Axis V in the *DSM-IV-TR* was called the Global Assessment of Functioning (GAF) (American Psychiatric Association, 2000). Its inclusion in the multiaxial diagnostic system acknowledged that the severity of a condition includes its impact on the individual's functioning. The GAF used a 100-point scale to quantify the individual's level of psychological and social functioning at the time of assessment. To supplement the GAF, *DSM-IV-TR* introduced two new measures of adaptive functioning for research: the Social and Occupational Functioning Assessment Scale and the Global Assessment of Relational Functioning Scale. Analyses suggested that the scales are reliable and valid (Hay, Katsikitis, Begg, Da Costa, & Blumenfeld, 2003; Hilsenroth, Ackerman, Blagys, et al., 2000).

DSM-5 has eliminated the multiaxial format (Gever, 2012). Axes I, II, and III have been combined. However, separate notations about psychosocial and contextual factors, formerly Axis IV, and about disability, formerly Axis V, are maintained. Although this change responds to the preference of many mental health professionals and simplifies reporting for insurance purposes, the decision is unfortunate if it narrows rather than expands the perspective of the treating clinicians. Careful consideration of medical history, intellectual and neurodevelopmental conditions, and psychosocial context of psychiatric disorders is essential in a comprehensive assessment. The *DSM-5* introduces dimensions to capture the variations in severity of the condition. Severity is a function not only of the individual's specific condition but also of his or her co-occurring conditions, psychosocial factors, and context. It remains essential to consider the important role of context in moderating the effects of the condition on outcomes and not to attribute variation only to intrapersonal factors. The use of multiple axes forced a disciplined approach to the complexity of mental health conditions. Time will tell whether the complexity is lost with the *DSM-5* changes.

Table 8.2. Application of the multiaxial assessment from the *DSM-IV* to the characters in A.A. Milne's Hundred Acre Wood (Shea, Gordon, Hawkins, Kawchuk, & Smith, 2000; p. 1558)

Character	Axis I	Axis II	Axis III	Axis IV
Winnie the Pooh	ADHD, inattention subtype; OCD provisional	Borderline intellectual functioning	Obesity, binge eating	
Piglet	Generalized anxiety disorder		Failure to thrive	
Eeyore	Dysthymia		Traumatic amputation of tail	Housing problems
Rabbit	—	Narcissistic personality disorder		
Owl	Reading disorder			Housing problems
Tigger	ADHD, hyperactive–impulsive type			
Christopher Robin				Lack of parental supervision, possible educational problems

Note: The Axis V (Global Assessment of Functioning) scale was deferred.

Key: OCD, obsessive-compulsive disorder.

International Guidelines for Diagnostic Assessment of the World Psychiatric Association Model of Multiaxial Assessment

A different method for multiaxial assessment was proposed by the IGDA Workgroup of the World Psychiatric Association in 2003 (IGDA Workgroup & World Psychiatric Association, 2003a) (Table 8.3). The IGDA system collapses the mental and general medical conditions into a single axis. It adds an axis of disabilities, and it specifies that disabilities could be encountered in one of several domains: personal care, occupational functioning, functioning with family, and broader social functioning.

Table 8.3. Multiaxial assessment proposed by the *International Guidelines for Diagnostic Assessment (IGDA)* of the World Psychiatric Association

Axis	Definition	Examples
I	Clinical disorders (mental and general medical conditions)	Attention-deficit/hyperactive disorder, obsessive-compulsive disorder, generalized anxiety disorder, obesity, failure to thrive
II	Disabilities	Inability to care for self, poor peer and family relationships, frequent school detentions and suspensions
III	Contextual factors	Inadequate housing, inadequate parental supervision
IV	Quality of life	Reduced in standardized assessment because of limited community recreational activities and poor social relationships

Source: IGDA Workgroup and World Psychiatric Association (2003).

These domains of function cross levels within the framework of the ICF (WHO, 2002), with one domain at the level of activity (personal care) and the three others at the level of social participation. In addition, the IGDA approach includes an axis for the quality of life, a multidimensional and global assessment of the individual's self-perceived well-being in areas such as physical and emotional state; satisfaction with independent, occupational, and interpersonal functioning, and with socio-emotional and instrumental supports; and the individual's sense of personal and spiritual fulfillment (IGDA Workgroup & World Psychiatric Association, 2003a). The IGDA Workgroup also recommends inclusion of an idiographic, or personal, diagnostic formulation (IGDA Workgroup & World Psychiatric Association, 2003b). The idiographic formulation recognizes that the individual may have elements of his or her unique experience that are important and meaningful in the diagnostic formulation. For example, the adaptation of an individual to a health condition or disability may depend in part on whether the person has relatives with the disorder and how those relatives coped with the condition. If the relative was happy and productive, then the individual may have optimism, whereas if the relative was isolated and limited, the individual may develop pessimism or hopelessness. Clinicians, the individual, and the family contribute to the idiographic diagnosis. Any discrepancies must be discussed to permit their resolution and integration into a shared understanding of the case at hand.

Limitations of the Current Multiaxial Models

Many mental health clinicians in the United States complain that the multiaxial assessment system of the *DSM-IV* is a bureaucratic requirement of insurance carriers rather than a meaningful clinical tool. Axes II–V add little beyond the primary diagnosis in Axis I. This critique exposes one perspective within the field of psychiatry: psychiatric conditions can be best conceptualized within the medical model that considers the psychiatric condition as an illness within the individual. From that perspective, the corollary is that treatment strategies are directed to the individual and not the context, and that the thrust of care is curing the individual of his or her disorder. When we consider mental health disorders as disabilities rather than as illnesses, when we acknowledge that cure may be beyond our current therapeutic reach and that consideration of the person in context is important in health care delivery, then the multiaxial approach to assessment has clinical relevance. Of the *DSM-IV* or IGDA approaches previously described, it is not clear which one has greater utility. To address that issue, research on multiaxial assessment and its link to treatment planning and longitudinal follow-up needs to be conducted (Chapter 12). In the situation of children with disabilities, the axes may need to be further adjusted to capture the factors important for them and for their families.

A NEW MULTIAXIAL ASSESSMENT STRATEGY FOR CHILDREN WITH DISABILITIES

In the care of children with disabilities, a multiaxial assessment system can capture in a single, organized document the complex interplay of issues that affect these children in their environments. Such a system should prove useful for children with physical, cognitive, or emotional conditions and would be appropriate whether the child has a severe or mild condition. Six axes are fundamental to offer a comprehensive understanding of the children; these axes incorporate features from the *DSM-IV* and IGDA systems previously described. For some uses, the entries within each of the axes could be described in plain language to facilitate communication with families and interdisciplinary team members, and for other purposes, such as the electronic medical record, the axes can be coded using an appropriate diagnostic and statistical manual. Whereas the traditional psychiatric multiaxial assessment focuses on clinical conditions and problems, the multiaxial system proposed here should include strengths or assets of the children and their environments because clearly positive factors influence treatment as profoundly as do problems. Table 8.4 shows the axes, an appropriate coding manual, and examples.

This proposed multiaxial system is similar to current psychiatric versions in that medical problems and developmental, emotional, and behavioral problems are retained in separate axes. The axes are kept separate because medical and developmental or mental health conditions typically have distinctive diagnostic categories, coding manuals, professional teams, goals and objectives, and treatments. Also, like the psychiatric model, it retains an axis for psychosocial and environmental conditions because of their profound impact on the severity of a condition and on the treatment planning process.

The proposed system is distinct from previous multiaxial assessments in that the axes are labeled but not numbered. This decision reflects an underlying assumption that one axis does not have primacy over others. The order of presentation of the axes is arbitrary and may be rearranged over time to indicate a shift in the primary issues. However, it retains the internal organization, so it is more useful than the problem lists described above. Additional features of this system are described in the following sections.

Table 8.4. Multiaxial assessment for children with disabilities

Axes	Coding manual	Examples
Long-term or high-severity medical conditions	*ICD-10*	Congenital heart disease, trisomy 21, neuromuscular disorders, autism
Health and wellness	*ICD-10*	Diet, nutrition, physical exercise
Short-term or low-severity medical problems	*ICD-10*	Acute infections, allergies, eczema
Developmental, emotional, or behavioral disorders	*DSM-IV* or *DSM-5* (or *ICD-10*)	Expressive language disorder, intellectual disability, major depressive disorder, attention-deficit hyperactivity disorder, anxiety
Psychosocial and environmental conditions	*ICD-10* V codes (within the *DSM-PC*) or ICF environmental codes	Family constellation, nature of the family relationships, stressors, poverty, food insecurity, parental unemployment, sibling with health or mental health condition
Function	*ICF*	Emphasis on activities and participation
Personal factors	NA	Idiographic factors affecting manifestations of the condition or function, such as optimism, cultural factors, specific motivations

Key: DSM-PC, *Diagnostic and Statistical Manual for Primary Care, Child and Adolescent Version*; *ICD, International Classification of Disease*; *ICF, International Classification of Functioning, Disability, and Health*; NA, not available.

Axes for Medical and Health Conditions

In the proposed multiaxial system, three axes are included for health and medical issues. The first is *long-term or high-severity medical conditions*. This axis would include Down syndrome or trisomy 21, cerebral palsy or middle cerebral artery stroke, hydrocephalus, seizure disorder, or neurofibromatosis. In many cases, the listed medical conditions represent the cause of developmental, emotional, and behavioral disorders; for example, trisomy 21 is associated with intellectual disability and cerebral palsy with learning disability. However, serious medical conditions may also include heart, lung, liver, or kidney diseases that may not be directly related to disabilities. A child with Down syndrome may develop leukemia, which would also be included on this axis. All of the medical conditions listed may have a team of professionals that oversee diagnosis, management, and treatment. What is important is that all members of the interdisciplinary health care team that serves children with disabilities and their families be keenly aware of all long-term and severe medical conditions. For example, the speech-language pathologist treating a young child with Down syndrome needs to be cognizant of the child's leukemia as it may affect the child's energy levels, persistence, and engagement, as well as the scheduling of therapy and the advisability of group versus individual treatment. (See the commentary below.)

The second axis is *short-term or low-severity medical problems*. On this axis, clinicians could list acute otitis media or mild eczema, allowing these relatively short-term and less severe conditions to be recorded and yet separating them from high-severity conditions. Using this separate axis allows focus and prioritization, depending on which clinician or therapist is reviewing the list. Again, different team

Commentary
Caught Off Guard

I work on an interdisciplinary team of physicians, physical and occupational therapists, public health nurses, social workers, and dieticians providing therapy and care coordination to children with severe motor and neuromuscular disorders. The team has been very active in following a young child with a severe muscle disorder. Despite average intellectual and language abilities, this gentle child has difficulty maintaining an upright position such as sitting or standing.

I was surprised at our regional collaborative meeting when one of the members of another community-based service organization asked my opinion about the cause and consequences of the child's diarrheal illness. Some in the collaborative knew that the child had been having this problem on and off for several months, but I was in the dark. When I had a chance, I went back to the records to learn about the onset and severity of this condition. Tucked deep in a paper file were the appropriate reports. However, nothing flagged them as new and important. I also checked the electronic record at our hospital, where she receives care. Again, the reports are there, but nothing indicates that the section of Outpatient Records or Gastroenterology Service notes have been updated with this new information.

So, in spite of an engaged interdisciplinary team, the lack of an integrated care plan was highly problematic. I find that it is far easier to find updates about my Facebook friends than it is to find updates about my patients.

members might find the information highly pertinent to their work. For example, if a physical therapist wants to try taping or a customized rehabilitation system worn under clothing as a strategy for treatment, then the child's eczema may be relevant to whether the child can tolerate either of these two treatments.

The final axis related to health is called *health and wellness*, and it may include information on diet, nutrition, and physical exercise. These core issues are as pertinent for children with disabilities as they are for the general population, and yet they are often overlooked in children with medical or neurodevelopmental problems. It is important to note when a child may require a nutritional assessment, weight reduction, or increased physical activity. In this axis, positive features of the child's overall health and wellness, such as a healthy organic diet or daily physical exercise, can be coded in addition to problems, such as feeding disorders. The status of the child's immunizations can also be included in this axis. (See the commentary below.)

Axis for Psychosocial and Environmental Conditions

A multiaxial assessment system for disabilities must include an axis to code environmental factors. The axis includes the physical and the psychosocial environments because both are relevant to understanding the severity of long-term conditions and their functional outcomes. The axis is deliberately labeled *psychosocial and environmental conditions*, rather than *problems*. Psychosocial problems, such as parental divorce and interpersonal violence, are highly pertinent to treatment planning. However, equally important are psychosocial assets and strengths, which can be marshaled in the planning process. For example, a child who is making very rapid progress may warrant frequent therapy visits to capitalize on this rate of improvement. A child who has strong verbal skills may be able to give herself step-by-step instructions to improve weak fine motor skills. Similarly, environmental conditions may include barriers or facilitators for a child or family. If the child lives in a home with sufficient space to allow for physical therapy to take place, then the physical therapist could teach the family techniques for home treatment. If the family lives

Commentary
Anthony

Anthony is the boy with attention-deficit hyperactivity disorder described in vignettes in Chapter 7. For 5 years, he took stimulant medication to control the symptoms of inattention and hyperactivity that define the condition, but he experienced a common adverse side effect of medication, severe loss of appetite. He never wanted to eat lunch. Consequently, he lost weight and slowed in growth. His doctor modified the dose and schedule of medication. His parents tried many different strategies to increase his interest in food during the day, including giving him high-calorie lunches from the fast-food restaurant he really liked, but even that approach did not entice him to eat.

The parents obtained a consultation from the dietician at the hospital, who reviewed a 3-day food diary, established the goals for intake, and helped the parents to increase the caloric and nutritional value of Anthony's breakfast and bedtime snack. Those interventions stabilized his weight and height gains and allowed him to continue on medication.

in close quarters that are not conducive to a home program, then the team might explore whether the exercises can be done at school.

Two systems for coding environmental and psychosocial issues of children with disabilities and their families are available. The first comes from *The Classification of Child and Adolescent Mental Conditions in Primary Care: Diagnostic and Statistical Manual for Primary Care (DSM-PC), Child and Adolescent Version* (Wolraich, Felice, & Drotar, 1996). The manual provides a comprehensive list of potential risk and protective factors that were conceptualized for that volume as stressors impacting children's mental health. The list can be viewed broadly as a set of factors that may affect health conditions and functional outcomes beyond the scope of mental health (Table 8.5).

Another listing comes from the environmental factors from the ICF-CY (Ellingsen & Simeonsson, 2011) and is shown in Table 8.6. This list includes environmental factors, such as products and technology for communication, education, recreation, and sport. It also considers the design of buildings and the availability of transportation. It is less detailed than the DSM-PC about psychosocial stressors, such as parental illiteracy, unemployment, inadequate housing, or crime. An integration of the two systems within a single coding scheme would capture the broad set of issues.

Axis for Function

An essential component of the multiaxial system is function. See Chapter 7 for more information on the overall importance of a focus on function in the health care of children with disabilities and a discussion of how function is not exclusively a listing of impairments and limitations but also a compendium of strengths and assets.

Table 8.5. Psychosocial conditions that may affect health and function of children with disabilities from *The Classification of Child and Adolescent Mental Conditions in Primary Care: Diagnostic and Statistical Manual for Primary Care* (*DSM-PC*)

Condition	Examples
Changes in caregiving	Foster care, adoption, institutional care; substance-abusing parent; neglect; physical abuse, sexual abuse; quality-of-nurture problem; mental disorder of parent; physical illness of parent; physical illness of sibling; mental or behavioral disorder of sibling
Other functional change in family	Addition of a sibling, change in parental caregiver
Community/social challenges	Acculturation, social discrimination, religious or spiritual problem
Educational challenges	Illiteracy of parent, inadequate school facilities, discord with peers/teachers
Parent or adolescent occupational challenges	Parent or adolescent occupational challenge, unemployment, loss of a job, adverse effect of work environment
Housing challenges	Homelessness, inadequate housing, unsafe neighborhood, dislocation
Economic challenges	Poverty/inadequate financial status, inadequate access to health or mental health care
Legal system or crime problem	Crime problem of parent or adolescent
Other environmental situations	Natural disaster, witness of violence

Source: Wolraich, Felice, and Drotar (1996).

Table 8.6. Environmental codes from the *International Classification of Functioning, Disability and Health, Children and Youth* developmental code set for children (Ellingsen & Simeonsson, 2011)

Code	Description
e1110	Food and drink (e.g., appropriateness, nutrition, amount, consistency)
e1101	Drugs (type of drug and amount for medical purposes)
e115	Products and technology for personal use in daily living (e.g., furniture, stroller, chairs, personal care equipment, adapted or specially designed devices, and orthopedic devices)
e120	Products and technology for personal indoor and outdoor mobility and transportation (e.g., family car, cab, bus, train, adapted chairs, walking devices, wheelchair, bicycle)
e125	Products and technology for communication (e.g., telephone, television and video, computers/e-mail, glasses and aids for sight and hearing, aids for writing)
e130	Products and technology for education (e.g., books, computers, educational toys, adapted material for learning such as computer software)
e140	Products and technology for culture, recreation, and sport (e.g., skis, musical instruments, adapted equipment)
e1152	Products and technology used for play (e.g., household objects; toys; other products like balls, games, puzzles, or adapted materials for play; indoor and playground)
e310	Immediate family
e315	Extended family
e330	People in a position of authority
e340	Personal care providers and personal assistants
e425	Acquaintances, peers, colleagues, neighbors, and community members
e320	Friends
e410	Individual attitudes of immediate family members
e420	Individual attitudes of friends
e150	Design, construction, and building products and technology of buildings for public use (e.g., entrees, elevators, door openers, signs, hearing devices, picture support, Braille, security equipment).
e5400	Transportation (services aimed at moving persons or goods by road, path, rail, air, or water, by public or private transport)
e575	Social support services, systems, policies (public assistance other than Social Security)
e580	Health services (e.g., access to early intervention, technical aids, other health services)
e355	Health professionals
e450	Individual attitudes of health professionals

From Ellingsen, K.M., & Simeonsson, R.J. (2011). *ICF-CY developmental code set for children six through twelve years* (6–12). Retrieved from http://www.icfcydevelopmentalcodesets.com/Page_3_KXVK.html; adapted by permission.

The axis for function in the multiaxial assessment is actually a set of axes and categories from the *ICF-CY.* For children with disabilities, a single dimension of function, such as what was in the *DSM-IV* Axis V, makes no sense: Children may be high functioning in some domains, such as social skills, but very limited in other domains, such as mobility or self-care. It is important for the treatment plan to appreciate the variation in ability across domains. The *ICF* is an exhaustive and comprehensive system and therefore is well suited for capturing such variations and nuances.

The very features that make the *ICF* attractive for coding function also make it daunting to use in daily practice. In most situations, clinicians need only a set of categories from the overall system. Following are two recommendations for how to encode function in a sensible and efficient manner.

1. Focus on activities and social participation. These areas of function are often overlooked entirely in the usual medical record. Thus, information about the child's learning, communication, social interactions, recreation, and leisure might not be incorporated into the assessment if not through this focus.
2. Use core sets. Research using the ICF is attempting to determine which categories or chapters of the ICF are most useful for defining the impact of particular conditions (ICF Research Branch, 2010). This research is primarily geared toward general categories of conditions, such as mental health or musculoskeletal conditions, and toward adults rather than children. However, the results are likely to shed light on childhood conditions as well. A current alternative is to create a core set of items based on face validity. Figure 8.1 is an example of a core set of functional problems that are likely to be associated with ADHD (Loe & Feldman, 2007).

Axis for Personal Factors

Personal factors are particularly central to an individual's function. Indeed, the ICF acknowledges that both personal factors and environmental factors are important contributors to function (WHO, 2002). The ICF has not yet developed a coding scheme for personal factors. In large part, the challenge is to determine which of the many distinctive features of individuals would be most important to include. Inspired by the quality of life and the idiographic axes of the IGDA multiaxial assessment system, an intriguing idea is to allow the individual child or the family to complete this axis. Without any constraints, the individual or family would be able to declare what is most important to them. For some individuals, their race, ethnicity, or religious backgrounds may be highly central to their interpretation of their health condition and to their functioning. They might want specific interventions or conditions met so that their cultural practices are not violated. For others, these factors may not be as important, whereas education and personal motivation may be most relevant to their functioning. The axis can also include the individual and family's evaluation of their personal situation, including the degree of stress they experience or their satisfaction with life circumstances, as well as their strategies for coping with stress. Including this final axis in the multiaxial system encourages active exchange between children, families, and their clinicians about the family's unique constellation of features.

THE INTEGRATED MULTIAXIAL PLAN

The most important reason to construct a multiaxial assessment is to create a corresponding multiaxial health care plan that can be shared across the interdisciplinary team, including the family. This can be referred to as the multiaxial plan (MAP). Importantly, the MAP brings together the care plans for both clinical conditions and functional status. All of the recommendations for all of the child's issues are combined into a single care plan to facilitate cross-referencing and integration.

The process of creating this comprehensive care plan requires establishing specific goals or target outcomes for the various conditions on the axes. Articulating the measurable objectives is so important in the care of children with disabilities because it increases the likelihood that children will make progress in the desired directions. This fundamental principle was incorporated into the Education for All

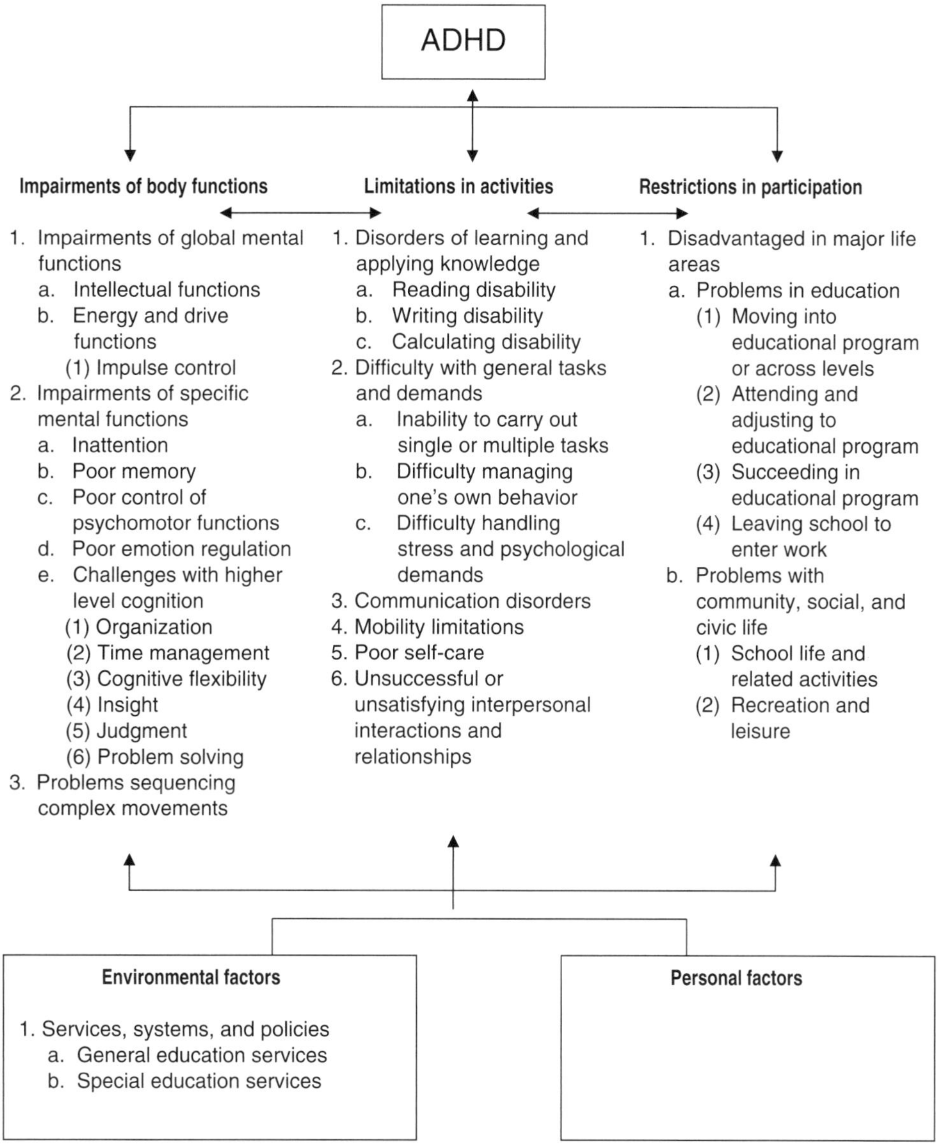

Figure 8.1. Core set of functional problems associated with attention-deficit hyperactivity disorder (ADHD), based on the *International Classification of Functioning, Disability, and Health* conceptual model. (Reprinted from Loe, I.M., & Feldman, H.M. [2007]. Academic and educational outcomes of children with ADHD. *Journal of Pediatric Psychology 32*[6], 643–654 and *Ambulatory Pediatrics 7*[Suppl. 1], 82–90. Copyright 2007 with permission from Elsevier.)

Handicapped Children Act of 1975 and Individuals with Disabilities Education Act, which required that children found eligible for special education receive an IEP that specifies objectives for each domain in which the child's performance is not at age or grade level. The objectives inform the educational approaches and form the basis of evaluation of both the child and the educators. Other disciplines, including physical and occupational therapy, speech-language pathology, and nursing, also write detailed objectives and care plans to guide their therapeutic interventions.

Establishing goals and objectives is particularly important in addressing long-term concerns. In health care for long-term conditions, multiple goals are possible. Different members of the team may disagree about which goals are most important as well as about which strategies are most likely to meet the primary goals. Therefore, establishing explicitly what the goals are is important for keeping the care focused and organized. For example, the target outcomes for treating one school-age boy with ADHD might be to improve academic output, whereas the target outcome for a different child with the same disorder may be to improve peer relationships. Clearly, although both goals are reasonable, they would lead to different treatment plans.

Creating goals is a shared responsibility of child, family, and the interdisciplinary team. The goals may need to be negotiated with input from all points of view to achieve the best plan for the child. Parents of a child with seizure disorder may want the child to be totally seizure free, but physicians may worry that using too many medications at too high doses might lead to long-term complications, such as liver disease. Through discussion and negotiation, a consensus about the plan can be achieved.

In addition to the target outcomes, the MAP includes the clinicians or therapists or coordinators who will oversee the care associated with that condition. It specifies the strategies that will be used and includes timelines for reevaluation. To return to the example of ADHD, one of the target outcomes for the primary condition may be to increase the child's time on task and completion of assignments. The strategy might be the use of stimulant medication. For this objective, the primary care or subspecialty physician may be the primary clinician. The MAP would lay out which physician is prescribing the medication and following up to determine whether the target outcomes are met. Another target outcome for that child might be to increase positive peer interactions and reduce impulsive aggression. The strategies for these functional conditions might involve behavior management at school. In this case, the school counselor or teacher would be primarily responsible for providing the care. The timeline for improvement would be different, and reevaluation would be planned accordingly. By explicitly agreeing on the person who will be providing the care, the roles of team members can be clear to everyone, including the family. Communication pathways and time points for follow-up can also be defined. Ideally, the use of the MAP reduces the possibility that important issues will be overlooked or forgotten.

The MAP may not be precisely the most efficient method for integrating conditions and treatments into a single integrated care plan, and other formats are of course possible. However, the need for a coordinated and integrated plan is incontrovertible. At a recent parent conference, I asked approximately 200 parents about how they organized the health information on their child. The majority of respondents had no systematic approach and/or were dissatisfied with their efforts. Those with a system generally used notebooks with copies of all reports in chronological order. They became extremely excited by the MAP construct as a way to organize their own records, prioritize their child's needs, and work with their child's care team. We have been using this approach to introduce pediatric residents to issues of long-term care for individual children and their families. Imagine all of the issues that need to be addressed in the care of a preschool-aged child with Down syndrome who develops leukemia. Table 8.7 is a MAP for that child. The residents like the way the MAP integrates the information and thereby simplifies the job of creating a plan and monitoring adherence and accountabilities.

Table 8.7. Multiaxial assessment plan for a 4-year-old child with Down syndrome and leukemia

Axis	Specific conditions	*ICD-9* or *DSM* code	Management coordinator	Goals/progress	Strategies	Timeline
Long-term medical conditions	Down syndrome Leukemia	758 204	Primary MD Oncologist	Follow guidelines Achieve remission	Double click for protocol	Next annual evaluation: June 2014
Acute or intermittent medical conditions	Eczema Acute otitis media	692.9 382.9	Dermatologist Primary MD	As needed As needed		
Health and wellness	Overweight	278.02	Primary MD	Weight for height <90% on DS charts	No eating except at table	Weight check every 3 months
Developmental, mental, emotional, and behavioral conditions and traits	Mild intellectual disability	317	Special education coordinator	Learn to read Learn all basic math	Special education push-in	Triannual evaluation for IEP
Psychosocial and environmental factors	Two-parent household Typically developing older sibling		Family with primary MD	Continue to participate in family–family support		As needed
Function						
Body function and structures						
Activities and participation						
Learning and applying knowledge	Preliteracy skills		Teacher Family	Learn rhyming and alphabet		Annual school assessment
Handling tasks and demands	Low frustration tolerance		Primary MD Behavior consultant	Delay implementation until after leukemia treatment		Discuss at conclusion of leukemia treatment (anticipated December 2013)
Communication	Strong verbal skills		School-based speech-language pathologist	Increased sentence length and vocabulary		Annual school assessment
Mobility	Walking, running		Swimming class	Defer until after leukemia treatment		Annual school assessment
Self-care	Not toilet trained		Family Teacher	Defer until after leukemia treatment		Annual MD and family assessment
Interpersonal interactions and relationships	Very social					As needed
Education	Integrated preschool			Promote regular attendance during leukemia treatment		Reevaluate at kindergarten entry
Community, social, and civic life	Participation in parent–child group			Promote regular attendance during leukemia treatment		As needed
Personal factors, self-defined	Dietary restrictions based on religious affiliation		Noted by Primary MD			

DSM, *Diagnostic and Statistical Manual*; DS, Down Syndrome; ICD, International Classification of Disease; IEP, individualized education program; MD, medical doctor.

Future research is required to determine whether this recommendation leads to systematic improvements in health care delivery for children with chronic conditions and may also inform the best format and delivery of the MAP (e.g., electronic availability versus paper).

IMPLEMENTATION CHALLENGES

The MAP should be conceptualized at this point in its development as a framework rather than a tool. Many important questions about how to implement the MAP have not been fully addressed: Who would complete the initial assessment? When would it be updated and by whom? What would happen if family members and clinicians differed in their assessment or in their priorities for the child? How would differences in opinions about priorities and plans within the health care team be handled? How would a clinician know if she were working from the most current version of the plan? Where would the plan reside and who would maintain it? The MAP can get extremely dense and complicated; how do we keep it simple and useful?

I envision that the responsibility for creating, updating, and maintaining the multiaxial assessments and plans should rest with the family, who would work with a designated care coordinator or the medical home. The *medical home* is the central coordinating unit that is available to families at all times and serves as the repository for information about the child, the conditions, and the treatments (AAP, 2005). The medical home and care coordination are discussed in more detail in Chapters 9 and 10.

Because the medical home should serve as the repository of all medical information, it makes sense that the MAP can become the primary tool for the medical home to integrate information about a child, establish the care priorities, and hold the various clinicians and organizations accountable for achieving their objectives within the plan's timelines. Professionals within the medical home, either physicians or care coordinators, could work with families to update goals and objectives on a regular basis or when appropriate because of status changes. However, at the same time, the MAP should belong to the family to ensure they can share it with everyone necessary, whether physically or via a Web site, so that it is accessible from many different locations. Layers of detail can be included by embedding details of a portion of the plan within the larger framework. The family can decide to share all or a portion of the plan with members of the team, including educators, by giving them explicit permissions. The child and family can use the integrated plan to organize their priorities and activities, monitor treatment, and establish responsibility and accountability.

OTHER USES OF THE MULTIAXIAL ASSESSMENT AND MULTIAXIAL PLAN

Multiaxial assessment can be used to characterize at the cohort or population level as well as at the individual level. Public health planners could use the collective MAPs from a region for planning resources.

If a health insurance plan wants to offer risk-adjusted rates for care of children with disabilities, it needs a way to establish the complexity of the care an individual child requires. The sum total of the codes may provide key information for the determination of rates. Health authorities could also use the assessments for planning at a population level. The effect might be the appropriate assignment of health care resources and expenditures, less waste, and better services.

SUMMARY

Previous chapters discussed that children with disabilities frequently have more than one long-term health condition or disability and that care is highly complex. Though disabilities can occur in any group, disabilities are more prevalent among families who live in poverty and experience psychosocial stress than in families who have adequate financial and social resources. The psychosocial conditions add to the complexity. Therefore, even for children with relatively mild to moderate disabilities, many different problems co-occur. In the current system, each professional and organization that sees a child with disabilities and his or her family maintains its own records and its own individual plan. This situation leads to unfortunate fragmentation and sometimes dangerous situations.

A multiaxial assessment is a tool for integrating multiple diverse issues facing children with disabilities and their families into a concise and usable format that can be shared and shaped by all those who are involved with the child and family. Importantly, the approach is designed so that the assessment informs treatment planning. A MAP ensures that care plans are comprehensive and coordinated, although many logistical issues remain about how to design processes for creating and updating the MAP that are efficient, timely, and effective. As a beginning, the plan can be a strategy within the family-centered medical home, the focus of the following chapter.

Exercises

1. Create a multiaxial assessment for disabilities for a child in your practice based on existing records. What information is readily obtained in the record? What information is missing?
2. Create a multiaxial assessment for disabilities for a child from a conversation with the parents. What information do they readily contribute? What information is missing?
3. From these multiaxial assessments, create a comprehensive and integrated care plan. How does the plan created though this assessment process compare with the plan already in place?
4. Consider how to integrate health care and educational plans. How can the multiaxial assessment help in the process?
5. Share a multiaxial assessment with parents. Ask them if they like the system. Determine what the possession of such a plan might do for them. Try the same exercise with a teenager with disabilities. What does the adolescent think of the plan?

9

Family- and Person-Centered Care

Teresa and Tim

Tim, a handsome and healthy newborn, was Teresa's second son. All went well during birth and delivery; however, at 2 weeks of age, he refused to eat and developed a high fever. His parents rushed him to the emergency room, where doctors feared that he had the flu, a devastating viral infection for a newborn. They also had to consider other possibilities, such as bacterial meningitis, a serious infection of the covering of the brain. When they went to do the spinal tap, a procedure necessary for determining whether bacteria had invaded the nervous system, they asked Teresa and her husband to leave the room. Teresa, worried and frightened, wanted to remain with her infant as his sole source of comfort. The doctors were insistent. She left the room but quickly turned back, longing to be with her baby. The doctors became furious, accused her of interfering with their work, and stationed a security guard at the door to prevent her return.

In the hospital, Teresa remained at Tim's side. On the third day, she became convinced that his breathing was deteriorating and called the nurses to reevaluate him. The nurses told her she was exaggerating because she was overtired. They contacted Teresa's husband and told him that Teresa had to go home to get some sleep. Teresa's husband decided to stay with Tim while Teresa rested rather than leave the baby unattended. Four hours later, he called Teresa to tell her that Tim's breathing had stopped, that he was in full cardiorespiratory arrest. He needed cardiopulmonary resuscitation and mechanical ventilation. They learned later that he had developed heart failure. The arrest caused multiple organs to fail, including his kidneys. His brain was severely damaged.

For 4 months, Tim remained hospitalized. In the ICU, Tim was tethered to a warming bed, with a ventilator tube in place and multiple intravenous lines in his arms and legs. Teresa searched for a way of communicating to him that she was there to support him. Finally, she settled on stroking the soft brown hair on the very top of his head. Sadly, she felt ridiculed by the clinicians who watched her.

When Teresa took Tim home, he had become an irritable child, difficult to engage and to soothe, far behind in his developmental path. The five primary care doctors she consulted told her that he had been through tremendous stress and would ultimately be fine. She remained unconvinced. Fortunately, when he was about 9 months old, an office nurse unofficially recommended that Teresa take Tim to a publicly funded early intervention organization. Their evaluators confirmed her fears that he was far behind age expectations. They enrolled him in a program with regular physical therapy, occupational therapy, and developmental services.

Today, Teresa works at a community-based family resource center and serves as the family representative in a training program. Her goal is to ensure that other families do not experience what she did as a young and frightened mother.

Over the last generation, the power dynamic within the U.S. health care system has undergone a sea change. In the not-so-distant-past, as Teresa experienced, professionals maintained, or at least tried to maintain, total control of the provision of health care. They determined who participated in the care and who was present during procedures. They meted out information to patients and their families as they thought appropriate. Professionals made the vast majority of major decisions, and they controlled the records. Since about the early 1990s, within pediatrics, the paradigm has shifted from profession-dominated to family-centered care. Within adult medicine, including geriatrics, the analogous shift has been labeled *person-centered care*; in situations in which an individual may not be able to make decisions independently, person- and family-centered care fuse. This evolution to family- and person-centered care reflects new values, beliefs, and attitudes about long-term illness, who owns the information about an individual's condition, and who makes the critical decisions.

When health care for children with disabilities becomes increasingly focused on inclusion and contribution, when attention to maintaining or enhancing the person's function is a primary focus, then the individual's and/or family's role in the decision-making process becomes even more central than it was in the past. It is the family or the person with disabilities who ultimately establishes goals, charts the course, and follows through on recommendations. The family or person bears responsibility for the decisions and experiences positive or negative consequences. Health care professionals play an essential role, not truly as caregivers but rather as technicians, teachers, consultants, advisors, reality checkers, and supports to the family and person.

This chapter begins with a definition of family-centered practice, with emphasis on its role in longitudinal care of children with disabilities. The discussion focuses on the history of the concept and why family-centered care is important, reviewing the scientific evidence that supports the approach, where it exists. The discussion then turns to person-centered care, anticipating that many children and adolescents with disabilities will arrive at adulthood and then will need person-centered care. The chapter includes strategies for implementing family- and person-centered care at the clinical level and at the organizational and policy levels.

FAMILY-CENTERED CARE

Family-centered care is the practice of welcoming families and children as equal partners on the health care team. Family-centered care operates at all levels and in all aspects of health care, including planning services, delivering care, and evaluating outcomes. Within clinical care, it is an approach that supports families' participation at every step: Families attend all health care encounters, acquiring basic and advanced information about the child's conditions and treatments, and decide for themselves whether to remain present for medical procedures; they participate actively in decision making; they learn how to administer health care treatments at home and in the hospital or community; and they contribute to the evaluation of those treatments on their child's health and functioning. Within organizations, families play key roles as providers of information from the consumer and family perspective, including participation at the highest levels of administration, on the boards of organizations, as decision makers and direction setters. Within the development of policy, families and the advocacy groups that represent them and their children also play an active role in articulating problems and evaluating proposed remedies within the public sector.

Family-centered care begins with the explicit acknowledgement that in the vast majority of situations, the family is the main source of stability, continuity, and care for children. The family provides social, emotional, and developmental support that is essential to the well-being of all children. Families have what can only be considered as expertise based on a lifetime of intimate, tender, and meaningful relationships. They have spent more time, expended more love, and provided more care to the child than any professional. The parents and family know the child's personality, preferences, sensitivities, and idiosyncrasies. They know which strategies are feasible for their child within their family life and circumstances. Their expertise is distinctive and a necessary complement to that of professionals. Their personal knowledge and relationships serve as a counterbalance to scientific information and technical skills that contribute fundamentally to health and well-being but can be rendered impersonally. Therefore, they should serve as their child's representative and proxy decision maker, consulting the young child and engaging the older child, adolescent, or youth in the decision making.

History

Attention to family-centered care is relatively new to health care. In the first half of the 20th century, health institutions did not appreciate the important role of family in the health and well-being of children, whether they were developing typically or had a disability. Many hospitals, even children's hospitals, limited parents' visits to their young children to a few hours a day. They misinterpreted children's illnesses and crying as moral failings to be corrected during a hospital stay, thereby justifying the separation of parent and child (Merkel, 2008). Fortunately, these institutions ultimately changed their policies to allow family members to be with their hospitalized child around the clock. A similar battle was fought over family presence during medical procedures. As illustrated in the vignette about Teresa and Tim, the argument was that parents would be distracting to the clinicians, prone to interference or judgment. Gradually, policies have evolved to offer parents the opportunity to remain with their child throughout procedures. Maternity wards routinely separated mother from newborn during neonatal hospitalization. Rooming-in, a practice that allows the baby to remain with her mother throughout the hospital stay, was radical during my own medical training and now is fairly common.

The early 20th century was also an era of institutionalization for children and adults with severe disabilities. With limited therapeutic options and a prevailing belief that families would do better if the child with disabilities were not a financial and emotional burden on them, most health care providers, especially physicians, recommended institutionalization. The family's major decision was whether or not to agree to that option.

Many contextual changes have stimulated a rethinking of the paradigms of care. In the last half of the 20th century, the number of biomedical treatments and technological options for children and adults with disabilities exploded. However, these treatments all come with their own complications. The anticonvulsant medications that treat seizures may themselves cause cognitive blunting. Surgery for intractable epilepsy may reduce the frequency of seizures but lead to severe neuropsychological disorders. Cardiac surgery for children with Down syndrome and congenital heart disease may improve the child's heart and lung function but is very risky. Given the complicated equations of benefit and risk, it is presumptuous for the health care team to make these monumental decisions without the input of the family. After all, it is the family and not the team who assumes the ultimate lifelong responsibility associated with these health care decisions. They are the ones to provide daily care, get the child to professional visits, give medications, and do the prescribed home exercises. They provide the love that supports healing and positive change.

The important role of families was recognized in the Education for All Handicapped Children Act of 1975. The law put families on the interdisciplinary team that created individualized education programs for children with disabilities who qualified for special education (U.S. Department of Education, 2007). The law also created a process by which families could contest the decisions of the team if they disagreed. The reauthorization of the law in 1986 set the legal standards for early intervention services for children birth to 3 years of age (US Department of Education, 2007). By this time, the role of families was so clear, particularly for infants and toddlers, that the customized plans to support the development of infants and toddlers were called individualized family service plans. The individualized family service plan incorporates parental priorities, preferences, and strategies. It also includes the supports and services that allow parents to participate in the delivery of early intervention to their children. The plan may include transportation for the family to the therapist's office or translation services so that the parents understand the treatment approach.

Within health care, the construct of family-centered care was formally introduced in 1987 as part of an initiative promoted by then U.S. Surgeon General C. Everett Koop for family-centered, community-based, coordinated care for children with special health care needs and their families. The initiative was unveiled at a conference sponsored by the American Academy of Pediatrics (AAP) and the Bureau of Maternal and Child Health and Resources Development, U.S. Department of Health and Human Services. In the speech at the conclusion of this conference,

Dr. Koop unveiled a seven-step program to improve the care of children with special health care needs and their families. (See the commentary below.) He reminded the audience that as a pediatric surgeon in clinical practice for about 40 years, he had witnessed the intense struggles of families of children with what he called special health care needs. He paid tribute to their remarkable equanimity under stress (Koop, 1987).

The AAP formulated a policy statement in 2003 in favor of family-centered care (Committee on Hospital Care & Institute for Family-Centered Care, 2003). Within this document were listed the core principles of collaboration between child health clinicians and families. This document served to bring the importance and characteristics of family-centered care to almost all of the practicing pediatricians in the United States.

Core Elements

The Institute for Patient- and Family-Centered Care (2010) has articulated four essential elements of family-centered care, as follows:

> *Respect and dignity*: Health care practitioners listen to and honor patient and family perspectives and choices. Patient and family knowledge, values, beliefs, and cultural backgrounds are incorporated into the planning and delivery of care.
>
> *Information sharing*: Health care practitioners communicate and share complete and unbiased information with patients and families in ways that are affirming and useful. Patients and families receive timely, complete, and accurate information in order to effectively participate in care and decision making.
>
> *Participation*: Patients and families are encouraged and supported in participating in care and decision making at the level they choose.
>
> *Collaboration*: Patients, families, health care practitioners, and hospital leaders collaborate in policy and program development, implementation, and evaluation; in health care facility design; and in professional education, as well as in the delivery of care.

Additional elements listed in the policy statement (Committee on Hospital Care & Institute for Family-Centered Care, 2003, p. 692) are as follows:

Commentary
The 1987 Initiative Regarding Health Care for Children with Special Health Care Needs

In the Surgeon General's report, C. Everett Koop embedded family-centered care within the context of the seven major steps to improve access to care and quality of life for the children. The steps were as follows (Brewer, McPherson, Magrab, & Hutchins, 1989; Koop, 1987):

> *(1) A pledge of a national commitment to all children with special health care needs and their families, (2) encouragement of localities in the building of community-based service systems, (3) assistance in ensuring adequate preparation of providers of care, (4) development of coalitions to improve the delivery of services, (5) establishment of guidelines to control costs of services, (6) encouragement and support of the development of adequate health care financing, and (7) continuation of research and dissemination of information.*

Honoring racial, ethnic, cultural, and socioeconomic diversity and its effect on the family's experience and perception of care

Recognizing and building on the strengths of each child and family, even in difficult and challenging situations

Ensuring flexibility in organizational policies, procedures, and provider practices so that services can be tailored to the needs, beliefs, and cultural values of each child and family

Providing and/or ensuring formal and informal support (e.g., family-to-family support) for the child and parent(s) and/or guardian(s) during pregnancy, childbirth, infancy, childhood, adolescence, and young adulthood

Empowering each child and family to discover their own strengths, build confidence, and make choices and decisions about their health

Dunst and Trivette (1996) created a model for what they called effective helping that serves as a useful conceptualization for family-centered care. The model uses an equilateral triangle to articulate the core elements (see Figure 9.1). The first side of the triangle is up-to-date scientific knowledge and competent technical skills. Clearly, health care professionals must be good at their craft. The second side of the triangle is compassionate, warm, and caring relationship. These traits are indicative of the dignity and respect that must be afforded to children and families. Many training programs for health professionals teach communication skills that meet this criterion. The third side of the triangle is information sharing and collaborative decision making. This key ingredient is not as emphasized in training as is good listening. Yet it is extremely important; it's what separates what could be called good bedside manner from true family-centered care. It encourages professionals to acknowledge that the family bears the major and long-term responsibility for a child and therefore carries the authority to accept or reject professional recommendations.

The word *family* in family-centered care refers to those individuals who are intimately related in any way to a child patient. Traditionally, the connections are biological. However, as family structures have shifted, the family may also be defined in terms of emotional rather than biological connections. For example, a child may have a very close relationship with her stepmother or neighbor. In some

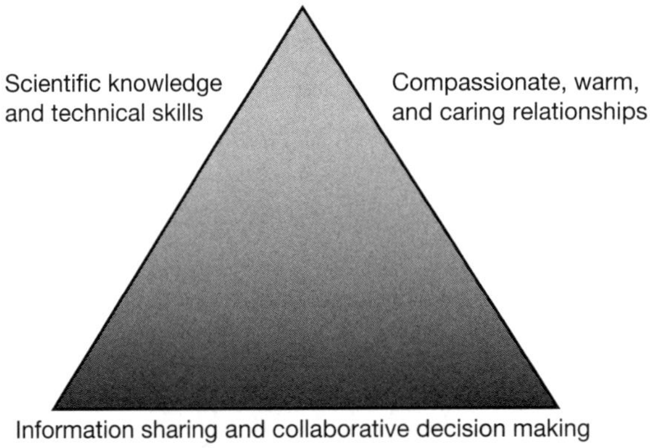

Figure 9.1. Components of helping behavior. (From Dunst, C.J., & Trivette, C.M. [1996]. Empowerment, effective help giving practices and family-centered care. *Pediatric Nursing*, 22[4], 334–337; reprinted by permission.)

situations, the family may be defined legally as well as emotionally, including guardians. What is critical is that whenever possible, individuals define their own families. In pediatrics, the definition of the family often falls to the parents. They can choose who comes with them to the clinic, office, or hospital, and what role that companion plays. Health care clinicians should make no assumptions about who is in the family and should be very comfortable in discussing the issue with children and adults. (See the commentary below.)

We often forget in pediatric health care delivery that children are also members of the team. Of course, their ability to participate in clinical processes varies as a function of their age, developmental level, and experience, as well as the issues at hand. Whenever a child is competent to understand their condition and to make decisions concerning their own health care, then the individual child must be consulted about what should be done. For example, a young teen should decide whether his parent remains in the examination room during his evaluation. An adolescent can weigh in on whether a schedule of treatments is feasible within the school day or week. Preschoolers and young school-age children with long-term conditions may also be able to contribute to decision making from their own perspective, despite

Commentary
Who Is a Family?

I remember as a resident in San Diego in the early 1980s treating a Hmong infant, about 2 months old, who was quite ill. All I knew at the time was that the Hmong were a group from the mountains of Northern Laos who had been armed to help the United States prevent incursions of North Vietnamese into Laos and South Vietnam. When the United States left Vietnam, the Laotians and North Vietnamese targeted the Hmong for retribution. Many immigrated to refugee camps in Thailand and eventually to the United States. One of their main ports of entry was San Diego.

This particular baby came to the hospital very dehydrated. We determined that the child was vomiting from pyloric stenosis, a constriction of the valve that allows food to leave the stomach. The usual treatment is to stabilize the infant with fluids and then to surgically repair the valve. The residents wanted to put an intravenous line into one of the scalp veins, the easiest veins to find in a dehydrated infant. A nurse warned that we should not proceed to put a needle in the scalp because damaging the head in any way was highly upsetting to Hmong families. So instead, the team decided to speed up the operation. We used the translators we had available to relay information to the family in a sequence of English to French, French to Thai, and Thai to Hmong. We explained the operation and the importance of acting quickly. The parents seemed to understand what we were saying but refused to sign the consent form. We made no headway after repeating all of the information a second time. We even considered whether a court order for treatment was the appropriate next step to proceed with necessary care.

It was then that the clan leader arrived. The distressed parents dutifully discussed the child's situation with the leader. The leader gave his verbal consent, and then the parents signed our written consent. I came to learn that the chief was the ultimate decision maker for this Hmong clan.

their young age. I know a 6-year-old boy with cerebral palsy who has strong opinions about whether it is worth him experiencing insomnia from wearing braces at night if his flexibility at the ankles is currently not diminished. In these situations, the clinicians may be able to give voice to the child who has yet to convince his family that he has a valid point of view.

Cultural Competence

Family-centered care implies respect for a family's distinctive beliefs, attitudes, values, styles, and preferences and recognizes that these factors are in part determined by the family's culture. Clinicians who seek to provide family-centered care must become aware of the cultural influences on the families they are working with. *Culture* refers to the integrated patterns of human behavior that include language, thoughts, communications, actions, customs, beliefs, values, and institutions based at least in part on the racial, ethnic, religious, or social affiliations of individuals.

The importance of understanding cultures has increased over the last several decades as the U.S. population, and especially the population of children, has become increasingly diverse in terms of its racial, ethnic, and linguistic composition. *Cultural competence* occurs when the behaviors, attitudes, and policies of professionals, agencies, or systems coalesce to allow effective work in cross-cultural situations. *Competence* implies having the capacity to function effectively as an individual and an organization within the context of the cultural beliefs, behaviors, and needs presented by consumers and their communities (Office of Minority Health, 2005)

The process of developing cultural competence begins by acknowledging one's own cultural roots and recognizing how these cultural forces affect clinical behavior and decisions (Campinha-Bacote, 2002). Cultural background includes race, ethnicity, religion, and economic background, as well as chosen profession. All professions have their distinctive language, beliefs, history, and practices. For many who study long and hard to earn professional degrees, that professional culture comes to override the culture of their youth. Some fail to recognize that their professions have come to influence their interpretations of the world, explicitly and implicitly (Kleinman, Eisenbery, & Good, 1978). (See the commentary on p. 141.)

Cultural competence requires that professionals learn about dominant cultural beliefs, values, or practices in the diverse groups that obtain care in the clinician's community while avoiding stereotyping. Patients and families interpret their physical symptoms and psychological experiences from their cultural perspective, so appreciating cultural beliefs aids in understanding their experience of the condition (Kleinman et al., 1978). Cultural competence also requires learning about the prevalence of various conditions and about distinctive features in treatment efficacy in that population (Campinha-Bacote, 2002). In many situations, a family's approach to disability or health care decision making may resemble the approach of others from the same racial, ethnic, demographic, or socioeconomic group.

It is important to note that variations within a group may be as great as the variation between groups. From outside, it is often difficult to determine with what cultures a family might identify. For example, the children and grandchildren of immigrants may not relate to their cultural origins in the same way as the first

Commentary
Professional Cultures

The diagnosis of sensory integration disorders and the appropriate therapy for such disorders are a flashpoint between two different cultures within the health care system: occupational and other therapists and physicians.

An occupational therapist, A. Jean Ayres, developed a theory that when sensory neurons are immature or inefficient, integrated sensory processing is defective (Ayres, 1979). According to the theory, this problem leads to deficits in other domains, including learning and emotional regulation. Since the 1970s, occupational therapists have used the theory to explain various clinical characteristics of children with disabilities, such as crying or withdrawal when exposed to loud noises or irritation at the labels in their clothing. The therapists prescribe sensory "diets" and specific approaches to modulate the input to the child's sensory systems. Techniques such as brushing and swinging are frequently applied. Occupational therapists use single case studies and family testimonials to document the effectiveness of the treatment.

The sensory integration approach makes sense to many parents, who willingly pay out of pocket for sensory integration treatments. They give moving accounts about the positive impact of sensory integration therapy on their child.

Many Western medical doctors, however, are skeptical about the diagnosis of sensory processing disorder (Section on Complementary and Integrative Medicine and Council on Children with Disabilties, 2012). In their approach, the clinical criteria for this disorder have never been established, and sensory symptoms are part and parcel of many disorders, including autism, attention-deficit hyperactivity disorder, and intellectual disability. They are also unconvinced that sensory integration treatment substantially improves the functioning of children who are treated with it, above and beyond the placebo effects of the warm nurturing relationship that develops between the child and therapist. They denigrate studies designed to show the efficacy of sensory integration therapy as lacking the scientific rigor of studies that show the efficacy of medications or other medical treatments. Occupational therapists counter that a single outcome measure chosen for large group studies may miss the individual positive impacts that they see in different children after sensory integration. Physicians counter that neutral parties, unaware of whether the child received the treatment or a control condition, must evaluate outcomes if they are to believe the results of such studies.

The cultures clash when physicians refuse to write prescriptions for sensory integration occupational therapy on the basis of their strong beliefs. Parents may be caught in the middle. They do not want to forego any treatments that might prove beneficial, and they cannot access occupational therapy directly without the prescription.

The American Academy of Pediatrics issued a policy statement about sensory integration therapy (Section on Complementary and Intergrative Medicine and Council on Children with Disabilties, 2012). It tried to find a middle road that acknowledges that the techniques may have value despite the current lack of scientific evidence. However, the statement fails to acknowledge that this ongoing debate is fueled by cultural differences between the professions.

generation. Economically successful families from any distinctive ethnic or religious community may have different beliefs, values, and language than low-income families from that same community. So, although knowledge of prevailing trends may be helpful, there is no substitute for developing clinical skills for collecting information about the family and its unique blend of cultural influences. Families may be hesitant to reveal their cultural beliefs to professionals. Clinicians need to demonstrate their true interest by asking them what they thought caused their condition, their concepts about the long-term course, and their expectations for treatment (Kleinman et al., 1978).

The term *competence* might not be quite right for the professional approach to culture. It usually refers to the mastery of a finite amount of information or a specific set of skills. However, in improving an approach to cultural variation, mastery may not be possible or desirable. More suitable is a lifelong process of self-examination and engagement with others. This openness can lead to an evolving understanding of the role of culture in health and health care delivery. Indeed, cultures themselves may change over time as the life experiences of the members change, requiring new constructs and new understanding. The construct of *cultural humility* has been offered as a contrast to cultural competence because it implies the need for continuous self-reflection and change (Tervalon & Murray-Garcia, 1998).

Positive Outcomes

It is easy to justify the need for family-centered care simply on an ethical basis. If the family bears responsibility for the long-term care of the child, then the family should participate in the decisions about that care. In addition, family-centered care promotes autonomy, responsibility, and dignity for every family member involved in the longitudinal care of a child with long-term conditions. It is important to know whether family-centered care actually improves health outcomes for children. If it does, that would be further reason to promote it, particularly in long-term health care.

The evidence that family-centered care is associated with positive outcomes is accumulating. Many of the positive outcomes are enumerated in a policy statement from the American Academy of Pediatrics that defines family-centered practice and links it to health care outcomes (Committee on Hospital Care & Institute for Family-Centered Care, 2003). Here are a few examples of positive outcomes.

Parental Presence During Procedures Parental presence during medical procedures leads to positive psychological and medical outcomes. Teresa in the opening vignette had the right instincts as a mother. Children whose parents remain with them during procedures exhibit less anxiety than those whose parents are not present. When parents are prepared, they do not prolong the procedure or make the provider more anxious (Blesch & Fisher, 1996). Quality improvement studies have documented that children who underwent surgery with their parents present cried less, were less restless, and required less medication than those who had a similar procedure when their parents were not present and unavailable to assist in pain assessment and management (Fina, Lopas, Stagnone, & Santucci, 1997). Children whose mothers were involved in their post-tonsillectomy care recovered faster and were discharged earlier than were children whose mothers did not participate in their care (Shelton & Stepanek, 1994)

Parent-to-Parent Support Evidence also supports parent-to-parent support networks as an important factor in increasing parental confidence, problem-solving ability, and mental health. In a multicenter study, parents assigned to a 2-month parent-to-parent support group had higher scores on measures of coping, attitude, and progress addressing problems than parents in a wait-list control group (Singer et al., 1999). Qualitative analyses have found that parents value support from other parents with whom they share demographic or situational features, who are readily available, and with whom they can establish mutual relationships (Ainbinder et al., 1998). A particularly impressive demonstration of the power of parent-to-parent support was a randomized trial of a program called the Family-to-Family Network (Ireys, Chernoff, DeVet, & Kim, 2001), in which half of the 161 mothers of children with long-term illnesses including diabetes, sickle cell anemia, cystic fibrosis, or moderate to severe asthma were assigned to the treatment group and paired with a parent mentor and a child life specialist, whereas the other half were simply given the name of another parent of a child with the same condition. After the 15-month intervention, mothers who received the support showed statistically significant reductions in anxiety compared with those who did not get the support. In contrast, only 3% of the control group contacted the parent whose name they had been given as a potential supporter (Ireys et al., 2001).

Parental Decision Making Although the evidence is still modest, the results of parental decision making are positive. One important study took place in King County, Washington, in a children's managed care program that was based on a family-participation service model. Families made the decisions about how funds would be spent for their children with mental health needs. The caveat was that a collaborative team that the family had convened actually created the comprehensive service plan that guided expenditures. The results were very positive. In the 5 years after the program's inception, the percentage of children living in family homes instead of institutions increased dramatically, from 24% to 91%, and the percentage attending community schools also increased, from 48% to 95%. What might come as a surprise is that the average cost of care per child or family per month actually decreased, from approximately \$6,000 to \$4,100 (Committee on Hospital Care & Institute for Family-Centered Care, 2003).

Challenges to Practicing Family-Centered Care

In rare situations, the family cannot participate fully in the clinical process, cannot make decisions in the best interest of their child, or cannot follow through on team recommendations, including their own commitments. These issues arise when the family experiences overwhelming stress or does not have coping strategies to meet their level of stress. Challenges occur when parents have mental health disorders, learning issues, or social problems such as separation and divorce. Many of these issues can be addressed directly and supportively to reengage the family meaningfully in their child's care (see Table 9.1).

Abuse and Neglect One of the most vexing challenges to practicing family-centered care is child physical or sexual abuse or child neglect. If clinicians uncover abuse or neglect, their primary responsibility is to report the findings to the appropriate agency. It is important to be open with the family when a child abuse report will be made. The information should be presented to them frankly and without judgment.

Parents who have abused or neglected their child usually want what is best for that child. They may even recognize that reporting is in the child's best interests. For example, abuse may be the result of poor impulse control and neglect the result of limited knowledge; parents may appreciate support to change their behavior or their caregiving. The rates of abuse increase during economic recessions and high unemployment when increased stress interacts with increased contact between child and parent. Alcohol or drug use may also disinhibit parents who otherwise would never harm their child.

Reporting does not necessarily need to end the clinician–family relationship. For example, a clinician could say, "I am concerned about how you are disciplining

Table 9.1. Addressing challenges to practicing family-centered care

Challenge	Description	Strategies for reengaging families
Overwhelming stress	Levels of stress exceed the family's ability to cope	• Reduce demands on the family • Identify other professionals or informal supports to provide care for the child • Give permission for the family to take a break, either appealing to relatives or friends for support or identifying respite care programs in the community • Help families meet their other needs for food, shelter, or safety
Weak coping skills	Coping skills that may be adequate for routine stress cannot meet high levels of stress	• Encourage families to remember how they handled other major stresses, such as death of a loved one • Identify sources of social support within their network • Identify families going through similar challenges to offer support • Address feelings of shame or inadequacy that compromise coping
Parental mental health disorders	Parental mental or emotional issues interfere with their ability to participate in decisions or provide care	• Evaluate parent's willingness and interest to receive help or referrals • Refer willing and interested parents for mental health care. Facilitate referrals by making calls and researching options • Continue to provide support for families who decide not to accept referrals to mental health professionals
Parental learning issues	Family's educational attainment limits their understanding of recommendations or treatments	• Ensure that family members understand by asking them to repeat what they have heard • Identify materials that match the health literacy level • Identify informal supports to assist with comprehension • Identify care coordinators or social services to assist with comprehension
Separation and divorce	Only one parent available or conflict between parents	• Encourage teamwork on behalf of the child • Contact the absent parent directly • Negotiate and consider mediation

your child. I will need to report the incident to the Child Protection Organization. I hope that we can still work together on behalf of your child." I have personally been gratified that families have been willing to return to my care after I have filed a child abuse report on behalf of their children. In some cases, they wanted to demonstrate to me that they had learned from the experience and changed their approach to discipline or stress.

Family–Team Disagreements

Professional members of the health care team may disagree with the family about the nature or intensity of the services a child should receive. In some cases, the professionals push for additional interventions that the family does not deem important. In other cases, the family demands treatment that the professionals do not think is indicated. It can feel like a tug of war if both sides rigidly maintain their stance, feeling justified in their position. Humility is in order on both sides. Recall that in the opening vignette, it was Teresa, the mother, who had the right instincts about her child from the moment his appetite declined until she had him diagnosed with cerebral palsy 5 months after his discharge from the hospital. Even well-trained and well-intentioned professionals can be wrong. At the same time, parental worries may be out of proportion to the situation, or their demands might be beyond what the system can provide.

Rather than entering into head-on confrontation, refusing to consider the parental point of view, or capitulating to parental pressure while feeling uncertain, the health care team can try negotiation. There is often a middle ground. Consider the mother of a child with mild cerebral palsy who demanded twice as much therapy as the child was receiving because she was concerned that one foot was turning inward while the other was not. The middle ground in this case might include a time-limited trial of increased therapy to determine whether an increased frequency of physical therapy would change the outcome. Alternatively, the middle ground might lead to a second opinion about the frequency of treatment. Open communication may not lead to consensus about these issues but may maintain the mutual respect of clinician and family. (See the commentary on p. 146.)

PERSON-CENTERED MEDICINE

The Institute of Medicine defines patient-centered care as "care that is respectful of and responsive to individual patient preferences, needs and values, and ensuring that patient values guide all clinical decisions" (Institute of Medicine, 2001, p. 6). As children with disabilities get older and enter adolescence and young adulthood, many will assume increasing responsibility for their own health care and health care decisions. Even those individuals with intellectual and developmental disabilities may be able to contribute their preferences, needs, and values to decisions. Thus, their care will evolve from family- to person-centered.

History

Several different strands in general medicine, rehabilitation, and assisted living came together to create the current concept of person-centered care; this chapter touches on only a few of these influences. Michael Balint, a Hungarian psychoanalyst coined the term *patient-centered medicine*. His life work focused on bringing together practitioners whose work together could support the integration of psychotherapeutic techniques into general medical practice (Johnson, 2001). A foundation of the approach is that patients must be understood as unique individuals, each with a story to tell that involves their life experience as well as their physical symptoms. The clinician's obligation is to explore the illness experience, understanding the person and not simply the disease, and to use supportive clinical skills to build a respectful clinician–patient relationship that addresses the patient's agenda (Beach, Saha, & Cooper, 2006). The approach can be summarized succinctly as seeing the condition through the patient's eyes (Beach et al., 2006). Family medicine in the United States has embraced the principles of patient-centered care. Program requirements for residency in family medicine state the following:

> The family physician assumes responsibility for the total health care of the individual and family, taking into account social, behavioral, economic, cultural, and biologic dimensions. Therefore, residents must learn to demonstrate cultural competence in caring for patients from varied ethnic and cultural backgrounds. (Accreditation Council for Graduate Medical Education, 2007, Section IV.A.5.a.(2).(b).(ii), p. 18)

Commentary
Dr. Cohen's One-Down Approach

William I. Cohen was a colleague of mine at the University of Pittsburgh for more than 20 years. Dr. Cohen had extensive education in family systems and clinical training in family therapy as well as pediatrics. He had extraordinary skills in family-centered practice.

Dr. Cohen had a special touch when he encountered a family who favored an approach at odds with prevailing clinical wisdom or his best judgment. As long as the family preferences did not put the child at significant risk, Dr. Cohen taught young professionals and colleagues alike to take the "one-down" position. Our usual approach as professionals, he would counsel, is to assume the "one-up" position. Going one-up is insisting that we know more than the family about the clinical condition, its causes, and its management. Often when we push as professionals, the family also digs in to their position as well.

The one-down position requires that the clinician abandon any investment in the decisions that the family makes. It encourages curiosity and humility. Dr. Cohen demonstrated how to assume this stance by asking lots of questions about the family's situation, their interpretation of the child or the child's condition, and their understanding of the options before them. He also advised that it was important to keep the lines of communication open. The child and family's needs might change or their take on the situation evolve.

To achieve these ends, he would make comments such as, "I trust you will know when another approach might become necessary" and "Why don't you try your plan between now and our next visit and then we can reassess the situation together?"

Without pressure, many families came around to Dr. Cohen's treatment recommendations; sometimes quickly, and other times more slowly. Along the way, Dr. Cohen learned new ideas, strategies, and clinical options from those families who stuck to their guns.

Another strand in this development was the Picker-Commonwealth Program for Patient-Centered Care, launched in 1987 with a focus on promoting a person-centered approach in hospital care and health services (Beach et al., 2006). The core principles of their approach operate at the level of interpersonal communication and health care organizations. Similar to the Balint approach to interpersonal communication, in this model clinicians use a biopsychosocial model to view the patient as a unique individual and to share responsibility in effective relationships. Clinicians remain keenly aware that they are individuals within the relationship and not strictly technicians. Expanding on the Balint approach, this model also includes the level of health care delivery. At the organizational level, services are aligned to patient needs and preferences. Services are therefore coordinated, accessible, and inclusive of health promotion and physical comfort (Beach et al., 2006).

Yet another contributor to the evolution of the concept was Tom Kitwood, a British psychologist at Bradford University who brought the concept of person-centered care to the treatment of dementia. He identified multiple factors that promote well-being and should be the focus in person-centered practice. They include understanding the person's identity; engaging the person in occupation and meaningful tasks; providing warmth, acceptance, and comfort; enabling attachments; and including the person in what is happening (Bradford Dementia Group, 2012).

Since these beginnings, the movement toward person-centered care has been accelerating and expanding. The Institute of Medicine issued a seminal report in 2001 entitled *Crossing the Quality Chasm: A New Health System for the 21st Century* (Institute of Medicine, 2001). Among the 10 principles for systems change within that report is the declaration that partnerships among professionals, patients, and families are essential to such a caregiving process. Though the term *person-centered care* was not used, among the 10 Rules to Redesign and Improve Care are several that are completely consistent with person-centered practice (institute of Medicine, 2001, pp. 61–62):

- Care is based on continuous healing relationships.
- Care is customized to patient needs and values.
- The patient is the source of control.
- Shared knowledge and the free flow of information.
- The need for transparency.

The transformation in how clinical care is delivered has become an international movement. Person-centered planning is mandated by government policy in the United Kingdom and other industrialized countries. WHO places people at the center of health care and public health across the globe, in developing as well as developed countries (WHO, 2010). It is no longer acceptable to resort to hierarchical, patronizing, impersonal, or professional-centered care.

IMPLEMENTATION IN CLINICAL ENCOUNTERS

For emerging professionals, one of the best ways to learn family- and person-centered practice is by working with experienced practitioners, observing their strategies in action and obtaining their feedback on early attempts to provide family-centered care. Several recommendations for education programs are included in Chapter 11. Below are some tips regarding clinical skills that demonstrate family- and patient-centered care:

- Demonstrating respect, promoting dignity
    - Use the child's or person's and the parents' names, as they would like to be addressed. Pediatric clinicians who work with parents are apt to substitute Mom or Dad for the parent's name. Their names are far more personal.
    - Acknowledge the family's or person's point of view.
    - Clarify what the family or patient means or wants. It is appropriate to say, "Let me see if I fully understand what you are saying."
    - Maintain strict confidentiality, particularly about sensitive information.
- Setting the agenda
    - Agree on the agenda for a visit. Make no assumptions about what the family/person wants or needs. Often what the family expects or wants is not obvious when their child has a long-term condition.
    - If more than one family member is present, ask each to contribute what they want to get out of the visit, remaining sensitive to the family's cultural style of communication.
    - If the family/person and clinician agenda are different, negotiate a plan of action. It is acceptable to ask, "How would it be after we discuss your issue, if we also address one of my concerns?"
- Opening up the lines of communication
    - Sit down with the family or person.
    - Listen without interrupting. Pause after providing information to allow the family/person to respond or react. Asking, "What do you think about that idea?" may allow them to appreciate that you want their input. Silence is active and effective. It is acceptable to follow an adage that has been attributed to many different clinicians: "Don't just do something, sit there!"
    - Check the level of understanding. You might try a question like this: "When you go home this evening and your extended family asks what happened at the visit, what will you tell them?"
    - Define medical terms or professional jargon in language the family/person understands. Use written information as much as possible so that the family/person can review the material beyond the time constraints of a visit. Be sensitive to the general and health literacy level of the family/person (Yin et al., 2009).
- Honoring observations and interpretations (see the commentary on p. 150)
    - Invite the family/person to share their observations and interpretations.

- Take a good history of others who have been involved in the child's or person's care. Ask what was said and what the family/person thinks about the recommendations or interpretations.
- Take a good history of the results of previous treatments so as not to repeat previously unsuccessful recommendations. If your inclination is to try an approach that had previously failed, clarify what will be different this time. It might be that the child is older, that the treatment will be more intensive, or that pacing will change. Explain how that change may bring about a different outcome.
- Ask families/individuals how they would like to participate in treatments.
- Discuss what approaches are likely to work for the family/person. Ask them how suggestions might fit into everyday experiences. For parents, discuss the importance of maintaining the intimate family bonds while doing exercises, homework, or therapy. Ensure that individuals can follow through with recommendations so that you do not set them up to fail.

- Providing unbiased information
  - Use handouts and information sheets. Have versions in all languages that are common in your community. Check that the recipients can understand the material (Yin et al., 2009).
  - Choose materials that have been prepared by neutral organizations or family support agencies where there is no conflict of interest.
  - Plan strategies on how to increase knowledge, understanding, and skill to prepare the family/person for increasing responsibility in decision making.
- Encouraging parent-to-parent or peer support
  - Encourage and facilitate support and networking.
  - Help individuals and families to connect with education and advocacy organizations around specific clinical conditions that can assist them with access to others. (See the commentary on p. 151.)
  - Find organizations where they may meet others of the same ethnic, cultural, or linguistic group, even if conditions are different.
- Sharing decision making
  - Ask the family/person what treatments or evaluation procedures they had expected.
  - Check in about their reactions to recommendations.
  - Refrain from pressuring if they are reluctant to accept a recommendation. Listen carefully to their reservations. Consider variations that allow them to adhere to the recommendations. Consider brief trials and close follow-up until they have a chance to evaluate the approach.
  - When multiple suitable options are available, allow the family/person to weigh the risks and benefits and make the final determination.

Commentary
Adaptive Practice

Several years ago, the interdisciplinary clinical team on which I worked became uncertain about how to provide family-centered care during the diagnostic process. We recognized that families often came to us when they were uncertain about their child's development or behavior; they had very limited information about the condition that their child might have. Under those circumstances, families could provide detailed information about the child's features and functioning. But how could the family participate in the decision-making process during diagnosis? These questions led to a self-reflective process and ultimately to a conceptual framework entitled Physician-Family Partnerships: The Adaptive Practice Model (Feldman, Ploof, & Cohen, 1999). Although the title specifies physicians, the principles can be applied to a range of health professions.

The inspiration for the adaptive practice model was a highly respected approach to leadership within the business world called situational leadership. The thesis in situational leadership is that good managers adjust their approach to workers on the basis of workers' abilities and their motivation. Managers are more authoritative when a worker is new on the job than when the worker is fully trained, and they give more leeway to workers with high motivation than to those with limited confidence or initiative. If a worker's job changes, the manager may need to return to the authoritative style until the worker is prepared for the new role.

Adaptive practice recognizes that health care professionals must similarly adapt their approach to families on the basis of the family's knowledge and ability to engage in the clinical process. The model posits four main styles of interacting with families. Clinicians use directing when the family has limited knowledge about the child's condition and when dealing with an emergency or crisis. The dialogue is limited, and information flow goes primarily from professional to family. This scenario may be appropriate for many families in the diagnostic process. Clinicians shift to teaching when it becomes appropriate to educate the family about a child's condition and begin a treatment planning process. In teaching, the interactions become longer and the dialogue more bidirectional. Families not only ask questions but also interpret the information the clinician provides in accordance with the child's individuality. This style of interaction may also be appropriate at the time of diagnosis if families are somewhat prepared to engage in discussion on the basis of their previous suspicions, reading, or personal style. Clinicians chose collaborating when the family has assumed responsibility and decision making for the child and yet may still need or want input. This type of interaction may work when a family has another child with the same disorder and can rapidly begin to apply the knowledge and skill they had acquired for the first child to another child. Finally, clinicians usually reserve supporting for long-term follow-up during which the family informs the clinician about their choices and plans and the clinician provides a reality check. Even after the professional has engaged in supporting, he or she may need to move back to another type of interaction if a new situation arises for which the family is unprepared.

- Becoming accountable
  - See them for follow-up visits as appropriate.
  - Do what you promise.
  - Establish realistic timelines for change.
  - Invite feedback about the feasibility or success of treatment recommendations.
  - Communicate with others on the health care team on the child's behalf.
- Managing disagreements and conflicts
  - Encourage specific actions that are important. Explain the reason for waiting if that is a good course of action.
  - Review the scientific evidence or practice guidelines that support the recommendations.
  - Ask the family/person specifically whether they think that they can adhere to recommendations or follow through with treatments.
  - If failing to provide therapy is likely to cause harm and the treatment carries little risk, share you concern; persuade without resorting to coercion or manipulation.

Commentary
Family and Parent Resources

Many conditions have organizations with the condition name in the title. Here is a list of just a few:

- *Angelman Syndrome Foundation (http://www.angelman.org)*
- *Autism Speaks (http://www.autismspeaks.org)*
- *National Down Syndrome Congress (http://ndsccenter.org)*
- *National Down Syndrome Society (http://www.ndss.org)*
- *National Fragile X Foundation (http://www.fragilex.org)*
- *Tourette Syndrome Association (http://www.tsa-usa.org)*
- *Unique – The Rare Chromosome Disorder Support Group (http://www.rarechromo.org/html/home.asp)*
- *Williams Syndrome Association (http://www.williams-syndrome.org)*

For children with extremely rare conditions, the National Association of Rare Disorders (http://www.rarediseases.org) assists families in reaching out to others across the globe.

Many states provide funding for parent support networks. For example, in California there are family resource centers in every county. Parents Helping Parents (http://www.php.com) is the family resource center in San Jose. It does an outstanding job connecting families within cultural groups well represented in northern California.

- If providing the treatment is likely to produce minimal gain and may be harmful, establish clear criteria for evaluation and cessation of the treatment.
- Suggest a second or third opinion. If the second opinion is different from the first, talk directly with the other professional to learn the reasons for his or her recommendations.
- Remember that unless the treatment or lack thereof will cause the child/person severe harm, parents have the right to refuse or reject medical recommendations or to practice alternative approaches. Court orders may have a role, but only when the parents' decisions are clearly harmful.

- Finding meaning
  - The care of a child with disabilities and long-term health care conditions sometimes brings a spiritual dimension to family life and can transform how families look at their world. Having a disability may also have enormous meaning for an individual. Acknowledging this meaning displays a respect for his or her worldview.
  - For some clinicians, the care of individuals with disabilities is more than a career. It becomes a calling. Finding this common ground gives meaning to both the clinician and the family or person.

IMPLEMENTATION BEYOND THE CLINICAL LEVEL

To sustain family-centered care requires more than a personal commitment of clinicians from the interdisciplinary team that serves children with disabilities and his or her families. It requires institutional guarantees and new models of health care delivery.

Family-Centered Care at the Organizational Level

Health care organizations, such as hospitals or managed care organizations, demonstrate their support for family- and person-centered care by including families and individuals on task forces, advisory councils, and committees, up to and including the level of the board of directors. Because the interests of families may differ from those of individuals with disabilities, consumer and family advisory boards allow both patients and their representatives to make regular and meaningful input to the hospital, facility, or agency. Consumers and family members can be further involved when special projects arise, such as a renovation, development of a new service, or planning for a research endeavor. They can also be participants in quality improvement initiatives and program evaluation.

Family- and person-centered care at the organization level requires that the family and individuals play substantive roles in setting directions and making policy. It is important to consider where the family advisory board, consumer advisory board, and quality committees sit in the organizational structure; who serves to facilitate them; to whom they report; and how much administrative support they receive. Minimal support or reporting to a person or office with a limited impact on the entire organization may indicate token rather than sincere involvement. Family participation built on volunteerism signals a peripheral role in the organization. An indication that the organization truly respects and values family and consumer input is that the representatives are paid for their efforts and that they have dedicated administrative support. (See the commentary below.)

Another example of organizational commitment to family- and person-centered care is including in job descriptions the expectations for this model of care. If that expectation is explicit, then new employees may require training to learn the organizational culture and practices. In addition, individual patients and families should be asked to provide systematic evaluations as part of the employee's performance appraisal.

Several prominent organizations have begun demonstrations of family- and person-centered care at the organizational level. In 2006, the Joint Commission on the Accreditation of Health Care Organizations, a private nonprofit organization that seeks to improve the safety and quality of health care through accreditation of health care organizations, convened its first patient and family advisory committee and published a book entitled *Patients as Partners: How to Involve Patients and Families in Their Own Care*. The Agency for Healthcare Quality and Research and the Centers for Medicare & Medicaid Services (CMS) in the United States have supported the development of the Consumer Assessment of Healthcare Providers and Systems (CAHPS) surveys, which measure the patient and consumer experience across the continuum of care, including health plans, medical groups, individual physicians, hospitals, nursing homes, home care services, and assisted living facilities. CMS publicly reports data from many of the CAHPS surveys on its web site. At the international level, WHO launched the World Alliance for Patient Safety in 2004. Patient and families are at the center of this effort to improve patient safety. Patients for Patient Safety, one of the six action areas of the World Alliance, is designed to ensure that the perspectives of patients and families are a central reference point in shaping this initiative (WHO, 2012).

Although these developments are all very positive, sustainable partnerships with patients and families will require additional profound changes in organizational culture and leadership. These partnerships may produce benefits and may also cause tension within the organization. Organizational change is usually slow

Commentary
Family-Centered Care at Lucile Packard Children's Hospital

I was so pleased when I joined the faculty at Stanford University and began working at Lucile Packard Children's Hospital (LPCH) at Stanford University and learned that family-centered care was both in its mission statement and its goals. The hospital has an impressive track record of living up to these standards.

LPCH at Stanford has an office of family-centered care.

The director of Family-Centered Care has an endowed position. The salary of the director is paid from the interest on a large investment. The program includes the Parent Mentor Program, the Family Advisory Council, the Parents as Educators Program, and the Parents as Policy Participants and Staff Training. Karen Wayman, Ph.D., currently holds the position.

and often painful. Senior leaders need to be on board with major changes within the organizations. When problems inevitably arise, the leadership must remain committed to partnerships, recognizing that these partnerships ultimately lead to the best outcomes and to improvements in quality and safety.

Family-Centered/Person-Centered Medical Home

The medical home is a health care delivery model that is designed to promote family-centered care. The medical home, by definition, ensures that continuous and comprehensive preventive, acute, and long-term care is delivered to individuals in the context of an ongoing relationship with a physician and/or health care team. The American Academy of Pediatrics was the first major health care organization to promote the medical home for all children, including children with disabilities and long-term health care needs (Ad Hoc Task Force on Definition of the Medical Home, 1992). The medical home is in the family's community, is often a primary care pediatric practice, and is therefore accessible to families physically and culturally. The medical home brings together evidence-based or scientifically supported approaches with compassion and warmth. Though shared decision making is not highlighted in the descriptions of the medical home, it is implied on the basis of the close longitudinal relationship between the clinicians and the family. The medical home is able to coordinate and integrate all of the child's health care needs and becomes the central repository for all health care information.

Family medicine organizations (Martin et al., 2004) have joined the movement and have been supporting a patient-centered medical home concept. Similar to the pediatric counterpart, these medical homes are designed to ensure that all of the patients' health care needs are met in an integrated and coordinated fashion. Implicit again is the concept of shared decision making.

The medical home health care delivery model makes important contributions to reducing fragmentation and poor coordination in health care delivery. Encouraging continuous relationships between a health care team and person or family reduces alienation and increases discussion and negotiation. The current models, however, may not go far enough. First, shared decision making in the models is not actually explicit. As currently described, it would be possible for the medical home to retain a power differential between health care providers and consumers, patients, or families. The impetus for the model must be the empowerment of families and individuals, not simply increased coordination or cost savings. Placement of the medical home in the community-based pediatrics or family medicine practice may be suitable for many families and individuals but may be burdensome or ineffective for others. Support from all members of the interdisciplinary team is necessary to ensure that the medical home is a repository for all health care information, including the MAP discussed at length in Chapter 8.

It is also important to note that despite the advocacy of the American Academy of Pediatrics over decades, only approximately half of families surveyed reported a medical home that met minimal standards (Data Resource Center for Child & Adolescent Health, 2012). The proportion of families has not increased over time. Approximately one third of families report that they do not experience family-centered care from all of their health care providers (Data Resource Center for Child & Adolescent Health, 2012).

Personal Health Records

Within the U.S. health care system, the integrated care plans may need to be in the hands of families and individuals, taking family- and person-centered care to a new level and new domain. No other central repository for information currently exists. The medical home model will need to expand substantially and develop new mechanisms before information with hospitals and other providers can be exchanged in an efficient manner. Although a radical departure from our usual practices, placing health records in the possession of families or individuals would indicate that the individual (and in the case of a child, the family) owns their health information. It also acknowledges that no single entity in the U.S. health care system has all of the information required for an integrated plan.

The shift would require the development of individual web sites for health care records. These web sites would need to be very easy to understand and use. It would be ideal if they supported the families or individuals in organizing the information, uploading new data as they come in, and updating status. Members of the health care team would be given permissions from the family to access the information. The family might choose to give some members of the team only limited access to parts of the web site. For example, a child's teacher might not need information about the family history of mental health disorders. On the other hand, care coordinators, working with the family, may need access to all of the information in order to be most effective. Families and individuals would need to be trained to use the systems, which would be user-friendly, sensitive to literacy, and available in multiple formats that can be used by individuals with sensory or motor disabilities. All of this change may seem unlikely; however, as of this writing, projects are under way experimenting with the use of mobile telephones for health care reminders and information exchange. Putting the entire comprehensive, integrated plan in a simple accessible application for telephones may not be far away. Regardless of the specifics, consumer-owned records with structures for information exchange, integration, and accountabilities should be developed. In keeping with the principles of family- and person-centered care, the primary users, the families and the individuals with disabilities, should be active participants in a planning process.

SUMMARY

Family-centered care has become a cornerstone in the health care of children with disabilities because the families bear primary responsibility for the consequences of care. The concept was introduced in health care in 1987 and promoted by the AAP and has been gaining acceptance since then. The key elements are dignity and respect, information sharing, participation, and collaboration. Family-centered care dovetails with cultural competence, the knowledge and skills to understand family beliefs, values, and practices that are based on cultural identity. The data that currently exist demonstrate that family-centered care leads to positive outcomes for child health and family well-being.

Person-centered care acknowledges that individuals, including individuals with disabilities, assume responsibility for their own health care. The construct has multiple historical sources. A welcome development is that many organizations, including professional family medical societies and WHO, are now promoting person-centered care.

Delivering family- or person-centered care requires new clinical skills as well as shifts in attitudes and beliefs. Family- and person-centered care is making inroads at the organizational and policy levels. Although the developments thus far have been extremely encouraging, it is likely that additional changes to health care organization and leadership will be necessary to sustain the progress. The family- or patient-centered medical home is an effort to integrate this perspective into an organized health care delivery model. The medical home is a health delivery system that is highly compatible with family- and person-centered care. Implementation of the model has been slow, and only about half of families describe primary care practices that meet the medical home standards. Moving forward, families and individuals may need to assume an even more central role to ensure that the care they receive is comprehensive and integrated.

Exercises

1. Implementing family-centered care is extremely challenging. How would you handle the following difficult situations in accordance with family-centered care?
    a. You are working in the outpatient setting. Parents of a 2-year-old bring the child in for consultation because he is delayed in language development and throwing disruptive tantrums every day. Your careful assessment reveals that the child meets diagnostic criteria for autism. When you gently and supportively offer this diagnosis, the parents become enraged. They refuse to accept your diagnosis and treatment plans.
    b. Both parents come for the evaluation of their child and tell you in the course of the visit that they are now divorced. In obtaining the history of the condition, the parents offer different information and different interpretations. When you prescribe a course of action, they disagree with each other. One supports your ideas; the other rejects them.
    c. You are the therapist for a young child whose family comes from a culture you are not familiar with. You explain to the parents that you practice family-centered care and that you want them to learn the techniques so that they can implement them at home. At the next visit, eight family members, including a 10-year-old cousin, come to the therapy session. The parents tell you that they are all important caregivers for your patient. The parents add that they don't feel comfortable teaching all of these folks what you are showing them.
2. Imagine you are part of a research team evaluating a new medical treatment designed to improve the functional capacities of adults with Down syndrome. How can you use the principles of patient-centered care to recruit and enroll participants in this study?
3. In rare cases, families may choose courses of action that put their child at risk. What would you do in the following situations?
    a. Parents demand that the surgeon promise not to transfuse blood even if the child requires a transfusion during the operation.

b. The extended family refuses to give permission for antibiotics although their infant has a life-threatening infection.

c. The mother of an 8-year-old girl with severe learning disabilities decides to homeschool her daughter, though she has no teaching experience.

d. The family of a 3-year-old child with autism confides in you that they have visited a doctor who has recommended using hyperbaric oxygen therapy as treatment. The treatment entails 10 sessions and costs $2,000 per session.

4. How might you handle the situation of suspected child abuse or neglect while honoring the principles of family-centered care?

10

Care Coordination

with Alexis Hansen

Susan and Eric—Part I

Susan and her husband found out during pregnancy that their third child had spina bifida, a congenital disorder of the spinal cord that leads to varying degrees of lower limb paralysis, bowel and bladder control problems, and orthopedic abnormalities. Susan asked many questions and never felt satisfied with the answers. Years later, she realized that no one could have told her exactly the extent to which her child would be affected. But someone could have offered a guidebook, a flow sheet, or a helping hand to lead her through the complex process she and her family were about to embark on.

From the day he was born, Eric required extensive medical attention and procedures, including multiple surgeries to repair his spinal cord and later to correct deformations in his legs, hips, and feet. Susan met therapists, teachers, social workers, nurses, and physicians in the community, all of whom contributed in meaningful ways to Eric's rehabilitation and educational needs. On top of all of that, she met representatives of Medicaid, the Social Security Administration, and her own private health insurance company to arrange payment for most of his care. With each new player or organization came a new case worker or case manager to help manage Eric's care.

Alexis Hansen, M.D., coauthor of this chapter, was a medical student at the Stanford University School of Medicine at the time she co-authored this chapter. She is currently a family practice resident with a strong interest in the care of individuals with disabilities. As a medical student, she conducted research focused on evaluating a noninvasive manual therapy for children with cerebral palsy and served as teaching assistant in an undergraduate course on developmental disabilities. As a family physician, she plans to work to improve the experience of these populations in the health care system.

Susan was keenly aware of how poorly coordinated Eric's health care was. His primary care physician saw him rarely and was not knowledgeable about treatments for spina bifida. The orthopedist who operated on Eric did not consult the community-based physical therapists that were treating him, and the therapists got no written instructions about how to modify their treatments after the surgery. His teachers were never consulted about how the timing of surgery might impact his studies or about how long was required for rehabilitation. Susan tried to intervene in many of these situations. She found enormous variation in how the various team members responded when she relayed therapists' observations or translated the surgeon's recommendations. Meanwhile, bills accumulated at the family home while the insurance company and Medicaid debated their respective financial obligations.

Eric, like many of the other children in this book, saw a wide variety of different clinicians because of his spina bifida and many resulting health care needs. Visits with individual specialists typically occurred in isolation. The physicians focused on medical issues; the therapists and educators, working at different sites, addressed function. There was certainly no multiaxial assessment or plan from which all professionals worked. From his mother's perspective, each clinician made minimal effort to communicate with other providers or to integrate the planning for Eric's overall health care goals. His mother tried valiantly to ensure that his care remained coordinated, but she sometimes lacked information about the issues and frequently lacked access to the professionals. When she was able to make contact, she often found it difficult to get the professionals to pay attention to her impressions about Eric's status or to request her input regarding treatment outcomes. She did know how to get them to share their long-term care plans with her, let alone with each other.

Addressing the need to fix this fragmentation, the Institute of Medicine has created a definition of *care coordination* that has been used in several of its publications, as follows:

> To establish and support a continuous healing relationship, enabled by an integrated clinical environment and characterized by the proactive delivery of evidence-based care and follow-up. Clinical integration is further defined as the extent to which patient care services are coordinated across people, functions, activities, and sites over time so as to maximize the value of services delivered to patients. Coordination encompasses a set of practitioner behaviors and information systems intended to bring together health services, patient needs, and streams of information to facilitate the delivery of care. (Adams, Greiner, & Corrigan, 2004, p. 47)

The Institute of Medicine made care coordination one of the top 20 priority areas for national action in 2003 (Adams & Corrigan, 2003). Almost a decade later, we have come to realize that though care coordination is a priority in care provision, its implementation is complex and strains the capacity of the current health care system.

Care coordination facilitates communication among the health care clinicians and between the health care system and other community-based resources and services. Without care coordination, the lines of communication required for well-coordinated and well-planned complex care are numerous and easily become unmanageable (Figure 10.1). Families interact individually with each service and also need to serve as an information relay among services that do not reliably communicate with each other. They have varying levels of success in this role.

Care coordination provides a communication hub, a central point or person who maintains the big picture and who understands how each service relates to the other and to the treatment plan (Figure 10.2). The care coordinator simplifies lines of communication greatly. The child and family still interact with each service, perhaps with the exception of administrators and case managers. However, the care coordinator ideally ensures that all services are well aware of the participation. The elevated number of clinicians in cases like Eric's is a major factor in the increased complexity of care for these children and increases the potential for error dramatically if not properly managed. Care coordination is a strategy to reduce complexity by reducing the number of steps in communication.

Care coordination also serves as a source of information about services and support available to children with disabilities and their families. A multitude of services are available to children with disabilities and other long-term conditions through governmental policies, public institutions, and private organizations. However, finding the right set for a child and navigating to and through these services is extremely challenging, particularly for families of children who have just received a new medical diagnosis. A care coordinator assists as a knowledgeable and well-connected guide, helping to get families clear, accurate, unbiased information to improve their decision-making abilities. Care coordination also facilitates the transfer of medical

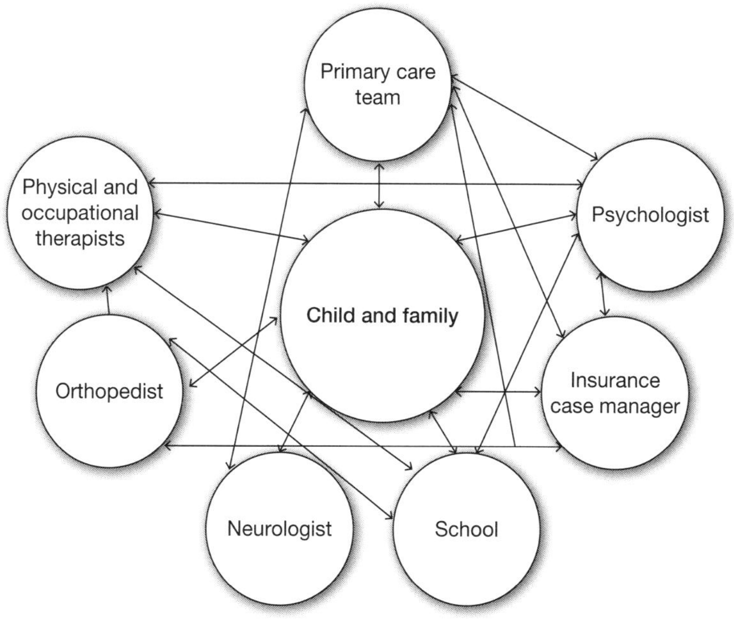

Figure 10.1. Schematic representation of lines of communication under current arrangements when they are working adequately. Note that the entire team communicates with the family. Although the physical and occupational therapists communicate with the orthopedist, the school, and the psychologist, they do not communicate with the neurologist. The neurologist communicates intermittently with the primary care team, but the neurologist does not communicate with the psychologist. The insurance case manager communicates with the family, some of the professionals, and with the primary care team.

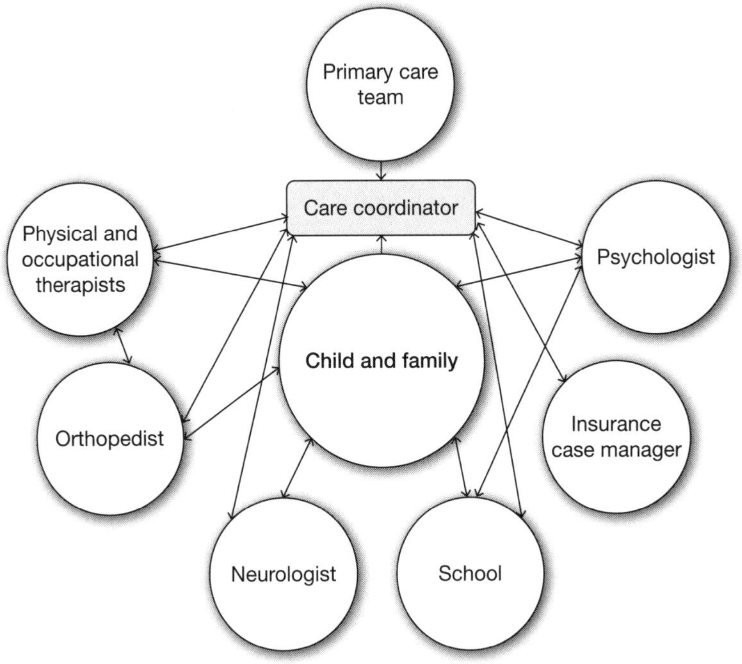

Figure 10.2. Schematic representation of the ideal lines of communication with care coordination. Note that the child and family continue to interact with all parties, except the insurance case manager, who now coordinates with the care coordinator only. Professionals communicate with all others either directly or through the care coordinator. The primary care team learns about all of the other parties through the care coordinator and the family. The number of lines of communication have been greatly reduced in this model.

information to and from these agencies to streamline the eligibility process, as well as to ensure that each clinician has sufficient information to take up his or her role effectively.

Within the health care system, a variety of new mechanisms are in development for coordinating the care of children when it becomes expensive, ineffective, and possibly dangerous. In this chapter, the current situation is reviewed, including calls to place the responsibility for care coordination within the primary care office. Although care coordination has not been fully implemented on a systems level, clinicians can begin to alter practices at the clinical level and evaluate proposals or plans at the policy level to address major inefficiencies of the current system.

THE CURRENT SITUATION

Since the 1990s, evolving U.S. policies have begun to include care coordination as an integral part of care for children with disabilities and other long-term conditions. A timeline of the developments is included in the commentary on the next page. The timeline demonstrates the increasing pace of development in line with the increasing sense of urgency in society and among families regarding this issue.

At the level of children and families, the results of the U.S. National Survey of Children with Special Health Care Needs in 2001 reinforced the need for a systematic approach. In that survey, only 40% of parents of children with special health

Commentary
Policy Developments in the Care Coordination Time Line

- *1935–Social Security Act Title V: States provide maternal and child health grants for federal and state partnerships to improve the care of women and children. At least 30% of funds must go to programs and care organizations supporting children with special health care needs.*
- *1989–Omnibus Budget Reconciliation Act (PL 101-239): Amended Title V of Social Security Act, extending its responsibility to cover children with special health care needs and facilitating the development of "community based systems and services" for these children and their families (Omnibus Budget Reconciliation Act of 1989).*
- *1992–The concept of a medical home is introduced and defined by the American Academy of Pediatrics (AAP).*
- *1992–Community Integrated Service Systems (CISS) grants are funded by the Maternal and Child Health Bureau. CISS projects seek to increase local service delivery capacity and foster comprehensive, integrated community service systems for mothers and children.*
- *1998–United States Maternal and Child Health Bureau defined children with special health care needs as "those who are at increased risk for a chronic physical, developmental, behavioral, or emotional condition and who also require health and related services of a type or amount beyond that required by children generally" (Mcpherson et al., 1998, p. 138).*
- *2002–AAP releases a policy statement on the medical home declaring that it should be a priority that every child have a designated medical home and for the medical home to serve as a care coordinator for children with disabilities and long-term health care needs.*
- *2009–Children's Health Insurance Program Reauthorization Act (PL 111-3): Contains provisions supporting state initiatives to strengthen medical homes for children with disabilities (e.g., Idaho and Utah receive quality demonstration grants supported by this act to implement electronic medical record systems and place medical home coordinators in both primary and subspecialty practices).*
- *2010–Patient Protection and Affordable Care Act (PL 111-148) section 2701 (Health Home for Enrollees with Chronic Conditions): Gives states a federal match for funding medical home services for children with disabilities.*
- *2011–Bundled Payments Initiative: Providers are invited to help test a new model of bundling payments that allows more flexibility for care coordination compensation.*
- *2012–Accountable care organizations (ACOs): Supported by the Affordable Care Act, providers organized as ACOs that voluntarily meet quality thresholds are able to share in the cost savings they achieve for the Medicare program, providing monetary incentive to provide better care coordination.*

care needs rated their care coordination as adequate, and 37% rated communication between doctors and other providers as very good to excellent. However, 32% reported that they received no help at all with care coordination (Strickland et al., 2004).

Important barriers to the implementation of care coordination are the lack of clear definitions and limited understanding of the possible ways it should work. Who should be the care coordinator for children with disabilities? What should their training consist of? Where should their offices be to be most helpful to children and their families? What modes of communication should be put in place? How should these positions be funded to minimize conflicts of interest? How many care plans can a competent care coordinator effectively coordinate? These fundamental questions have not yet been adequately answered.

Care Coordination in the Medical Home

The AAP has been promoting the concept that the primary care office is the most appropriate locus for care coordination. Care coordination was included as an essential component of the comprehensive medical home model of care, first introduced by the AAP in 1992 (Ad Hoc Task Force on Definition of the Medical Home, 1992). The AAP elevated the construct in 2002 by creating a policy statement promoting the medical home that was published in 2002 ("The Medical Home," 2002). The AAP defines a *medical home* as a provider, office, or organization offering medical care that is "accessible, family-centered, continuous, comprehensive, coordinated, compassionate, and culturally effective" (p. 185). Inclusion of the term *coordinated* in the list of characteristics signals the AAP's interest in placing care coordination in primary care. They note that coordination of care must operate both *vertically* (among medical services) and *horizontally* (among community services and agencies).

The argument for this model is that the primary care clinician is well known to the child and family and should already be managing essentially all aspects of pediatric medical care. The office is likely to have considerable pertinent information and would indeed be well positioned to coordinate care. The primary care office has the requisite medical knowledge and clinical skills to assist families in obtaining unbiased information about a child's condition and in evaluating recommendations for intervention, unlike consulting professionals, who may have an implicit conflict of interest when they recommend their services because they stand to benefit if the family agrees.

Though many primary care physicians report they are providing care coordination, one study showed that only 24% are always involved in the hospital discharge planning for their patients, and only 19% involve or inform schools when coordinating medical and educational needs of these children (Antonelli, Stille, & Antonelli, 2008). Primary care physicians describe the main barriers to care coordination as limited time, staff, and reimbursement. However, care coordination requires many skills, including familiarity with services and resources in the community, that are not routinely taught in medical school or residencies (Antonelli, Stille, & Antonelli, 2008).

Another major obstacle to setting care coordination in the primary care office is that many children with disabilities, like Eric, have more frequent contact with their subspecialists than they have with their primary care clinician. Visits to the primary care physician may be only for acute intermittent illnesses and immunizations, contact that is generally brief and problem focused, different from the extensive and open-ended dialogue required for identifying and evaluating treatment options or addressing the emotional context of the decisions.

If the primary care office wants to transform and incorporate care coordination, then several changes need to take place. First, health maintenance and counseling appointments for children with disabilities need to be longer than similar appointments for typically developing children are. This change would allow clinicians and families to establish rapport and trust as well as provide opportunity to discuss important issues. Second, other professionals such as mental health, social service, and rehabilitation specialists would be located within the practice to complement the medical orientation of primary care clinicians. This expansion of the model from strictly medical to rehabilitative and social would increase the therapeutic potential of the practice. Third, the practice would need to either hire knowledgeable care coordinators or designate and train others within the practice to assume the critical role.

Care Coordination in Community-Based Organizations

Some public agencies and private organizations that serve children with disabilities designate a case manager for children and families. For example, state organizations that serve individuals with intellectual disabilities assign a case manager to all who are eligible—adults and children. These case managers serve to assist in determining the needs of children and in accessing appropriate services within the system. Case managers vary widely in their degree of knowledge about disabilities, long-term health conditions, and the services available to children and families; they vary widely in the degree to which they assist children and families in accessing the services. They do not necessarily facilitate access to services beyond their own organization and often have large caseloads that make it impossible to complete even the paperwork for ensuring services and supports. Case managers rarely serve as a communication hub across systems. They are often ill prepared to provide families with comprehensive information about a child's conditions or about treatment possibilities, especially within the domain of health or medical care. For example, they could not offer a second opinion about the need for surgery or the advisability of a medication.

In many organizations, the principal role of the case manager is to minimize agency expenditures. As such, they ensure that participants do not receive redundant or cost-burdensome care; they direct children and families to low-cost resources and services. Although it is important to evaluate the effectiveness and cost-effectiveness of the care the patient is receiving to ensure that resources are used appropriately, there is little motivation for persons in the role of case manager with this type of job description to suggest additional care and services that could be beneficial. In fact, these case managers also have an implicit conflict of interest when they advise families because they have a role in protecting the financial health of their organization over the clinical health of their client. This problem becomes acute when children or their families need expensive interventions, such as applied behavioral analysis for the treatment of autism. The families often need to battle with the case manager and his supervisor in the agency, wasting time and money that could have been dedicated to the provision of care.

Parents and Caregivers as Care Coordinators

This situation leaves the family or other primary caregivers with the primary responsibility of coordinating care for their children with disabilities. In Eric's case, his mother eventually embraced the role of care coordinator, recognizing that she was in the best position to bridge the gaps among all the different organizations and health professionals who participated in her child's care. (See the commentary below.)

In many ways, it makes sense for the parent to take this active role. It instantiates family-centered care. The parents are likely the only people who have a complete picture of the care team, including the doctors, therapists, school programs and teachers, community services, and community-based informal supports such as coaches or religious leaders. Families cherish their children. They maintain complete records of information relevant to their child's care (including a record of services) that they make available to each provider. Given the difficulty in transferring personal health information under current U.S. confidentiality laws, the information parents provide can be extremely helpful to providers across different offices or systems. Through their caregiving experience, parents are typically experts regarding their child's unique health needs beyond the diagnoses; they are keenly aware when their child is happy or sad, comfortable or afraid, progressing or stagnating. They are often the first to recognize when the child's health status changes, and they often have cogent hypotheses about the change. Parents join parent-to-parent support networks and condition-specific organizations; they often receive information about treatment breakthroughs via these networks before the information is widely

Commentary
Susan and Eric—Part II

As Eric entered preschool, Susan suddenly recognized that she had become an expert in the care of her son. She also realized that the clinicians and caseworkers she had met were familiar with their own system; however, none of them knew all of the systems involved in Eric's life. No one had that broad view but Susan. It was then that she realized that she was an integral and important part of Eric's health care team, not only as his primary caregiver but also as his care coordinator. She officially designated herself as such. Once she had done so, she knew she had to become even more knowledgeable and assertive than she had been. She began to systematically research treatment options and community services that Eric needed. She introduced herself as care coordinator whenever she met with anyone involved in Eric's care. She improved the organization of her notebooks with Eric's medical records. The professionals responded well to her on the basis of her command of the information and her impressive advocacy skills.

Though Eric is now approaching adulthood, Susan continues to take her role seriously—sending information from the physicians to his teachers and therapists and from them back to the physicians. She researches all of the potential resources in the community that could help Eric, and she is planning for his transition to adulthood. She now needs to educate Eric about how to assume this role for himself when he is fully an adult and must consent to his own procedures.

available in the medical literature. Many parents recognize, implicitly or explicitly, that they are serving as their child's care coordinator.

Despite the advantages of parents as care coordinators, there are significant problems at several levels. It is really asking a lot of family members. Parents may not have full knowledge about their child's condition, skills to understand and evaluate medical information without support, or familiarity with community-based resources and services. Their strong emotional bonds to the child, limited energy and finances, and other demands may complicate their understanding and decision making. Parents and/or extended family may also disagree on what is needed. It may prove difficult to resolve those conflicts without a third party providing additional information, support, and mediation. Many families appreciate the opportunity to address their child's issues with an impartial participant with whom they can do a reality check. For many families, it is often overwhelming to bear responsibility for identifying all of the treatment options for their child, coordinating all of the care components, and dealing with the emotional consequences of any resulting difficulties.

At the systems level, parents are often not recognized as the care coordinator. Their advocacy efforts are sometimes not understood, not encouraged, or undermined—intentionally or unintentionally—by professionals. This situation proves to be highly frustrating to both the family and to the professionals and can damage the relationship. Those parents who take on this responsibility are not paid for their role, but the time and effort required may be enough to compromise their ability to work or at least require significant time off from work. Thus, although parents remain crucial partners and decision makers in their child's care, it is reasonable to expect that they should not be solely responsible for the effective coordination of their children's complex needs.

PARENT-SUPPORT ORGANIZATIONS

Community-based organizations that provide information and support to parents of children with disabilities offer elements of care coordination. They often take advantage of parent expertise and provide a forum for parents to support each other. Parent to Parent USA is one such organization that promotes connecting parents to parents to facilitate free "emotional and informational support for families of children who have special needs" (P2P USA: Parent to Parent USA, 2012). It promotes statewide organizations across the country that train support parents and match them to families seeking support in their day-to-day lives, as well as with recommendations for community resources and help navigating the health care system. Through peer support, the parent-to-parent model has proven effective in helping parents to make cognitive adaptations toward increasing acceptance, to cope more effectively with specific problems arising in their children's care, and to pursue the goals they have for their child (Singer et al., 1999).

Parent support groups can also be found through the child's hospital, school, or religious institution. These groups are an invaluable source of information about services, programs, and other resources. Parents benefit from emotional support from peers, sharing of experiences with specific providers and treatment protocols, and even equipment exchanges between families to facilitate access to needed devices. Often centers that facilitate these family groups also provide informational materials and training in advocacy and communication skills for parents.

A limitation of community-based organizations and parent-to-parent support groups is that they have no official standing within the health care system. They provide informal support that must be funneled to the health care team via the family. Members of the parent-to-parent network may have idiosyncratic ideas about the right approach to care for which the scientific evidence is limited. Pushing parents in the direction of scientifically unsupported approaches can put parents and other family members in an uncomfortable position when they interact with their health care team. Some organizations train parents for their roles as support agents in order to reduce any bias they may bring to the counseling role that they play. Nonetheless, because the parents do not receive the same degree of training, it may be challenging for them to abandon a favored position. Thus, although these connections are extremely important, they are not an adequate solution to the issue of care coordination.

Evaluation of the Current Situation

Placing care coordination within a medical home has advantages for integrating information about health with information about other community-based services. The medical home may have less bias and conflict of interest than the case managers in various agencies. However, the primary care physician is unprepared to serve all of the roles required of meaningful care coordination. One very realistic solution is to evolve primary care offices into interdisciplinary teams. Nurses, social workers, and/or parent advocates could become essential members of the medical home team. Working with physicians, these team members might be able to take up the responsibility of supporting families in home management of medical conditions and in identifying community resources and services. The records within the office become an integrated compendium of health and other information pertinent to the care of the children. Under the leadership of social workers or parents, the office can create a community map of relevant resources. Members of the community could write reviews about these services that are posted on a web site, much as we have come to expect when we browse for restaurants or services on the Internet. If the system moves in this direction, it is still important to recognize and address the challenges, as described in the next section.

ADDRESSING THE CHALLENGES

Many additional challenges have limited the development of care coordination systems. These barriers must be addressed in any emerging models of care coordination.

Ownership

At the center of the concept of care coordination is the idea that a single point of contact acts to keep track of the care that the child is and could be receiving. The care coordinator could be a clinician, family member, or family designee. It could also be a new specialized position, a prepared and activated care coordinator who assumes these responsibilities. However, because of limits in expertise, time constraints, and lack of financial support, most parties are reluctant to assume ownership of the role. The solution requires an explicit commitment to and financial support for assuming the role. It seems highly unlikely that any one profession or organization can serve this expansive role in isolation. Team approaches are necessary, as proposed for the medical home in Chapter 9. Financial models must support the team, as discussed in Chapter 13.

Time

Attending to the activities involved in care coordination takes time beyond traditional clinical visits. The more complex the patient, the more time required to fully attend to their complex needs. Primary care clinicians and subspecialists alike already have time pressures without the additional time and financial support required to coordinate care among the various agencies and organizations involved. Scheduling systems for patient visits are poorly designed to differentiate among visit types, such as brief visits for acute problems, longer visits for complex problems, and extended visits for counseling and care coordination. Adding to the issue is that time spent in care coordination and care for complex health care needs is inextricably tied to cost in the health care system. Regardless of who provides the services, the time required must be adequately reimbursed.

Cost

Within the current system, one of the biggest barriers to implementation of care coordination is inadequate reimbursement for care coordination activities. Although it is well understood that children with disabilities and long-term health care needs require more time for both care of complex health issues and care coordination, the fee-for-service model still dominant in the United States does not support care coordination activities. Where codes to bill for these services are available, insurance plans rarely reimburse them. Thus, clinicians who provide these services are at an economic disadvantage. Families requiring extra coordination, such as Eric's, seek out those practitioners who are known to provide coordination, further pulling these practitioners from activities for which they can bill insurance organizations. Therefore, caring clinicians can quickly be overwhelmed by unreimbursed costs. At the level of the clinical office, it is difficult to determine whether the addition of a care coordination team member is financially advantageous or not.

Further complicating the issue, the structure of insurance billing does not allow primary care clinicians to bill for certain aspects of treatment. Insurance "carve outs" often give responsibility of all treatment for a group of diseases to specialists. This decision forces the hand of each provider to care exclusively for one set of health issues. The result is that even given the time and flexibility within the practice to provide more comprehensive care, the primary care clinician must make referrals for care associated with specific conditions or face absorbing unreimbursed service costs. The issues of integrating information and coordination are thus made more difficult, and fragmentation of care becomes more likely.

Evidence suggests that care coordination leads to increased primary care and specialist utilization by children with disabilities and long-term conditions, at least within the very short term (Lawson, Bloom, Sadof, Stille, & Perrin, 2011). Increased utilization leads to increased spending. The increased costs are most likely the result of the child receiving necessary or desirable services for health needs that would otherwise be left unmet. Increased costs are associated with simultaneous improved health outcomes. However, it is not clear whether these costs are ultimately recovered in a favorable outcome, such as decreased hospitalizations or, importantly, increased functional capacity. Studies to evaluate these questions need to be long term, conducted over many years. The financial benefits of care coordination may not be realized in the health care system at all. However, if children and families who receive care coordination make more substantial contributions than do those who receive no care coordination, then the positive impact may be reduced spending for education and social service or increased income from employment and taxes.

Challenges to Entering the System

As it stands now, children enter the system in many ways. For example, one child with autism might initially present to an early intervention agency on the basis of a parental request for evaluation. That child may not receive a diagnosis of autism but rather a program designed to address her developmental needs. She would therefore not get a medical evaluation of autism or other health service that might prove beneficial. Another child might go directly to a medical subspecialist who makes the diagnosis of autism. If that child finds his way to a developmental-behavioral pediatrician, he is highly likely to get referred to community-based early intervention or special education. If he ends up in neurology or allergy-immunology clinics, he might not be referred for community services. Thus, depending on multiple factors, such as acute needs, family education, parent recommendations, and availability of informed and activated primary care practice teams, children enter through different routes. Exacerbated by the lack of communication among care organizations, agencies and clinicians are not necessarily aware of other services the child and family are using. Practice guidelines or protocols for comprehensive care and interagency communication are not available or, when they are, are not widely used. The result is that no one agency or organization is accountable for guiding the children and families through the system.

Training for Care Coordination

A challenge to putting care coordination in the primary care office as medical home is the lack of preparation of the physicians in those practices. Many pediatricians report having received no training in treating prevalent childhood disabilities. For example, 20% reported no training about treating physical disabilities (Sneed, May, & Stencel, 2000), including arranging for therapies and durable medical equipment. In fact, most thought that prescribing these elements of comprehensive care was beyond the scope of their practice (Sneed et al., 2000). Pediatricians also report inadequate preparation for treating many other prevalent conditions such as learning disorders and ADHD (Camp, Gitterman, Headley, & Ball, 1997). Though the AAP and pediatric residencies around the United States have tried to meet these needs, directors of continuing medical education programs report that topics in developmental–behavioral pediatrics are always at the top of the list for requested presentations. The first step to getting primary care practitioners to serve as care coordinators is to educate them about this large population of children with disabilities.

The next step, whether the care coordinator is a professional or paraprofessional, is to educate that person to meet the requirements of the role. The education should include strategies for assessing functions, mechanics for creating integrated care plans, knowledge about services and supports, and advocacy skills. There are certificate programs for paraprofessionals to become care coordinators, but the duration of training, prerequisites for enrollment, level of education, and scope of the training vary across programs. Standardization of such programs would allow families and team members alike to begin to depend on a skill set for the care coordinators. It would also be appropriate to create programs targeted to professionals, who would then serve either as the direct care coordinators or as supervisors for preprofessional care coordinators.

Facility Inaccessibility

Unfortunately, despite the American with Disabilities Act, many facilities remain inaccessible to persons with disabilities. Ramps and wide doorways, waiting room accommodations, clinic room accessibility, and staff training in accommodating people of all abilities are essential to facilitate regular office visits for children with disabilities and their families. People with disabilities may not get the medical care they need because offices and equipment are inaccessible. For example, individuals in wheelchairs may not be weighed if the office lacks an accessible scale. In addition to the obvious issues regarding physical disabilities, children and families with cognitive, sensory, or social–emotional disabilities may also require accommodations to receive care and to make health decisions. Financial, linguistic, and cultural barriers all add to the problem of accessibility for all patients.

A Canadian study documented that individuals with disabilities experience severe disadvantages in accessing health care (McColl et al., 2008). Physicians were aware of the barriers to basic primary care for persons with disabilities. They were often unable, untrained, or unwilling to provide the necessary assistance for a comprehensive evaluation (McColl et al., 2008).

MODEL ORGANIZATIONS

Fully addressing care coordination will require a major restructuring of the health care system, but acknowledgment of the need for improved coordination has led to the development of new model organizations that have care coordination at their center. Although there is clearly much work remaining, there are examples of organizations that are restructuring care to fit this need.

Primary Care Practice Medical Home Models

As discussed previously, the medical home model is an approach that places care coordination within the primary care physician office ("The Medical Home," 2002) and that many organizations are starting to follow. One example, the Pediatric Alliance for Coordinated Care, is a group of six pediatric practices that introduced interventions within their practice in an attempt to implement the medical home for children with disabilities and long-term health conditions. The implementation consisted of several key features: a designated nurse practitioner within each practice serving as case manager/care coordinator, a parent consultant, individualized health plan development for each patient, and continuing medical education for health care professionals within the practice. In a study evaluating the success of this model, the results showed improved health and decreased disease burden on parents, increased parent satisfaction, and decreased hospitalizations, all with a relatively small financial investment (Palfrey et al., 2004).

Hospital-Based Models

Several hospital-based comprehensive care programs were developed in the early 2000s, and their popularity is growing. These models have the benefit of offering provider expertise and organizational efficiencies of all services located at one center. A recent study conducted a systematic review of 33 care programs that were based at least partially in a hospital setting, including categorical (disease specific) and noncategorical (not disease specific) programs. Children were assigned a multidisciplinary team located at the hospital that included subspecialty physicians, therapists, and social workers; a pediatrician or nurse practitioner acted as the care coordinator. Most of the studies reported positive results in multiple areas including effectiveness, efficiency, and degree of family- or patient-centeredness (Cohen, Jovcevska, Kuo, & Mahant, 2011).

Home- or Community-Based Care Coordination Models

A third model of care coordination uses providers other than medical professionals to provide these services to families of children with disabilities and long-term conditions. In these structures, nurses or social service workers work with families through home visits, phone, e-mail, and attending medical appointments. In one such program, Oregon's CaCoon program, public health nurses are trained and positioned as CaCoon Care Coordinators in each of Oregon's 36 counties. Eligible families are served by the CaCoon Coordinator, who trains the families to make appointments, fill prescriptions, and arrange transportation to medical visits; they also provide support for coordination of care through follow-up phone calls (Lucile Packard Foundation for Children's Health, 2009). A second example is Illinois's Division of Specialized Care for Children. This program provides care coordination through regional offices, where two-person teams (such as a nurse and social worker) collaboratively provide care coordination services. Through collaborations with the family, physician specialists, and other clinicians, the staff assist in developing the most appropriate program of care for the child by helping to arrange, coordinate, and pay for the child's specialized medical treatment (Lucile Packard Foundation for Children's Health, 2009).

Care Coordination for Adults with Disabilities

In adult medicine, disability care coordination organizations (DCCOs) are setting an example for cost-efficient care. These organizations differ from other models in that they support the individual's functional capacity in his or her environment rather than focus strictly on medical needs (Palsbo, Mastal, & O'Donnell, 2006). The support extends to all settings and is designed to help the individual develop self-efficacy skills for participation and contribution. Two defining features of these organizations are 1) they are accessible to and educated about the specific needs of individuals with disabilities and 2) they use a nurse–social worker partnership for care coordination. The organizations promote equality across all professionals and paraprofessionals, resulting in mutual respect, essential to the care coordinating team. In a study of six different DCCOs across the United States (Palsbo et al., 2006), six core clinical activities were common among all the organizations: comprehensive assessments of new participants on enrollment; self-directed, individualized service plans; care coordinator support at clinical visits; centralized medical–social record; engagement with community resource providers; and constant, proactive communication with clients. Evaluation of these programs has been very positive: Clinical outcomes for participants have improved, emergency department utilization has declined, and self-reported quality of life has risen (Palsbo et al., 2006).

Ambulatory Intensive Care Unit

Another model that has come from the world of adult medicine is the ambulatory intensive care unit (ICU). This model is based on improving the quality of medical care while at the same time reducing per capita spending. It targets the adults who use the most health care services. One example is a pilot project Boeing Companies called the Intensive Outpatient Care Program (IOCP). Patients enrolled in this program were connected to a care team that included both a physician and a nurse care manager. On enrolling, the individuals received a comprehensive intake interview, physical exam, and diagnostic testing. A comprehensive care plan was developed with the input of the person. The plan was implemented using in-person, telephone, and e-mail contacts. The program placed emphasis on the nurse case manager providing patient education and proactive outreach. The patients also had access to care coordination by the team and specialist care in direct communication with the IOCP team. Twelve months after implementation of the IOCP program, multiple outcomes were improved compared with baseline: functional status scores, depression scores, patient experience of care scores, and employees' absenteeism scores. Interestingly, the unit price per capita spending also dropped by 20% when compared with controls (Milstein, Kothari, Fernandopulle, & Helle, 2009).

Other Countries

Internationally, care coordination remains a challenge in other countries with different health delivery and health care financing systems. Results from a survey of 11 countries found distinctive strengths and weaknesses in the models used by different countries. Patients in the United States and Canada were most likely to receive duplicate tests because centralized records and integrated care plans are not available. Patients in France and Germany were much more likely to report lack of communication between primary care clinicians and specialists. Patients in France and Norway experienced significant gaps in hospital discharge planning (Schoen et al., 2011). No country seems to have developed a sound system for coordinated care for children or adults with serious disabilities. (See the commentary on p. 174.)

THE EFFECTS OF CARE COORDINATION

In order to effect change on the scale necessary to implement care coordination as a health care priority in the United States, we need evidence that the change would result in positive outcomes for children, their families and communities, and the health care system. The evidence that coordinated care results in better health outcomes is accumulating. An Australian study demonstrated that emergency department presentations and hospital admissions decreased, and hospital stays were significantly shortened (Peter et al., 2011). Studies have also shown repeatedly that individual and family satisfaction are increased in settings where a care coordinator is involved (Farmer, Clark, Drewel, Swenson, & Ge, 2011).

Unfortunately, care coordination is expensive and not easily reimbursable in the current system in the United States. The broad view suggests that improved health outcomes, particularly in groups who use more health services than the general population, would more than pay for the increased cost of coordination of care. For example, hospital admissions and emergency room visits are the most expensive form of health care; if care coordination reduces hospitalizations, then it is likely to lead to net savings. Unfortunately, with the structure of the U.S. health care system, the benefits of reduced hospitalization go to insurance companies, whereas increased expenditures for care coordination are borne by health care providers or hospitals.

Few studies have evaluated the costs and cost savings of care coordination for children with disabilities. One study estimated the direct costs of providing care coordination within a general pediatrics practice at $22,000 to $33,000 per year of unreimbursed care for staff time spent in care coordination activities (Antonelli et al., 2008). Whether this cost is prohibitive is a function of how many children are served and resulting decreases in other components of pediatric practice, such as

Commentary
Strategies in Other Countries

- Australia: *In this fee-for-service structure, practitioners may bill for involvement in multidisciplinary care planning, mental health care, and the development of management plans for children with eligible disabilities (Department of Health and Ageing, Australian Government, 2011).*
- United Kingdom: *In this centralized system, Primary Care Trusts (PCTs) take responsibility for providing ambulatory care as well as paying for hospital care for their local populations. One way PCTs save money is by encouraging preventative care and coordination. A community matron who has clinical expertise and training in care coordination, patient communication support, and advocacy helps to build individual care plans. The matron is also the central contact point (Hofmarcher, Oxley, & Rusticelli, 2007).*
- Cuba: *In this single-payer system organized by geographical area, the neighborhood* consularios *are responsible for the health of every person in the neighborhood and are connected with a polyclinic, organized into internal medicine, gynecology, and pediatrics. Polyclinics house all clinical and laboratory services, psychology, physical therapy, speech therapy, social work, and other services such as gyms and massage. Subspecialists meet patients at the polyclinic, and often the primary physician is present. Care is coordinated because individuals receive all of their medical care within one centralized facility, at which the team follows the individual and all records are available (Fitz, 2011).*

unnecessary office visits. In a hospital-based model, cost of care to the system was evaluated independent of the cost of implementing care coordination. Although outpatient claims and prescriptions increased, inpatient care claims decreased, resulting in a net decrease in total Medicaid costs of $1,179 per patient per month (Casey et al., 2011). Cost savings for the care of children are consistent with the findings in adults (Milstein et al., 2009)

SUMMARY AND MOVING FORWARD

Care coordination is extremely important to the care of children with disabilities and their families. Many different approaches are currently available for providing care coordination. Many models are being tested at the systems level within the United States and internationally.

The most appropriate model for children with disabilities may vary by circumstance. In low-density geographical locations, hospital-based programs that are far from the families' homes are impractical. In cultures that display deference to health care providers, it may be untenable for families to assume the role of care coordinator and advocate. For children whose care relies heavily on medical subspecialties, the best option may be at the hospital rather than the primary care office.

It is important that while systems are investigating different models and their outcomes, individual professionals working with children with disabilities and their families begin to improve care coordination. The process begins by acknowledging that care coordination is an absolutely essential part of health care. Together, the health care team and family should decide on a plan. Some families who have the resources—financial, educational, and social–emotional—may choose to assume responsibilities for care coordination. These families may nonetheless need additional support or information. Other families may choose a community representative, a health care professional, or a health care team. That person or team must recognize that their responsibility goes beyond narrow professional role definitions to include learning about the child's general condition and the community resources that child may need. The use of integrated health plans (Chapter 8) can greatly assist with care coordination.

Care coordinators need and deserve education and training for the role. Parents who choose the role of care coordinator definitely deserve specific training. Many basic skills and responsibilities involved in care coordination can be taught without a large investment of time. Family members may be able to use parent-to-parent support networks and national organizations such as Family Voices to increase their knowledge, skills, and comfort with care coordination.

Regardless of particular organizational model, in order to have a positive effect on coordination of care, the designated care coordinator must also be recognized by the clinicians as an important partner in providing quality care. Care coordinators, be they parents, nurses, social workers, or other physicians, must have access to communication with the clinicians on the child's health care team. They must have the support of the entire team and have access to health care records. The care coordinator must be granted power to be a part of the care decision-making process for these children. Ongoing research will be necessary to compare results of different models and refine the processes.

Exercises

1. Interview the family of a child with multiple disabilities about care coordination. How do they manage to navigate the system? Who is their main source of information? Who is their main source of support? How do they decide who to call if a problem arises?
2. Interview another family of a child with multiple disabilities from a different social class about care coordination. Contrast the experiences of the two families. What are the likely explanations for any differences? How can other factors such as race, ethnicity, language, country of origin, or family composition affect care coordination?
3. Develop a handout designed for families of children with Down syndrome in your state or region that helps them to identify all of the potential services that their children may need for care. Use the Health Supervision Guidelines for Down Syndrome to prompt the kinds of medical, therapeutic, educational, and social services that are routine for these children and their families (Bull & the Committee on Genetics, 2011).
4. Consider how to design care coordination for a young adolescent with sickle cell anemia who suddenly developed stroke and expressive aphasia after many years with no medical complications. The child had been routinely followed by medical subspecialists at a tertiary hospital 45 miles from the family home on an annual basis and saw the family physician in his hometown primarily for acute and intermittent problems, such as ear infections and for health maintenance visits. The adolescent was in his last year of middle school and had been an average student, receiving no special help. Who would make a good care coordinator? Who should be on the team? How can the team communicate effectively?
5. How does the Affordable Care Act encourage care coordination? What pathways are available? How will these pathways and strategies be evaluated at a public health and public policy level?

IV

Implementing Change

11

Changing Professional Education

The University, Community, Leaders, and Individuals with Disabilities Center

In the beginning, we called the new program the University, Community, Leaders, and Individuals with Disabilities (UCLID) Center at the University of Pittsburgh. We intended to signal a strong commitment to collaboration and partnership. Our funding was a Leadership Education in Neurodevelopmental Disabilities (LEND) grant from the Maternal and Child Bureau of Health Resources and Services Administration, U.S. Department of Health and Human Services. As per grant requirements, the faculty represented many different disciplines: medicine, nursing, psychology, speech-language pathology, audiology, social work, occupational and physical therapy, dentistry, public health, and special education. Many of us met for the first time when we came together to prepare the grant, even though we had worked for years at the same institution. The faculty identified a group of community leaders, including several with disabilities, who joined the LEND program as community partners in education, research, and advocacy.

Once the grant was awarded, the faculty established a Friday seminar series to educate ourselves and the first interdisciplinary wave of professional and preprofessional trainees about this interdisciplinary team. We quickly learned that many of us did not even know the basics about the other disciplines represented on the faculty. How does medicine or pediatrics differ from nursing and from rehabilitation specialties—such as occupational, physical, and speech-language therapy—in terms of conceptual framework, professional roles, skill set, and approach to children with disabilities? What is the purpose of public health as distinct from clinical pediatrics? How are occupational and physical therapists different in their history, orientation, conceptual foundations, and clinical practices? What are the different career paths for students in a graduate program of social work? Our first seminar course gave representatives from each of the disciplines a 2-hour block to educate the rest of us about their respective fields. The course, so simple in its design, was a great success that led us to a new level of understanding and respect for the team. We went on to repeat it annually for new trainees and new faculty.

Children with disabilities and their families should be able to count on a health care system and on related services that support their inclusion, contribution, and health through integrated, coordinated family-centered, culturally competent interdisciplinary care. Sadly, as so many of the stories in this book illustrate, health care often does not rise to these standards. Of course, we can make excuses about the failings. After all, medicine and science have progressed so rapidly that health care systems have hardly had enough time to keep pace. Many more children with disabilities are surviving once-fatal conditions compared wth a generation or two ago, and their need for ongoing services is swamping the evolving systems. The team of professionals required for comprehensive care for this population is so diverse that it defies meaningful integration. Unfortunately, explanations and excuses are not comforting or helpful to children and families in need. Health care and health care systems must rapidly overcome these shortcomings to meet the needs of the population.

An essential ingredient for improving the health care system for children with disabilities is to educate a new generation of professionals who are prepared, skilled, and committed to delivering functionally focused, coordinated, family-centered health care. Fortunately, educational programs that can deliver this type of education are in place in many settings. As the vignette above demonstrates, LEND programs and the closely allied University Centers of Excellence in Developmental Disabilities (UCEDDS) deserve particular mention. They are both federally funded programs that have been on the cutting edge of interdisciplinary education for more than 40 years. The LEND programs emphasize leadership and clinical training to prepare trainees to articulate the mission, vision, and values of interdisciplinary practice; set the directions for programs or policies that meet the needs of the constituency; respond efficiently to changing situations that affect the children or the systems that serve them; and rally others to work together toward the same vision. The UCEDDS coordinate creative community-based programs for children and adults with disabilities that serve as models for students and for the community.

Professional education and training are often directed to a single discipline, and programs vary in the degree to which they expose students to the interdisciplinary team and to the principles of function-focused, coordinated family-centered care. Continuing education programs for practicing professionals are also frequently geared toward a single discipline and tend to emphasize providing new knowledge and sometimes improving practitioner skills. They often do not encourage mature practitioners to reevaluate their beliefs and attitudes, to develop skills in working across disciplines, and to modernize their approach to practice.

This chapter offers recommendations on the preservice education of professionals preparing to serve children with disabilities and their families as well as suggestions for continuing education programs. It includes several model programs and concludes with recommendations for professional organizations on requirements for and maintenance of certification that emphasizes function-focused, integrated, interdisciplinary family-centered care.

PRESERVICE EDUCATION

Regardless of a student's discipline or course of study, professional education should be based on an adult-education model. Malcolm Knowles articulated the principles of adult education, sometimes called *andragogy*, beginning in the 1950s (Clardy, 2006). Adult education begins with the premise that the students want to learn. It acknowledges that learners have relevant prior experiences that they bring to the learning situation and recognizes that education must be relevant to the learner's goals and objectives. Therefore, rather than a rigid standardized program, adult education favors a flexible curriculum, individualized to the learners through a collaborative planning process between teachers and learners. The process may initiate with an assessment of the learner's interests, experiences, and accomplishments, on the one hand, and needs on the other hand. On the basis of this assessment, customized learning objectives are developed to complement the general learning objectives for the entire student class. The set of courses and/or activities within the program may need to be modified so that the learners can achieve their specific objectives. At each step in the educational process, the learner reevaluates his or her own learning objectives while also evaluating the quality of learning experiences. A flexible, iterative process allows for modification of the plans to accommodate the learner's development.

The adult learning model is particularly well suited to professional preparation for clinicians who plan to care for children with disabilities and their families because it mirrors the desired outcomes of that education. First, adult learning incorporates a respectful, collaborative, flexible process, customized to the needs and strengths of adult learners; this process is very similar to the process of family-centered, culturally competent clinical care. Second, the relationships that develop in adult learning are nonhierarchical. A learner, experienced in a particular area or skill, may become the teacher for a mentor whose expertise lies in different areas. This feature, too, is reminiscent of the nonhierarchical approach of family-centered care; families are experts about their child, whereas professionals are experts about specific conditions or treatments. Third, within the adult-learning model, even in formal courses, the teacher functions more as a guide than an expert; the teacher leads students to their own conclusions and models skills that the students acquire. This humility is an outstanding preparation for teaching, collaborating, and supporting families as opposed to directing care. (See the commentary on p. 182.)

The Curriculum

The curriculum for the preparation of professionals for the interdisciplinary team that serves children with disabilities must address explicitly all of the areas that are required for that professional role. The curriculum should cover family-centered care and cultural competence in addition to scientific knowledge and technical skills. The educational program cannot assume that learners will intuit the principles of family-centered care because they grew up in families, any more than education assumes that learners will understand cardiology because they grew up with a beating heart.

During training, students must apply the knowledge they acquire in the classroom. Lectures and readings alone do not assure that students can use that knowledge in real-life situations. The most effective learning takes place when the learning experiences are as close as possible to the ultimate real-life application of the skills. Ideally, clinical skills, such as family-centered communication and shared decision making (Chapter 8), should be addressed simultaneously with technical skills, such as casting or modeling, so that the two naturally flow together in practice.

To adhere to the principles of adult education in acquiring clinical and technical skills, learners should complete assessments of their level of competence and their needs early in the program. From the results of these assessments, they and their mentors can formulate their individualized learning objectives and the courses and activities needed to achieve them. Students who have had introductions to particular topics or skills can begin their education at advanced rather than basic levels. Evaluations, also ideally a collaborative process, serve to indicate the learner's

Commentary
Richie Sapp, Stanford Undergraduate

Richie first requested a meeting with me during his freshman year. He was one of approximately 20 students in a student-initiated, one-credit course about developmental disabilities. This evening course attracts freshman and sophomore students who are interested in volunteering for a service group called Kids with Dreams, an organization that supports children with disabilities in the community. I presented a seminar for one of their sessions. Richie was so engaged and curious during my presentation that I was not surprised when he asked to meet with me individually. Since then, I have served as an informal mentor for this talented and passionate student.

I learned that Richie's twin brother has disabilities and that Richie had made an unwavering personal commitment to serve children, adolescents, or adults with disabilities as his life's work. He had begun this path before I met him. While in high school, he and a few buddies organized a summer camp for high school students with disabilities, including his brother. The counselors took the campers throughout the community, from public swimming pools to fast-food restaurants, providing for them a fun-filled summer while helping them to refine the social skills required for community life.

Richie has a deep, personal understanding of the issues of living with a family member with a disability. I have a serious scholarly approach to the issues of disability and a long track record of teaching. We have developed a meaningful and bidirectional relationship. For example, when he became a junior, he stepped up to organize the same course in which I had originally met him, the introduction for volunteers for Kids with Dreams. He had ideas about what he wanted his students to get from the course. I helped him formulate those ideas into learning objectives and a curriculum that would blend professional presentations with personal stories from individuals with disabilities and their families. When I again gave my lecture in this course, I could sense the excitement that the course had engendered in another group of highly motivated undergraduates. One of the students in that group approached me after class to declare that after my presentation, she knew that what she wanted to do was become a developmental-behavioral pediatrician.

progress toward objectives and determine whether and what additional learning experiences are required.

Topics for the Curriculum

Continuous Long-Term Relationships To be prepared to deliver longitudinal care to children with disabilities, students must develop continuous long-term relationships with children and their families during their training. Professional training programs tend to offer students relatively short rotations in a variety of different settings. Students spend only days or weeks to months on various services and teams, allowing exposure to the breadth of their field. However, this schedule limits the ability of the student to observe the twists and turns that children with disabilities and their families experience as conditions change, children develop, circumstances evolve, or service systems change. It is difficult for students to develop long-term relationships with children and families when they are constantly on the move.

Voluntary programs in several professional training programs address this shortcoming by providing the students with longitudinal experiences during training. One approach is to pair students with children or adults with particular conditions, who then serve as patient or client mentors for the students over time. At the University of Pittsburgh, a group of faculty and medical students developed an elective Area of Concentration entitled *Disabilities Medicine* for medical students, recognized by the school's curriculum committee as a certificate program. Students who volunteered for the program participated in a series of academic and experiential learning opportunities throughout their 4-year education to probe the issues of disabilities in health care. The program included lunchtime seminars and early evening workshops. In addition, the program connected each participating student to an individual with disabilities. Students were expected to meet with the individual at least three or four times each year in more than one setting—home, work, school, or community—as well as in hospitals and clinics. Evaluations by the

Commentary
Lauren Weintraub, University of Pittsburgh Medical Student

During her medical school education at the University of Pittsburgh, Dr. Lauren Weintraub participated in the Disabilities Medicine Area of Concentration. As part of this program, she was assigned to a community mentor, a school-age child with fragile X syndrome and autism. She made a strong connection with him and his family; she observed him at school and attended clinic visits with him. In all of these settings, she saw his substantial challenges with social communication. At one point, his family invited her to a seder, a structured ceremonial family meal with many specific rituals and prayers that is part of the observation of the Jewish holiday Passover. At the family's home, Lauren saw her community mentor in a new light. He was flawless in reciting the prayers and blessings. Even though his spontaneous communication was limited and stilted, learning the prayers played to his strengths in memorization and repetition. In this setting, he was the expert at the table.

students regarding this component of the comprehensive program was that the community mentor was extremely valuable to their education because they got to know an individual rather than a clinical condition; they got to appreciate that individual's strengths as well as their needs. (See the commentary on p. 183.)

Another example of assigning a patient mentor to students is pairing medical students with pregnant women who they follow through pregnancy, labor, delivery, and the early stages of raising a child. The students learn how a pregnancy may evolve for the woman both physically and emotionally. They get to witness the birth and the family's transition to care for the child. They also get to witness health care from the patient perspective, increasing their appreciation of the critical benefits of patient- and family-centered care. (See the commentary below.)

Although programs such as these are outstanding strategies to provide professional students with longitudinal experiences during their education, they have limited impact because they are elective courses. Moving forward, continuity experience should be required of all students who want to serve children with disabilities and their families. Details of the program can be developed on the basis of the

Commentary
Women and Children Special Interest Group at Stanford University School of Medicine

At Stanford, the "Mommies and Babies" course is a student-initiated program that pairs first- and second-year medical students with pregnant women. The students join the women for obstetrical checkups, remain available to them for questions by phone or e-mail, attend the delivery if at all possible, and then visit the mother and baby at home. During this course, they also meet weekly with professors who provide information about women's health and child development. I agreed to provide one of the lectures on child development.

Before the start of my lecture, as per protocol, each of the students updated the group on the status of her patient–mentor. One of the students reported on a woman who was hospitalized in late pregnancy for the development of very high blood pressure and other clinical signs of potential problems for mother and infant. This student learned about the profound emotional impact of an unexpected and adverse turn of events in such an important life process. Another student observed a physician–patient interaction in which the doctor wanted the woman to have an additional diagnostic procedure midway through the pregnancy. The woman, who was predominantly Spanish speaking, did not understand the brief and technical explanation that the doctor offered. She received no handouts or pamphlets to explain the procedure and, importantly from her perspective, got no information about what she could do to improve her situation while waiting for the procedure. The student assigned to this woman spent hours in the aftermath of the visit trying to make up for the shortfalls in the clinical process. She searched the Internet for information in Spanish and consulted doctors and nurse midwives about health promotion for this woman.

We went through these situations in depth. It seemed to me that the students' abilities to process the complexities of clinical care were far more important than my planned presentation about child development. I wonder whether the insights that develop from these relationships reverberate in the students' careers as professionals.

profession, school, and learners' backgrounds, as well as respect for local conditions and constraints. The requirement could be satisfied with a weekly clinical experience, a home visitation program, or the development of an informal relationship within and outside of the health care system. The essential feature is that the student follows the child and family over time. In this way, students can observe the natural history of the condition, witness changing needs, evaluate the responses to treatment, and appreciate the role of health care professionals in the life of the individual. It may be ideal to encourage the student to make contacts in many ways, including face-to-face encounters in health care settings and in the community, and via telephone calls or social networking. Evidence that the student has absorbed the unique features of the child and family and the evolution of the individual over time could come from diaries and journaling. Patients and their families should contribute to the evaluation of the student's skills in family-centered care and cultural competence via explicit written evaluations.

An important warning for teachers and administrators is that these programs take considerable time and resources to administer. First, patients or patient mentors must be identified and prepared for their roles. During the program, students need supervision and mentoring to help them make sense of their experiences and to ensure that they develop the target skills. Senior members of the profession are best able to provide this supervision because they have accumulated a vast repertoire of experiences. Family members who are trained for the role may also be able to provide supervision. If these family members are part of the teaching staff, then they should be reimbursed for their efforts. Evaluations based on reflections and diaries take more time to complete than do multiple-choice questions, for both the student and the faculty member. Program evaluation and improvement must also occur on a regular basis. Thus, the educational program and professional school must commit the necessary resources to create a high-quality, meaningful educational experience.

Experiencing the Value of Inclusion and Productivity It is important that the professionals who work with children with disabilities and their families embrace inclusion as a fundamental goal of health care. Regardless of discipline, they must ensure that these children receive all of the rights, privileges, and protections of the society at large. Professionals must acknowledge their important role in supporting children with disabilities so that the children experience a life of human dignity and meaning, enjoy equality of opportunity, and make meaningful contributions to society (Chapter 4).

As our society continues to evolve toward greater inclusion and contributions from individuals with disabilities, chances are that in everyday life, students will have many experiences with individuals with disabilities in a wide range of roles and community settings. However, many students may not have had such exposures. In their training, students often meet the children when they are ill, highly dependent, or unhappy about yet another clinic or therapy visit. They may mistakenly believe that children with disabilities are always in a negative or "sick" state, even when they are in a very healthy state at home with their families, at school with their friends, and going about their daily lives in the community. They run the risk of seeing the child as a patient or diagnosis first and, as a result, may not appreciate the possibilities of inclusion, contribution, and full personhood. Thus, another critical experience in preservice education is getting trainees to see children with disabilities in inclusive, everyday settings with other children, such as in their neighborhoods, in clubs, and participating in activities. (See the commentary below.)

I strongly recommend getting students to visit inclusive classrooms or recreational activities to evaluate inclusion in action. Observing, or better yet, participating in actual experiences breaks down preconceptions and prejudices that may have developed from social indoctrination and limited exposure. In my experience, opportunities to visit inclusive schools remind students of the basic humanity of the children. Diagnoses fade in importance while personalities and abilities rise in importance. It becomes clear that children with disabilities may participate in academic and social settings differently from the way typically developing students participate. Yet everyone—with and without disabilities—has opportunities to share and enjoy. Students see firsthand how accommodations and supports increase opportunities for interaction and satisfaction.

Family-Centered Care and Cultural Competence Previous chapters emphasized the importance of family-centered care and cultural competence in health care for children with disabilities (Chapter 9). Skills and characteristics of high-quality integrated care for children with disabilities, family-centered care, and cultural competence should be part of training, along with other technical and interpersonal skills required for integrated care of children with disabilities.

Commentary
Observations at Abilities United

As part of the undergraduate course I teach called Developmental Disabilities: From Biology to Policy, I assign students to visit Abilities United, a community-based organization that supports inclusion and community participation for children and adults with disabilities, and prepare a reflection about their visit. Here are quotes from two student reflections from 2012:

- *Jill (student): This morning I visited Abilities United to observe the [inclusive] preschool class.... I have no knowledge of the nature or extent of the students' disabilities, nor even do I really know how many of the students present today had disabilities, but I could tell that each child's needs and preferences were well understood, and that each child was receiving both personalized yet also standardized care and instruction.*
- *Elise (student): My visit to the Milestones Preschool at Abilities United was really wonderful.... I was extremely impressed by the patience and poise of the four teachers of a class of eight children.... [One] boy...did not make eye contact...and needed prompting...to form even simple word answers.... His difficulty sitting still did not seem to interrupt the focus of the other children at his table...what struck me as the biggest difference [between this school and another campus nursery I visited] was the warm hands-on approach of these teachers. One teacher in particular was extremely interactive with the children, seeking out two children when they were wandering around the play space alone. She used smiles, touch, and speech to connect with them.*

This training begins with an honest self-assessment. The goal is for the students to identify strengths and weaknesses in their own personal communication or treatment styles to inform the learning objectives, specific strategies, and activities for improving skills. Family Voices has published a set of assessment tools, including the Self-Assessment Provider Tool (Family Voices, 2008), that can be used in this way for individuals or teams. The Institute for Patient- and Family-Centered Care makes available several toolkits, though several are geared for the institution rather than individual clinicians (Institute for Patient- and Family-Centered Care, 2012). The National Center for Cultural Competence includes on its Web site the rationale for self-assessment and a variety of tools for use by professional and other organizations (National Center for Cultural Competence, n.d.).

One strategy for teaching family-centered care is the use of simulations. Simulations have become central to educating students about cardiopulmonary resuscitation or challenging procedures because they allow the student to learn without risk to actual children or families. In the realm of family-centered care, simulations allow students to try out various clinical approaches and styles, without fear of upsetting or insulting a child or family. The student not only gains experience but can also obtain feedback on the impact of his or her choices.

In one variation of simulation, trained actors play the role of patient or family member, and students play the role of professionals. Actors are particularly well suited to simulations because they can realistically portray the details of another's life. They are also trained to pay close attention to their own reactions to people and situations when they are in a scene and are highly skilled at tracking and remembering their emotional reactions throughout the simulation. They can provide detailed feedback to the students about how they felt when the student said or did something during the interaction. Using actors for simulations, however, also requires financial resources. (See the commentary below.)

Commentary
Reflections on Actors as Simulators

At Children's Hospital of Pittsburgh, we hired actors to teach pediatric residents the fundamentals of family-centered communication. I remember one extremely moving session in which a senior clinician on the faculty served as the student while other faculty and residents observed him interview a mother and her teenage daughter. The case was riveting; the mother and daughter had grown apart, held secrets from each other, and were locked in a complicated and unproductive cycle of recrimination. All of us, both the experienced and the novice clinicians, learned a lot in the session.

At the conclusion of the exercise, I found myself in the elevator with the actors. The young one, the teenager, complimented the older one, the mother, on her acting, recalling a few of the subtleties the mother had used to reflect her continued affection for the daughter. Although I knew throughout the simulation that the two were actors, it was only in the elevator that I realized that they were not really mother and daughter. They had played their roles so successfully that I had just assumed that they were actually related.

Other inexpensive models for simulation are possible. For example, students or faculty may assume patient and family roles in the simulations. However, classmates may have a more difficult time staying in character for the exercise when it is a friend or teacher in the role of child or parent. Parent volunteers can also be used. However, if their participation becomes routine and expected, then they may need training to be able to vary their roles in different scenarios, to give feedback to students, and to maximize student learning. In addition, reimbursement for their contribution should be considered.

Another way to teach family-centered care is through modeling and direct observation. Students can sit with experienced clinicians to observe their skills with children and families. After the visit, the student and teacher can compare notes about what skills and strategies the experienced clinician used and their impact in that particular case. As students acquire knowledge and skill, they can gradually assume greater responsibility for the conduct of the visit. The process of feedback and evaluation engages the student in self-reflection and the teacher in observation.

Shared Decision Making For many health professionals, it is a major challenge to allow children and families to exercise control over health care decisions to the degree that they choose. Health care professionals have allowed patients and/or families to make the final decision in a few areas of medicine, for example, through informed consent for surgery or participation in research studies. However, shared decision making stretches the traditional medical model far beyond the standard of informed consent (Center for Mental Health Services, 2010). Informed consent ensures only that the consumer understands the treatment, including potential adverse effects. Shared decision making ensures that the consumer has a role in developing and deciding on the treatment plan. Professionals need to be highly flexible in the roles they play, recognizing that some families need direction and teaching and others need support for independent decision making.

Modeling, supervision, and feedback are all strategies for training students in shared decision making. Training for shared decision making is slow and time consuming because it challenges the students' very notion of what it means to be a professional in their discipline. The principle that helps students to relinquish a paternalistic approach is that the final decision maker should be the individual or group that bears primary responsibility for the outcome of the decision. When the issue is health care, families and children bear the responsibility for the long-term outcomes. So when families choose to make decisions, the professional role is to ensure that they are aware of benefits, risks, costs, and implications of their various options, and to provide this information in a balanced and unbiased manner, free from manipulation. Unless the family's decision may cause harm, it trumps professional advice. It is also wise for students to learn how to leave the door open for the family to change their minds, particularly when they do not achieve desired results. The key to learning how to practice shared decision making is to practice in both the educational and clinical settings. As students become more comfortable with decision making in their own education, informed by self-assessment, individualized learning plans, and continuous process improvement within their educational programs, their ability to generalize this approach to the clinical setting increases. (See the commentary on p. 189.)

Commentary
Jared

Jared was a 7-year-old second-grade student I evaluated who met criteria for attention-deficit hyperactivity disorder. His symptoms were very severe, but his parents refused to consider medication as part of the management plan. I counseled them about behavior management techniques and referred them to several highly respected community-based psychologists for ongoing behavior management therapy. They followed this recommendation and added dietary changes and herbal remedies to the treatment plan.

I received an urgent telephone call from Jared's parents when he was 8 years old and had just entered the third grade. His teachers were recommending an evaluation for special education on the basis of a severe emotional disturbance. Although Jared's improvements over the last year were noticeable, he was having persistent problems with inattention, hyperactivity, and increasing oppositional behavior. His parents agreed to a trial of medication, which reduced symptom severity enough that Jared was not placed in a different classroom, although he did receive enhanced behavior management at school. I was gratified that they knew that they could return to see me and change their minds without fear of judgment. I was also gratified that we could keep Jared in an unrestricted school environment.

Interdisciplinary Teaming Health care for children with disabilities requires the smooth functioning of an interdisciplinary team. The definition of *team* for these purposes is two or more professionals who have specific roles and perform interdependent tasks or work toward shared goals for the assessment or treatment of children with disabilities and their families. Teams may form to treat specific conditions, such as cerebral palsy; may coalesce around a delivery setting, such as early intervention; or may focus on specific functions, such as feeding programs. Families should be conceptualized as the central members of these teams.

Preservice education must prepare students to participate in effective interdisciplinary teams. Within such teams, the expertise of each team member is valued and leadership is shared. Decisions result from consensus, derived from effective communication, negotiation, and conflict resolution. The team functions optimally when its members share the overarching goals of intervention; those goals are improving the child's function and supporting her ability to participate and contribute to her family and social world. Making these goals explicit allows all members of the team to stand on common ground.

In aviation, military action, police work, and firefighting, teamwork reduces risks. Teamwork has comparable benefits in health care (Lerner, Magrane, & Friedman, 2009). The absence of effective team work may have disastrous consequences, as discussed at length in an influential report by the Institute of Medicine entitled *To Err is Human: Building a Safer Health System* (Lerner et al., 2009).

A term that has emerged to highlight the need to educate the next generation for collaboration and integration is *interprofessional* education. The concept is that interprofessional education produces a workforce schooled in collaborative practice and naturally leads to strengthened health systems and improved health outcomes (Health Professions Networks, Nursing & Midwifery, Human Resources for Health,

2010). Interprofessional education occurs simply when students or practitioners from two or more professionals learn about, from, and with each other (Health Professions Networks, Nursing & Midwifery, & Health, 2010). Interprofessional education is an essential strategy for delivering collaborative professionals to health care settings, reducing the fragmentation of health care, and ultimately improving the health status of individuals and communities.

In interprofessional education and training, students work together with other professionals in order to learn how to function effectively on an interdisciplinary team. The education begins with an assessment of the learner's knowledge of the role and practices of various team members and their experiences on interdisciplinary teams. On the basis of these assessment results, students can be assigned to interdisciplinary courses and to participation on teams that meet their educational objectives. If our early experiences in the UCLID Center are any basis, team members may initially have very limited understanding about the roles of their teammates.

The Maternal Child Health Training Grantee Network has enumerated knowledge and skills involved in interdisciplinary team building (MCH Training Grantee Network, 2011). Knowledge required includes stages of team development, practices

Commentary
Barbara Bentley, Psy.D.: In Her Own Words

I became a LEND trainee during my psychology internship. When I enrolled, I had intended on doing grief work and psychotherapy. I had not even decided that I would focus on children. My experience in the LEND program opened my eyes to an entirely different scope of practice. Our training included team discussions and case conferences with an interdisciplinary team. My mentors for policy projects and clinical research were from neuroscience and nutrition. The policy project was a review of the adequacy of primary and preventative care for children with developmental disabilities in the Lanterman Regional Center catchment area. I was the psychologist on the interdisciplinary team that evaluated 100 children over the course of a year. We were all shocked to learn that very few children had a true medical home; access to health care was inconsistent, and most of the families did not have support for their behavioral concerns related to the child's special needs. We also learned that educational services were often generic, not individualized; that dental care was significantly lacking; and that feeding problems were pervasive.

I became committed to addressing at least some of these important issues. So I requested to train with the feeding team and learn to provide interdisciplinary feeding evaluations and treatment services. Our team designed many new treatment options for families, including a formal g-tube transition program; this day-rehabilitation program supported the transition to oral feeding in a naturalistic way to avoid hospitalization. We also developed group treatments and parent training materials, and provided telemedicine through a grant to the California Regional Centers to provide technical assistance and support about feeding to rural Regional Centers.

My interests settled on children. I did a fellowship that focused on young children, especially those who are medically fragile. I expanded my work to include other specialty clinics in the hospital (such as gastroenterology, endocrinology, and hematology–oncology) and started working with the Neonatal Intensive Care Unit.

for teamwork, and managing team dynamics. Various approaches from multi- to inter- and transdisciplinary practice are reviewed. Team members need to understand the roles, competencies, language, and culture of their teammates. Basic team skills include assembling a team for a specific task, such as conducting clinical care or building a program; developing a shared vision; and fostering collaboration and cooperation in making decisions. (See the commentary on p. 190.)

Challenges to interprofessional education have increased as clinical practices have deemphasized interdisciplinary team evaluations of children with disabilities. At present, the interdisciplinary team for a child is customized, composed of the particular set of professionals who are needed to meet the child and family's needs. The team does not necessarily meet concurrently or even colocate in the same building. As the size of the team shrinks, team members may need to stretch beyond narrow disciplinary boundaries as they function adaptively and creatively to meet the child and family needs. Community-based professionals may serve as ad hoc members of the team if they have involvement with the child or family. The time allotted to face-to-face meetings has shrunken because of the high expense. Often the standing team meeting has been abandoned.

Given these challenges, preprofessional training must ultimately prepare the members of the interdisciplinary team to communicate and cooperate across time and place. I think that training programs should continue to use a concurrent interdisciplinary team to ensure that preservice students are competent in interdisciplinary teamwork before they find themselves in complicated dispersed teams. The problem arises when clinical revenues are the only source of support for team functioning. Current revenues are insufficient to cover the time for team preparation and team meetings. Clinical revenues also do not cover interprofessional education. Additional funding from grants and contracts, such as the LEND and UCEDD programs for interprofessional education, alleviate the pressure in many institutions. However, the institutions themselves, if they studied the situation, might find that supporting the team process saves time and money in other ways.

Single-discipline preservice education programs must find opportunities for their students to participate in interprofessional education. One simple and inexpensive strategy is to invite other disciplines to teach in their courses. For example, one course in the Special Education curriculum at the University of Pittsburgh introduced the students to all of the members of the interdisciplinary team that evaluates and treats children with disabilities in the health care system. However, the more important strategy is to assign students to work as active members of interdisciplinary teams, such as the feeding team or cerebral palsy team. It is difficult for students to learn team skills from coursework and reading alone. Participation on the interdisciplinary team is of mutual benefit, because the student contributes and learns from the other members of the team. The challenge is designing the supervision, performance support, and meaningful evaluation and feedback for the students in this form of training and service. In certification processes, professional organizations may need to allow supervision by other disciplines on interdisciplinary teams, particularly regarding the student's communication and team skills, in order to ensure that the students receive this essential experience.

Students should be evaluated for their performance in interdisciplinary team function. Such evaluations should sample specific knowledge, skills, and attitudes that enable individual team members to coordinate (Baker, Salas, King, Battles, &

Barach, 2005). A student's willingness to cooperate for a shared goal can be defined by behavioral indicators and evaluated. Specific measurable and scalable team competencies can be used to assess performance in health care at different levels from novice to experienced practitioner (Baker et al., 2005). The Accreditation Council for Graduate Medical Education has established a required core competency in interpersonal and communication skills that results in effective information exchange and teaming with patients, families, and professional associates. This competency is a clear indication that medical residencies are moving away from the idea of the physician as a self-sufficient and independent decision maker to a concept of the physician as an interdependent and cooperative member or leader of a health care team.

Integrated Functional Assessment and Integrated Care Plans Although the interdisciplinary team members often come together to conduct initial assessments and to design broad treatment goals, after that phase, clinicians often return

Commentary
Christina's Weight

Christina was born prematurely and had a rare and severe genetic disorder associated with intellectual and motor disabilities. During a prolonged neonatal hospitalization to address her slow and uncoordinated feeding pattern and a swallow study that suggested high risk for aspiration, a feeding gastrostomy tube was placed. Christina received 100% of her nutrition directly into her stomach. After she was discharged at 4 months of age, the gastrointestinal service and dietician at the hospital followed her progress. She was also referred to early intervention, in which weekly occupational and physical therapy was arranged in the community.

When Christina was approximately 9 months of age, the treating physical and occupational therapists in the community became increasingly alarmed as her weight rose to far above the 97th percentile for age while her stature remained at about the 3rd percentile for age. They noted that the child's awareness of her surroundings had dramatically improved and that her weight was a severe obstacle to sitting with support and bringing hands to the midline. Christina's mother shared their concerns about the child's weight and remained confused as to why the child continued to get a continuous infusion of food throughout the night when she was being fed every 3 hours during the day. A primary care physician referred the mother back to the dietician to ask these questions. However, the dieticians noted that the child had a planned follow-up visit 3 months later and so did not make another appointment.

An energetic pediatric intern, observing the early intervention setting, decided to try to bring the teams together virtually to reconsider the plan for diet and nutrition. This required several calls over several days. She finally connected with the dietician, who remembered the initial challenges in getting Christina to gain weight. The dietician was more concerned that Christina might lose weight than she was about the child failing to gain motor milestones. Through active negotiation and appeals to the principles of family-centered practice, the dietician agreed to move up the planned return visit for the purposes of adjusting the feeding schedule. At the same time, the therapists identified a public health nurse to accompany the family to the visit in order to advocate for a reduction in calories.

to their offices and clinics to treat children individually. Those interventions then address narrow disciplinary goals without reference to the broader context of global care plans. For example, an occupational therapist may participate on the interdisciplinary team that evaluates young children with developmental delays. A child who is diagnosed with autism receives recommendations for interventions to improve social skills and communication. However, if the child sees the occupational therapist individually, the therapist may decide to work on fine motor skills or on reducing the child's strong reactions to sensory experiences. The focus of the individual treatment is not necessarily subjugated to the overarching objectives established by the interdisciplinary team of improved communication and social skills. (See the commentary on p. 192.)

To encourage enhanced coordination, preprofessional students from all of the disciplines that serve children with disabilities and their families should receive training in the implementation of integrated care plans (Chapter 8). The plans should emphasize supporting the child's functional capacities (Chapter 7), not in piecemeal fashion, but as an integrated whole. For a child with autism, the treatment goal may be for him to participate actively in reciprocal peer social relationships. If that child is slated to receive speech-language-communication therapy, then the speech-language therapist might create specific objectives for verbal interaction among peers. The occupational therapist might work on fine motor skills or sensory processing in a social setting. If the child's aggressive behavior compromises reciprocal peer relationships, and aggression has persisted despite behavioral approaches, then medication may be an appropriate intervention to address the primary objectives. However, if the child's main barrier to peer relationships is poor verbal skills, medications are unlikely to improve social function (Huffman, Sutcliffe, Tanner, & Feldman, 2011).

Learning by co-treating a child with disabilities is one way that different disciplines can come to understand how to forge an integrated approach for a child. Different professionals would bring their distinctive expertise and skill set to the same child and would thereby discover ways of working toward the same objectives with their distinctive approaches. Standing teams, such as the infant feeding team, composed of physician, psychologist, occupational therapist, dietician, and social worker, have developed strategies for integrating care plans and working toward common objectives. These teams make outstanding training sites as they model integrated care.

Practice Guidelines and Standardized Approaches Introducing students to practice guidelines facilitates education and training and increases the likelihood that they will adopt these guidelines when they leave the educational setting. Students can come to appreciate how practice guidelines help to standardize care, ensure comprehensive treatment, and avoid errors (Improving Chronic Illness Care, 2011).

Many practitioners, whose training predated the increasing use of guidelines, remain skeptical about the role of guidelines in clinical care and feel constrained by the recommendations. Younger clinicians are more likely to accept the guidelines as they are introduced early in their education. They should become proficient in recognizing typical scenarios in which the guidelines are appropriate and unusual scenarios when they are not appropriate.

Maximizing the Use of Technology for Communication Modern technology for communication is changing how the interdisciplinary team records information, communicates among its members, and communicates with children and families. The electronic health record is becoming the norm rather than the exception. Families increasingly request e-mail communication rather than telephone calls so they can access information more easily. They realize that e-mail is not secure but value ease of access over assured confidentiality. Personal web sites are coming online as repositories for medical and personal information. Clinical reminders about record keeping or medication can be delivered automatically via text messaging.

Students will need to focus on learning the information technology at their office, clinic, or hospital. If reimbursement moves away from fee-for-service reimbursement to bundled payments, electronic communication will be a powerful strategy to reduce the number of visits and hospitalizations and improve interdisciplinary communication. It will be impossible to prepare students for all of the new capacities of the information age before their invention. However, it is important to prepare students with a sense of openness and a spirit of experimentation for new communication technology.

CONTINUING EDUCATION AND INSTITUTIONAL APPROACHES

Continuing education programs, like preservice education, can promote change in health care delivery for children with disabilities and their families among mature clinicians and the institutions in which they work. Such programs should include the same topics that must be integrated into preservice education: family-centered care, cultural competence, interdisciplinary teaming, practice guidelines, and new technologies.

Several features of continuing education, as it is typically presented, limit its power to affect changes toward interdisciplinary practice and function focused care.

- Many programs, such as conferences and grand rounds, are directed at a single professional group, such as physicians or nurses or occupational therapists. They do not bring together the interdisciplinary team that must work together in the new models.
- Many educational programs use traditional methods, such as lectures, or reasonable modern facsimiles, such as webinars. They are good for imparting information, but these didactic forms do not address the application of that knowledge to the clinical situation.
- Continuing education programs typically do not use the adult-learning model. Everyone gets the same program, presented in the same way at the same time. Learners are passive recipients.

Continuing education does not have to have these limitations. The following models encourage interdisciplinary teaming and practice change.

Interprofessional Case Review

Case reviews are an excellent way to learn collaboratively; they bring together colleagues from various disciplines to discuss and critique actual clinical cases. This design conforms to the principles of adult education. Done well, the case reviews tap the expertise of the entire group, as each participant has the opportunity to add information or insights from his or her vantage point. To make such case reviews supportive and effective, it helps to organize a stable group of participants who meet on a regular schedule under supportive leadership. The group then develops mutual trust and respect that facilitate honest and open exchange.

The Mortality and Morbidity (M&M) conference is a traditional form of interprofessional teaming. By design, the M&M conference focuses on bad outcomes (Orlander, Barger, & Fincke, 2002). The discussions often carry an implicit assumption that adverse outcomes are the result of errors or failings within the health care system rather than the fault of an individual. If those errors can be corrected, then the errors should not reoccur. In many cases, the conference reviews the clinical and technical aspects of the cases, with a focus on how to manage challenging cases. However, interdisciplinary discussions can be not only instructive but also opportunities for participants to release and share their emotional reactions to adverse outcomes, a focus, often neglected in medicine, which can further unite the team. Unfortunately, M&M conferences can be critical and intimidating to clinicians due to the judgmental climate they create and the unwillingness to look beyond individual culpability. Teams need constructive ground rules to work effectively.

A different model for case review is called the Balint Group, an approach in which a "group of clinicians...meet regularly in a leader-facilitated group to present and discuss clinical cases in order to better understand and utilize the clinician-patient relationship in a therapeutic, professional way" (The American Balint Society, 2012). These reviews focus not on technical aspects of the case but rather on the clinical process and especially on the relationship between the clinician and patient. These case reviews allow clinicians to reflect on their own experiences as care providers and to improve their care of individuals or families they find challenging The reviews are less focused on interdisciplinary communication and care planning; team members are used to help explore the relationships from different perspectives. In this model, the relationship among the participants is key. Without a safe, supportive environment, participants are unlikely to open up and share.

Recently, I have been involved in an exciting case review process called International Collaborative Office Rounds. Collaborative Office Rounds are an interdisciplinary discussion group composed of general and subspecialty pediatricians and child psychiatrists who meet regularly to discuss the process of care, particularly around the issues of child mental health, family functioning, and professional–family relationships. The Maternal Child Health Bureau has been funding Collaborative Office Rounds for many years. Our team is developing a variant using distance education methods to expand the team to multiple sites. Three centers are participating: Yale University, Stanford University, and the National University of the Health Sciences in Singapore. Although we use videoconferencing and although each team meets at a different time of day, the discussions have been extremely rich for all participants. We were pleased at how quickly the group created a safe and nurturing environment for the discussion. Our case reviews blend discussions about technical information regarding children with disabilities and clinical-process reflection regarding communication, family-centered practice, and cultural competence. The success of International Collaborative Office Rounds is a testament to the power of the model for continuing education. To improve the care of children with disabilities, a model that invites in a wider diversity of professionals would allow education and assessment of care processes across the team. (See the commentary below.)

Single-Profession Conferences

Professional organizations, such as the American Academy of Pediatrics (AAP), the National Association of Pediatric Nurse Practitioners, the American Occupational Therapy Association, the American Speech-Language-Hearing Association, and American Academy of Audiology, offer continuing education at the annual meetings for their membership. These professional organizations can play a major role in improving the care of children with disabilities.

Annual meetings should prioritize information on the care of children with disabilities within their educational offerings. Because the organizations cater to a single discipline, they should focus on specific strategies that promote family-centered care and interdisciplinary team approaches. When I served as Chair of the Program Committee of the Section of Developmental and Behavioral Pediatrics of the AAP, I hosted a panel of family members at the large national meeting to discuss the care of children with disabilities and the role of early-intervention services from the family perspective. I did not provide any specific training for the presenters; I simply asked them to tell their stories. The session was powerful. Parents described events and their reactions to those events without anger or judgment. The professional audience was transfixed as they considered the events from a parent's perspective. I strongly recommend inviting parents and consumers to participate in such single-profession meetings as one strategy for promoting family-centered care. I have also

Commentary
International Collaborative Office Rounds

In 2011, Dr. Carol Weitzman wrote a successful grant proposal to the Maternal and Child Health Bureau for a new model of Collaborative Office Rounds. The innovation was collaboration across three sites, two in the United States (Yale and Stanford University School of Medicine) and one in Singapore (National University Health Systems). A group of approximately 10 clinicians at each site meet monthly by teleconference. The sites rotate the responsibility for presenting the cases for discussion. Any clinician with a pressing issue is free to ask for consultation during the call.

I have been amazed at the power of the Collaborative Office Rounds model. Dr. Weitzman and her colleagues at Yale, who have participated in a local Collaborative Office Rounds project in New Haven, Connecticut, for many years, quickly established a safe and nurturing environment for the participants. Sufficient time was allotted for each case discussion to allow a deep reflection of the issues. Variations in the presentation of conditions in the different sites, as well as the approaches of different clinicians, could be discussed at length. Even though we are having the discussions electronically, the model promotes a sense of intimacy and trust. Fellows and seasoned practitioners have indicated high satisfaction with the discussions in their annual review.

invited panels of interdisciplinary professionals and representatives of community-based organizations to hospital grand rounds. These sessions have been uniformly well received.

Professional organizations play a key role in developing, publishing, and promoting practice guidelines. Their continuing education sessions are an important vehicle for the dissemination of those guidelines. Certification or recertification within that discipline can include a careful assessment of the clinician's technical and clinical skills in providing care to children with disabilities and should emphasize the importance of working with other disciplines.

Interprofessional Organizations

Professional organizations composed of an interdisciplinary membership play an extremely valuable role in educating the team about care of children with disabilities and their families. The Society of Developmental and Behavioral Pediatrics serves pediatricians, psychologists, nurses, and others who work together in developmental–behavioral pediatrics. The American Association of Cerebral Palsy and Developmental Medicine serves physicians and surgeons and physical and occupational therapists who work together for children with motor disabilities. The meetings of such organizations thereby support interprofessional education and training. Meetings that bring together parties interested in particular conditions, such as the International Meeting for Autism Research, also attract many different professional groups united in their commitment to support individuals with the condition.

Professionals who have limited time or funding to attend national meetings must make difficult decisions about whether to go to their professional meeting or to an interdisciplinary organization. On the basis of this discussion, my hope is that professionals will choose the interprofessional organizations to improve and reinforce critical inderdisciplinary team skills at least on a regular schedule.

Beyond the United States

Worldwide, WHO estimates a shortage of 4.3 million health workers, leading to a call in 2006 for a rapid scaling up of the health workforce preparation (Health Professions Networks et al., 2010). Interprofessional education is a key strategy for addressing the shortage because it brings to health care delivery a group of professionals ready to work together on behalf of individuals and communities. A survey designed to assess the status of interprofessional education globally found that it was in place in a wide range of developed and developing countries, but mainly at the undergraduate level. Therefore, WHO has published a framework that encourages member nations and local health authorities to support a shift to interprofessional education, using one or more of the following mechanisms:

- Institutional support mechanisms, including structured protocols, shared operating resources, appropriate personnel policies, and supportive management
- Working culture mechanisms, including communications strategies, conflict resolution policies, and shared decision-making processes
- Environmental mechanisms, including creating facilities and space design that support interprofessional communication and collaboration

State and national certification bodies must consider how to incorporate standards and requirements that reflect the importance of family-centered care, cultural competence, and interdisciplinary teamwork in the health care setting. The requirements should be reasonable and respectful of the practicing professional and be meaningfully integrated in the larger learning experience.

SUMMARY

Changing health care for children with disabilities requires educating a new generation of health care clinicians and helping the current generation of health care providers to understand, practice, and value the new integrated approach. Adult learning approaches emphasize that training should be relevant, respectful, and organized around the learner's individualized goals. Preservice education must include the topics previously covered in this book, including functional assessment, family-centered care, cultural competence, and interdisciplinary teamwork. The education programs must impart more than knowledge; they must provide opportunities to put the skills into place. Interprofessional education must become the norm for professionals who want to work on the interdisciplinary team caring for children with disabilities, and continuing education programs must prepare practicing clinicians for the new approaches. Though continuing education is often discipline specific, interdisciplinary or interprofessional approaches can be incorporated locally, nationally, and internationally.

Exercises

1. Compare the tables of contents of textbooks in related disciplines, such as physical and occupational therapy or speech-language pathology and audiology. How is the content similar and how is it different? Consider various explanations for the similarities and differences.
2. Create an interprofessional course entitled "Feeding and Disorders of Feeding, Eating, and Nutrition" designed for the team that cares for infants and young children with feeding issues. Which professions should be targeted to take this course? What are the core concepts that every participant should understand? What are differences among the approaches of the participants that may need to be reconciled during the course? Discuss how the class prepares students for active participation on feeding teams.
3. Create an interprofessional course titled, "Transition to Adulthood for Adolescents with Intellectual Disabilities." Which professions should be targeted to take this course? How does the composition of this team compare with the team targeted for disorders of feeding, eating, and nutrition? Anticipate conflicts that might arise within the team as it supports the youth and their families through the transition process. Anticipate conflicts that might arise between the parent and the young adult. How can you prepare the students for these challenging issues in this class?
4. Design a clinical scenario to educate students or practicing professionals about care of children with disabilities. Change the racial, ethnic, or language

background of the family in the case and assess how the changes influence the discussion and plan of care. How do the differences educate the students about health disparities?

5. Create a seminar or workshop for your professional association meeting to update practitioners about new models of care for children with disabilities and their families. How would you organize the session to make professional change compelling to members of your discipline?

12

Research

with Nathan J. Blum

Studying Treatments for Attention-Deficit/Hyperactivity Disorder

The Multimodal Treatment of Attention Deficit/Hyperactivity Disorder Study (MTA) began as a carefully planned, multisite, 14-month randomized clinical trial in 579 children 7–9 years old with attention-deficit/hyperactivity disorder (ADHD), combined type. The study addressed three questions:

1. *How do long-term medication and behavioral treatments compare to one another in the management of ADHD?*
2. *Are the benefits increased when the two modalities are used together?*
3. *How do experimental treatments delivered by researchers compare with routine care delivered by community practitioners?*

Initial reports emphasized that both the combination of medication and behavioral treatment and medication treatment alone were significantly superior to behavior treatment alone and community care in reducing the core symptoms of ADHD (The MTA Cooperative Group, 1999). Combination was found to be no better than medication for core symptoms but was superior to medication alone for some

---

Nathan J. Blum, M.D., coauthor of this chapter, is Professor of Pediatrics in the Perelman School of Medicine at the University of Pennsylvania. He is a board-certified developmental-behavioral pediatrician and directs the developmental-behavioral pediatrics fellowship training program at The Children's Hospital of Philadelphia. Dr. Blum also directs the Leadership Education in Neurodevelopmental Disabilities Training Program and the Network Coordinating Center for the Developmental-Behavioral Pediatrics Research Network.

outcomes, including decreasing oppositional, aggressive, or internalizing symptoms and improving reading performance, parent–child interactions, and social skills. In children with anxiety disorders as well as ADHD, behavioral treatment was better than community care and no different from medication and combined treatments ("Moderators and Mediators," 1999).

After the trial, investigators continued to monitor the participants over time. A report about them 6–8 years later found that children with ADHD fared more poorly than a comparable group of children in the community without ADHD on almost all of the measures collected. Differences across treatment groups based on the initial assignments had completely disappeared. Medication use decreased after the trial phase ended, but even after adjusting for duration of medication use, the pattern of results did not change. Within the group with ADHD, children with behavioral and demographic advantages had the best long-term prognosis (Molina et al., 2009).

This book espouses change in health care systems and health care delivery to promote inclusion, contribution, and health for children with disabilities. Case studies throughout the chapters are designed to demonstrate the rationale, methods, and results of this new direction. Convincing practitioners and health care systems on a broad scale to change their model of health care delivery requires more than heart-wrenching stories and educational programs. It requires compelling scientific evidence that the changes are beneficial to children and families and to the community at large. Such evidence is accumulated through scientific study.

This chapter begins with a discussion of the role of science in medicine. It reviews traditional research methods, like the randomized clinical trial method that was used in the MTA study described in the opening vignette. The randomized clinical trial has proven highly valuable for understanding causes and evaluating treatments for many health conditions, including disabilities like ADHD. However, these methods are challenging to apply to complex clinical problems, such as the long-term outcomes of medication and behavior management for ADHD, as the MTA study discussed in the opening vignette. In addition, they are frequently impractical for studies of health care delivery. The chapter then turns to alternative research methods that may be used to demonstrate effectiveness and cost-effectiveness of health care delivery for children with those disabilities. Health services research has far-reaching implications for improving child and family outcomes. For example, through our participation in a research network, we have learned that large variations occur in how services are provided, even among clinicians who know well the results of clinical trials. It is unlikely that all these variations are equally safe, effective, and cost-effective. Research networks can study these variations and can rapidly conduct high-quality clinical trials to speed up the acquisition of new information that improves clinical care and service delivery. To achieve maximal productivity for research on the care of children with disabilities, these networks must carefully choose outcome measures that are meaningful to children and families, including functional measures. The development of these outcome measures is such an important national priority that the Affordable Care Act of 2010 (U.S. Department of Health and Human Services, 2012) created a research institute with the goal of developing these measures, The Patient-Centered Outcome Research Institute.

SCIENCE AND MEDICINE

For over a century, the foundation of medical education and research has been the scientific method. It was not always so (Beck, 2004). The stimulus for change was an influential report published in 1910 by Abraham Flexner, a professional educator, who took up the study of American medical education at the request of the Council on Medical Education of the American Medical Association and the Carnegie Foundation for the Advancement of Teaching. The report recommended that medical schools affiliate with universities, that faculty members become full-time clinical professors, and that matriculating students meet minimal standards of education. Another fundamental recommendation, important to this discussion, was that medical schools adhere strictly to scientific principles in both teaching and research (Flexner, 1910). In the early 20th century, scientific evidence had simultaneously shown the futility of many traditional treatments, such as "blistering, bleeding, and purging," and the efficacy of practices such as "antiseptic surgery, vaccination, and public sanitation" (Beck, 2004). As the Flexner report was implemented, the intimate connection of medicine and science was assured.

Basic medical research uses objective data to prove or disprove specific hypotheses or answer specific questions. The research pipeline to investigate diagnostic assessments or treatments often begins in the laboratory, using test tubes and petri dishes, then proceeds to animal models, small-scale tests in humans to assess safety, and ultimately to large clinical trials with adult and then child participants to prove efficacy and further document safety. This scientific method has been responsible for generating a vast body of information that has radically changed diagnostic and therapeutic methods in health care. Despite this success, it often takes many years for proven treatments to become incorporated into practice by a high percentage of clinicians.

Evidence-Based Practice

An interest in reducing the long delay in the implementation of proven treatments has led to emphasis on the practice of evidence-based health care. Evidence-based medicine has been defined as the "conscientious, explicit, and judicious use of current best evidence in making decisions about the care of individual patients" (Sackett, Rosenberg, Gray, Haynes, & Richardson, 1996, p. 71). It requires systematically accumulating strong scientific support for clinical decision making, especially from patient-centered clinical research on diagnostic methods or "therapeutic, rehabilitative, and preventive regimens" (Sackett et al., 1996, p. 72). Other health care disciplines also accumulate information about their diagnostic and therapeutic approaches using the scientific method in order to achieve the high standards of evidence-based practice (Dollaghan, 2007). Ph.D. programs in these health care disciplines are flourishing to support the training of researchers who acquire scientific evidence and to accumulate sufficient support for their specific contributions to the health care team.

Randomized Clinical Trials

The randomized clinical trial (RCT) is a specific experimental design that is considered the gold standard for investigating the efficacy of health care treatments.

Potential subjects must meet strict eligibility criteria. Once they are deemed appropriate for the study, they are randomly assigned to receive one of the treatment methods. The decision about who gets which treatment is a bit like tossing a coin or picking a number from a hat. The method minimizes the chances that the division of individuals into treatment groups is somehow biased in ways that complicate the interpretation of the results. Once the participants are assigned to their respective group, the only difference in the care they receive is the particular treatment that they get (Figure 12.1).

Using the MTA study as the example, the key features of the RCT can be readily demonstrated:

- The study population was defined in detail. Participants were restricted to children ages 7–9, in Grades 1–4, in residence with their primary caregiver for 6 months, who all met the criteria for ADHD combined type in the *DSM-IV*

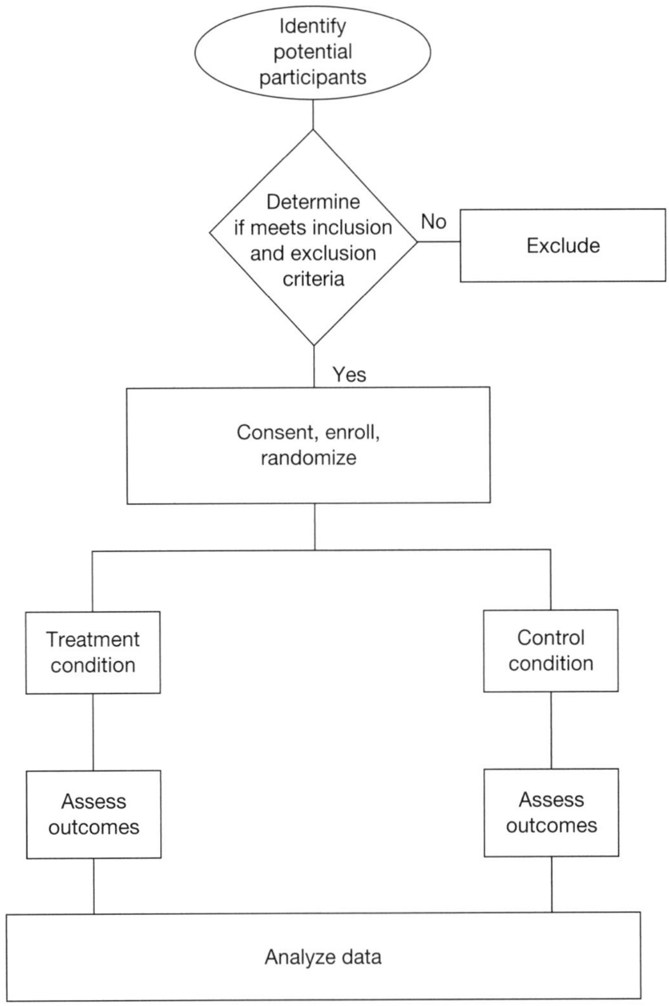

Figure 12.1. Methods used in a randomized clinical trial.

(American Psychiatric Association, 1994). Children with coexisting conditions that frequently occur with ADHD, such as oppositional defiant disorder, internalizing disorders, and specific learning disabilities, were not excluded from this study in order to establish whether the treatments worked similarly across subgroups.

- The treatments to be assessed were compared with alternatives. Medication, behavior treatments, and a combination were pitted against each other. All three were compared with the usual and customary care children received in the community.
- Participants were randomly assigned to one of the four groups at each site. As expected through randomization, the four treatment groups were very comparable in terms of subject characteristics, such as age.
- The identical and predetermined outcomes were assessed in all groups. Core symptoms of ADHD were the primary outcome, and many additional measures, such as parent–child interactions and social skills, were secondary outcomes.

Although the MTA was well planned, it nonetheless faced significant challenges in design and execution. The most rigorous randomized clinical trials compare actual treatments to a placebo, a treatment that looks as much like the treatment being tested as possible but is thought to be completely inert in the treatment of the condition. In the MTA, a no-treatment group was not included because the experimenters decided it was unethical to leave children with ADHD untreated for the 14-month duration of the study. Instead they used a comparison group of children who continued with community-based care as it was practiced at each of the sites. Though the decision was very reasonable, if the study had found no differences between the treatment groups and community control group, it would have been impossible to determine whether medication and/or behavior management improved outcomes. (See the commentary below.)

Ideally, in randomized clinical trials, the experimenters and the participants remain unaware of what treatment the participants are receiving, earning the designation *double-blinded*. This precaution reduces potential bias in the evaluation

Commentary
Testing New Medications for Attention-Deficit/Hyperactivity Disorder

In the evaluation of new nonstimulant medications for the medical management of attention-deficit/hyperactivity disorder, the requirement of the U.S. Food and Drug Administration (FDA) is to test new medication against a placebo. Using this model, many medications appear to be highly effective for treating ADHD and become FDA approved. They are then marketed to professionals and consumers on the basis of those study results. However, when these new medications were compared with existing stimulant medications used to treat ADHD, the stimulant medications have consistently proven more effective. Nonetheless, the medication manufacturers are not obliged to share that information with the FDA or the public.

of the treatment. The MTA could not be a double-blinded study because participants could not help but know the group to which they were assigned. In principle, the testers might have been kept in the dark about which child was in which group (a single-blind study). However, in such cases, it is very easy for participants to inadvertently reveal what treatments they received when interacting with assessors.

Participants do not always receive only the treatment they are assigned. For example, when participants, aware of their group assignment, think that the alternative is a better option, they may change the treatment on their own, without experimenter knowledge or approval. In other cases, the investigator may allow individuals to change treatment because it may be unethical to withhold a potentially effective treatment if the alternative treatment a patient is assigned is not working. In the MTA, 38 children crossed over to medication from one of the other groups (The MTA Cooperative Group, 1999, p. 1078). The experimenters then need to make decisions about handling these participants in data analysis. In the MTA, the experimenters used the initial group assignment in the analysis. This analysis is known as an intent-to-treat analysis. Although it typically decreases the chances of finding differences between groups, it is commonly done in randomized clinical trials because changing group assignment would invalidate the randomization and potentially introduce unknown biases into the study. (See the commentary below.)

Commentary
The Child Development/Otitis Media Study

For several years, I was an investigator in a large study designed to determine whether placement of tympanostomy tubes, or grommets, improves developmental outcomes of young children with persistent otitis media with effusion or chronic ear infections (Paradise et al., 2001, 2007). This study was a designed as a randomized trial. A total of 6,350 children from eight participating pediatric practices were enrolled and monitored monthly to determine which child accumulated 3 months of continuous bilateral ear infection or a bit longer for unilateral ear infection in order to meet the criterion for randomization. Once the criterion was met, children were assigned to receive the tympanostomy tubes immediately or to wait at least an additional 6 months and receive tubes only if the infection persisted throughout that wait. All children received comprehensive developmental assessments at 3, 4, 6, and 9–11 years of age.

The experience of this study also demonstrates the complexities of conducting a randomized trial. In this case, the participants could not be blinded to their group assignment. It would have been completely unethical to do a sham operation on children who would not actually receive the tubes. However, the evaluators did remain unaware of group assignment, so this study was single-blinded.

Another complexity was that those children assigned to the immediate treatment group had to be evaluated by an otolaryngologist who would perform the operation. By the time the children could be evaluated, some no longer had the ear infection and thus did not undergo the treatment. Other children, assigned to the no-treatment condition, did actually get tympanostomy tubes placed despite their study group assignment.

In this case, we used an intention-to-treat solution to assign children to groups: The children were included in the group to which they were assigned even when they did not follow the precise procedures for that group. We conducted a secondary analysis based on what treatment the children did receive and were assured that the children whose treatment violated group assignment were responsible for the findings.

The results of the study showed absolutely no differences in any outcome measure between the children who received the tubes and those who did not. We were very confident about these results because of several features of the experimental design. The sample size was large, adequate to detect small differences between the groups. The design was longitudinal, allowing us to replicate the findings with the same and different measures over time. The results were highly consistent across ages.

The treatments may have different effects on primary and secondary outcomes. In the MTA, this complexity turned out to be the case for management of core symptoms versus functional outcomes of ADHD. Treatments may also be effective only in subgroups of the participants. Fortunately, the MTA had a sufficiently large sample size to allow the experimenters to review the results in selected subsets of the sample as well as the entire group. Even for studying one of the most common disabilities, the MTA study required multiple sites to obtain a sufficiently large sample to look for subgroups in whom the treatment was most effective. For the MTA study, the investigators had to form a research collaboration across sites. A research network has the advantage of developing an ongoing collaboration than can carry out multiple studies, often simultaneously. (See the commentary on p. 208.)

Limitations of the Randomized Clinical Trial

RCTs may be inappropriate or impractical for addressing many important questions about treatments for children with disabilities. For example, when a condition is extremely rare, such as an unusual genetic variant, then accumulating an adequate sample size to compare groups may be exceedingly difficult. If a condition is dangerous or life threatening, such as a neurological complication of a surgical procedure, then a randomized trial would not be ethical if participation would delay participants getting treatment.

For long-term outcomes, such as the effects of a treatment initiated during elementary school on high school graduation rates, it is unlikely that individuals would agree to random assignment to treatments over such a long period. Maintaining contact with individuals over the necessary period is difficult and expensive, and consistently implementing many treatments over a long period is challenging for both participants and investigators.

If the topic of study involves determining whether variations in the intensity, schedule, or timing of therapy change the outcomes, then the RCT may become impractical unless experimenters can control these variables carefully and randomly assign participants to groups that vary on these dimensions.

Perhaps the greatest limitation of RCTs is that although the highly controlled nature of the design is very powerful for informing us about whether an intervention can work (efficacy), it does not tell us how the intervention will work when it is widely implemented in clinical practice. Typically, the investigators doing the

Commentary
Rationale for the Crossover Design

A significant barrier to the randomized clinical trial (RCT) is the unwillingness of potential participants to enroll if they learn that they or their child may receive a placebo or sham treatment rather than the promising treatment under study. For this reason, researchers may choose to use a crossover design. In this experimental model, participants are randomly assigned to which treatment they will receive first. Halfway through, they are reassigned to the other arm of the study. By the end of the trial, they have experienced both the placebo and the treatment. Such modifications to clinical trial methodology need to be carefully considered in light of the mechanism by which the treatment may work and the duration of benefits anticipated. When appropriate, this design may assist in recruiting participants. However, such designs are rated as lower quality than classic RCTs in systematic reviews of treatments.

studies know more about the interventions than most of clinicians who will use the interventions, and participants are often monitored more closely and seen more frequently in the trials than they are in clinical practice. For example, the MTA was conducted by some of the leading U.S. experts on pharmacological and behavioral treatments, and patients on medication were seen monthly, much more frequently than is recommended by clinical practice guidelines. Furthermore, although the RCT may have very specific inclusion criteria for who can participate, clinicians will often want to use the intervention in situations that seem similar, but not identical, to those of the participants in the study. For all of these and other reasons, an intervention may perform very differently in a randomized trial than it does in the real world. Studies of how well interventions work in the real world are known as *effectiveness studies.*

RCTs are almost impossible to use for studies of health care delivery systems, quality, finance mechanisms, or other system variables. In such cases, the opportunity to randomly assign children to treatment groups is usually beyond experimenter control. For example, it might be ideal to contrast the impact of different models of care coordination on clinical and functional outcomes and health care utilization. However, the experimenters usually are not in a position to establish a complicated system for care coordination, and most individuals are unlikely to consent to random assignment to a whole health care delivery system. However, naturally occurring experiments happen frequently. States decide to implement different models for the delivery of health insurance, and hospitals and clinicians care for patients in different ways. When one can evaluate the outcomes of these variations in care, one can often learn about which methods for the delivery of health services are most effective and/or most efficient. This type of research, known as *health services research*, is often the best way to address questions about how interventions work in the real world.

HEALTH SERVICES RESEARCH

Health services research is a multidisciplinary field of scientific inquiry that investigates how health services are delivered and the impact of those services on various constituencies or conditions (Martin, 2008). It focuses on how "social factors, financing systems, organizational structures and processes, technologies, and personal behaviors affect access to health care, the quality and cost of health care, and ultimately, our health and well-being" (Stephens, Levine, Burling, & Russ-Eft, 2011, p. 1). In 1966, the term was formalized when the federal government established a federal research study section to review grant proposals of this ilk. In 1969, the field was catapulted to greater recognition with the establishment of the National Center for Health Services Research and Development within the Department of Health, Education, and Welfare. Although health services research may improve health at both the individual and the population level, it is more likely to inform decisions about health systems rather than about individual treatment options (see Figure 12.2).

Health services research incorporates a wide variety of experimental methods, integrating paradigms not only from evidence-based medicine but also from clinical informatics and quality improvement activities (Scott & Campbell, 2002). It encompasses qualitative and quantitative approaches. Here are a few examples of health services research:

- *Effectiveness research*, as mentioned previously, describes the outcomes of treatment in real settings. Effectiveness research asks what is the right thing to do in a given clinical situation (Scott & Campbell, 2002) or how an intervention works when it is implemented across a population. At the population level, measures of effectiveness include measures such as quality-adjusted life years, years of life saved, or diseases prevented.
- *Comparative effectiveness* contrasts the effectiveness, safety, and/or outcomes of different treatments on specific conditions for a set of patients being treated in a naturalistic environment. The definition does not exclude randomized trials if they compare treatments and are conducted in naturalistic settings. (See the commentary on p. 211.)
- *Implementation research* aims at identifying the methods to allow clinicians or managers to implement research findings into actual practice. This type of research can investigate, for example, whether lectures, small group meetings, or audits with feedback are effective in changing clinician practices, and if so, which method has the greatest impact.

Use of Large Data Sets

Health services researchers often take advantage of modern information technology and statistical methods to study extremely large samples. This approach is extremely powerful for the study of rare events. For example, in the early 2000s, case reports of children on stimulant medication experiencing sudden death raised concerns that stimulant medication might increase the risk of this extremely rare event. Health services researchers were able to study large insurance databases for hundreds of thousands of individuals and could identify from claims data children diagnosed with ADHD, children prescribed stimulants, and children who died suddenly. Using these data, researchers have been able to demonstrate that stimulants do not seem to increase the risk of sudden death (Cooper et al., 2011). This question could never have been addressed in a clinical trial, as it would have required enrolling thousands of children in the trial.

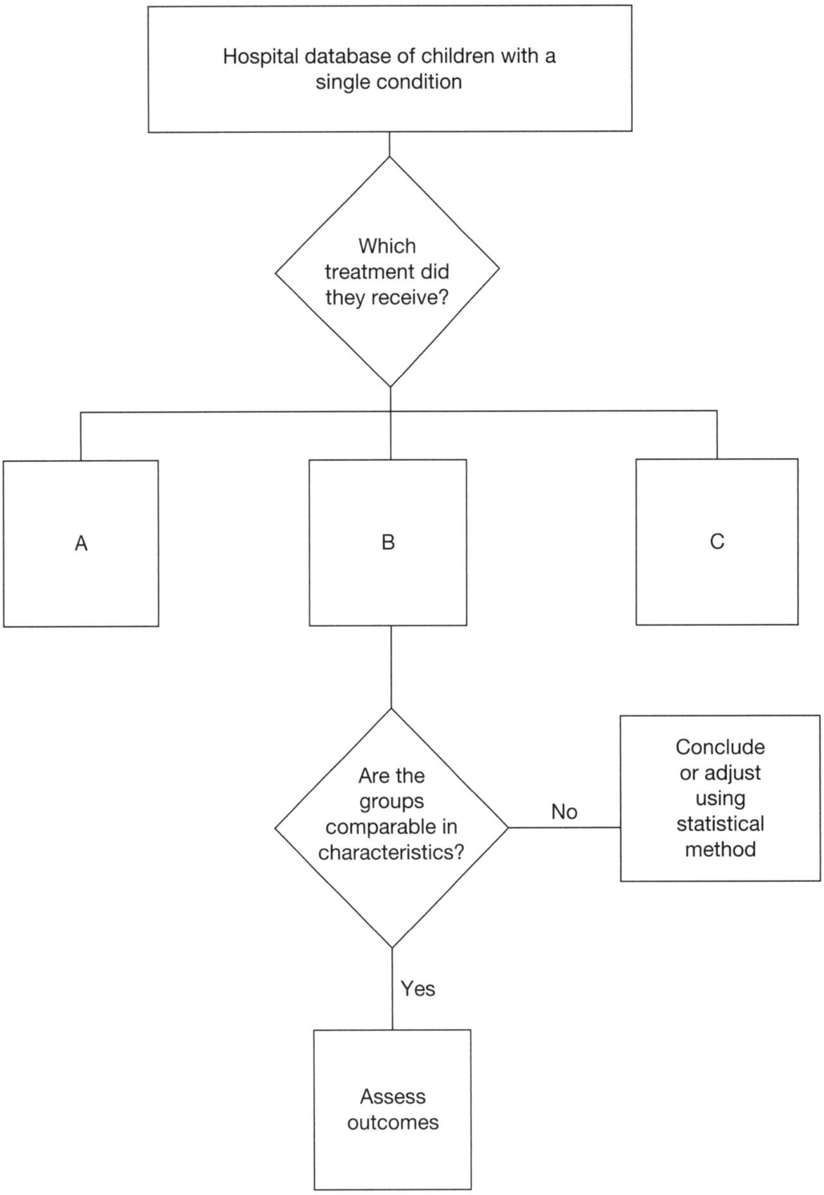

Figure 12.2. Methods that might be used in an effectiveness study.

Large sample sizes can also help address some of the problems related to the lack of experimental controls. Although RCTs usually enroll a relatively small sample of individuals thought to represent a broader group with a disorder, use of large databases may allow researchers to study almost every member of a group. For example, if the specific cases in which a treatment was used can be accurately identified from hospital records or insurance claims, then studies may be able to evaluate that treatment for every individual who received it within the hospital or insurance plan. With large sample sizes, the outcomes can be analyzed for the group as a whole and for multiple subsets within the sample, such as males versus females,

Commentary
Comparative Effectiveness Studies for Individuals with Disabilities

The federal government decided to invest $1.1 billion in comparative effectiveness research as part of the American Recovery and Reinvestment Act (PL 111-5) funding in 2008. The act established the Federal Coordination Council for Comparative Effectiveness Research to promote organization and integration of the efforts. The act required a report to the President and Congress in 2009 (Federal Coordinating Council for Comparative Effectiveness Research, 2009). This report is publicly available and extremely interesting to professionals who serve children and adults with disabilities.

The report targeted people with disabilities as an important focus for comparative effectiveness research. It highlighted that individuals with disabilities are often excluded from clinical trials, even when there is no compelling scientific reason for the exclusion (Federal Coordinating Council for Comparative Effectiveness Research, 2009). The report recommended that all research related to disability should include outcome measures that address "functional abilities, people's abilities to participate in daily activities, and quality of life" (p. 19). The report went on to emphasize that comparative effectiveness research should evaluate community-based models of care, including care coordination/care management to help individuals with disabilities to live independently in their communities with added years of quality life. Because care coordination models are underdeveloped and the definitions vary across settings and models, the effectiveness of different approaches has yet to be fully established. Finally, the report encouraged comparative effectiveness studies of rehabilitation interventions to restore or maintain functioning or minimize loss, including "speech-language, physical, and occupational therapy interventions" (p. 20). Children in general, and children with disabilities in particular, were mentioned as appropriate targets for comparative effectiveness research because results from adult studies cannot be simply extrapolated to children and because children's response to treatments may lead to improved functioning for the rest of their lives.

children versus adolescents and adults, or individuals with different underlying conditions. The treatment could also be evaluated as a function of features of the delivery of care, such as whether the clinician was a nurse, doctor, or therapist; whether the treatment took place in hospital, clinic, or home; and whether the intervention was provided in one or two visits or over several different sessions. Given this potential, health services studies of large samples and whole populations may speed up the process of scientific discovery.

Health Services Research on Children with Disabilities

Health services research has particular relevance to studies of children with disabilities. Four factors pertinent to research on children challenge traditional study designs, especially for children with disabilities: developmental changes, dependency, differential epidemiology, and demographics (Simpson, 1999). In terms of developmental changes, children of different ages develop at different rates. It may be challenging to determine whether treatments function similarly across the age range. It is also difficult to know whether changes after treatment can be validly attributed to the treatment or to developmental progress without a very large sample size. Large sample studies that hold the child's age or developmental status at entry constant can begin to tease apart treatment effects from developmental change. Health services research with large databases may be able to disentangle age, stage, development, and treatment effects when smaller studies cannot.

In terms of dependency, parents, as patient representatives, provide the consent to enroll children under the age of 18 years in the study. Parents are understandably cautious about subjecting their children to the unknown risks that are often associated with studies of new interventions. This concern may be particularly acute for parents of children with disabilities for whom the risks of rare events may seem high because children with disabilities have often already experienced a rare event. Further, children with disabilities may have already undergone many different treatments, leading to hesitancy to expose the child to further treatments and related monitoring. Thus, relatively few treatments for children with disabilities have been rigorously evaluated in clinical trials.

In terms of differential epidemiology, children are more likely to have rare health conditions than are adults. Depending on the condition, accumulating an adequate sample size may be difficult and may limit the motivation of pharmaceutical or educational companies to study interventions for a group when there will not be a large market for the product. In terms of demographics, several conditions are more prevalent among children who are poor, from underrepresented minorities, from single-parent households, and from families with other psychosocial characteristics that tend to be associated with low rates of participation in research. The time commitments of research and lack of understanding of research may be particular barriers for these families, as are the concerns of vulnerable populations that they may be mistreated by researchers as has occurred in the past. For all these reasons, health services research that can evaluate existing data, collected in the course of clinical care, may yield information about interventions that may not be obtainable from a clinical trial.

Limitations of Health Services Research

Of course, health services research, like all research methods, has limitations. These include the enormous variability in how care and how research is conducted. These issues are highlighted in systematic reviews and meta-analyses, both techniques that attempt to extract systematic data from multiple different studies. In systematic reviews, the researcher usually hones in on studies of high scientific quality. This requirement may result in elimination of as many as 90% of studies on a particular treatment or condition. However, focusing on the outcomes or adverse effects in these high-quality studies provides powerful evidence about what works and what does not. Meta-analysis combines the results of multiple studies of a particular treatment to evaluate the treatment or intervention over many different individuals and settings. In meta-analyses, the need to identify a common metric for improvement also means that many studies cannot be integrated into the methodology. However, again, if several studies use the same outcome measures, then pooling the data increases the chance of finding statistically significant effects.

Despite these limitations, these methodologies may be used to increase scientific evidence in support of current practices for children with disabilities. Many different professional groups that serve children with disabilities could conduct studies like those described. Interdisciplinary teams can also use these methodologies to evaluate their procedures or outcomes.

RESEARCH NETWORKS

Research networks bring together a large group of researchers and clinicians across multiple sites to collect large databases to answer important questions. Unlike existing hospital or insurance databases, which do not collect data for research purposes and thus contain limited types of data, these networks are able to address a wider range of questions. Many medical fields have turned to clinical research networks to simultaneously advance the underlying scientific basis of their specialty or subspecialty and to rapidly translate the scientific discoveries into effective clinical care.

Clinical research networks typically consist of a stable cohort of investigators who collaborate in research. The network has multiple sites so that it can engage a large and diverse pool of participants as needed and typically has an infrastructure that supports the conduct of the studies across sites. A governance structure defines leadership, membership, and processes by which the group identifies the research projects, collects and shares data, analyzes and interprets findings, and disseminates results. Mature and well-functioning research networks efficiently conduct large studies.

Research networks can be designed to conduct RCTs. Within pediatrics, one of the oldest and most well-respected research networks is called the Children's Oncology Group. This network consists of over 200 different treatment sites internationally and conducts about 100 clinical trials every year (Children's Oncology Group, n.d.; Slora, Harris, Bocian, & Wasserman, 2010). The vast majority of children with cancer in the United States are treated under protocols of this network. Another impressive research network with a long history is the Neonatal Research Network, established in 1986 by the Eunice Kennedy Shriver National Institute of Child Health and Human Development. This network also conducts multicenter clinical trails designed to reduce infant mortality and morbidity for children who require hospitalization in the Neonatal Intensive Care Unit (NICHD Neonatal Research Network, n.d.).

Alternatively, research networks may use the network to conduct health services research rather than clinical trials. In this model, the network may begin by identifying differences in procedures and outcomes across the participating sites. It then attempts to understand which factors are associated with positive outcomes and which with negative outcomes. The variation initially across sites is not a barrier to scientific inquiry but rather the focus of the research.

The Developmental Behavioral Pediatrics Research Network

In 2011, the Developmental Behavioral Pediatrics Research Network (DBPNet), a research network of developmental-behavioral pediatrics practices, was launched through a cooperative agreement of the Maternal Child Health Bureau of Health Resources and Services Administration of the U.S. Public Health Service (Blum et al., 2012). The mission of DBPNet is to "conduct collaborative, interdisciplinary research in developmental-behavioral pediatrics that advances clinical practice, supports research status of children with developmental and behavioral concerns and disorders, including children with autism spectrum disorders and other developmental disabilities" (pp. 509–510).

DBPNet is an exciting opportunity to expand research on health care and health care delivery for children with developmental disabilities. The network comprises 12 research sites and a data-coordinating center. Each of the sites has an interdisciplinary clinical team—at least a developmental–behavioral pediatrician and psychologist—in place for clinical care, training, and research. Many sites have several other faculty or staff from other disciplines that serve children with disabilities and their families. The sites are located across the United States and collectively see thousands of children with disabilities annually. The network is poised to address many questions that pertain to interdisciplinary care for children with disabilities within subspecialty programs across the country. It can also serve as a model for other networks that may form to investigate the care of children with disabilities.

The first face-to-face meeting of the network, convened shortly after funding, established an organizational structure that guides the operation. A steering committee includes the site directors at all 12 sites, plus several consultants from other research networks, the Society for Developmental and Behavioral Pediatrics, and a parent representative. An executive committee of five, including the principle investigator, allows for efficient decision making. The Data Coordinating Center is at the institution of the principal investigator. Members of the Executive Committee lead two other committees. The Research Project Development and Review Committee reviews proposals for research projects and full research protocols for the network. It assigns mentors from the Steering Committee to each proposal so that the researcher has a guide and support in the application process. The Dissemination Committee reviews abstracts, manuscripts, and grants prior to submission to assure the quality of the products. The Dissemination Committee also oversees the network's web site.

DBPNet's first study was a qualitative evaluation of the research priorities of the interdisciplinary teams at the participating centers (Blum et al., 2012). Four participants at each site—the DBPNet steering committee member, a physician, a psychologist, and a parent—were asked to complete questionnaires about their top priorities for clinical research in developmental-behavioral pediatrics. After the list of responses was organized to avoid duplication and edited to remove ambiguities, the respondents again reviewed the items to establish priorities and their weightings. The final list includes topics in several areas, listed below in order of the number of specific priorities identified:

- Efficacy and effectiveness research (14 priorities)
- Comparative effectiveness research (five priorities)
- Determinants or risk factors in conditions treated by DBP pediatricians (five priorities)
- Incidence and prevalence of disorders (three priorities)
- Tests or technology assessment (three priorities)
- Outcomes research (three priorities)
- Diagnostic processes (one priority)
- Practice variation (one priority)

At the time of this writing, the network has just completed data collection on a study of practice variation across the network. Pediatricians were asked to complete detailed surveys about the information that they gathered or had available in order to diagnose or treat children with autism spectrum disorders or with ADHD. For example, the survey asked about whether other professionals were part of the evaluation and which measures were used. What we have learned thus far is that there are very different delivery models in place at our different sites to evaluate and manage these common conditions. Going forward, it is hoped that the network will begin to identify the most effective and cost-effective approaches. Alternatively, we may see that each model has its own advantages and that the choice of model is dependent on the priorities of the center.

Future Directions for the Developmental Behavioral Pediatrics Research Network

Paper and pencil survey studies, such as the one that DBPNet completed, are extremely taxing on clinicians whose priorities are patient care. Oftentimes they require clinicians to enter data twice (in the medical record and the survey) and then another person to enter the survey data into the research database. Each of these steps could introduce potential errors into the data. Collecting data from electronic health records (EHR) limits some of these problems, as clinicians only have to enter the data once into the EHR and not the research database. Furthermore, if all patient encounters are documented in the EHR, then it is possible to collect data from all encounters, which would allow the network to use health services research methodologies to answer questions about the care of children with disabilities. As we have seen with other research methodologies, however, this approach has its own set of problems. The data collected in this manner will only be as accurate as the data entered into the medical records; some data may not be entered into the EHR, or if entered, it may not be entered in a way that is easy to extract. Further, within DBPNet, the 12 participating institutions are currently at different developmental points in the implementation of the EHRs, and they use a variety of different EHR systems that are not designed to communicate with each other.

Even more important than the diversity in health records is the variation in the data included within each record. To facilitate comparisons of data across sites and across conditions, it would be very useful to require common data elements that all participating centers and clinicians include in every encounter. To compare and contrast the results of different assessment or treatment practices, the most sensible choice for common data elements would be assessment and outcome variables. If, for example, all of the follow-up visits of children with autism included the nature and intensity of their treatment program and a common outcome measure, then the network could evaluate which treatments at which intensity were associated with the most favorable outcome. Given the size of the network and the number of cases that could be included in the study, the research could address the issue for children of different ages and different severity of the condition.

Two years into operation, DBPNet has just begun to explore the possibility of choosing a common outcome assessment for the network to use in some or all cases. Choosing the common assessments and outcome elements strains the collaborative process. Experienced clinicians who have practiced independently for many years have established their own protocols for clinical evaluations and report preparation.

The goal of becoming a research network must add value for these clinicians so that they are willing to adapt and conform to the network's recommendations.

TOWARD A RESEARCH AGENDA

The overall approach for the care of children with disabilities and their families—an emphasis on inclusion, contribution, and health, in that order—and the specific recommendations to focus on function, use integrated health plans, practice family-centered care, and implement care coordination—must be put to the empirical test. Without research, it is unlikely that the concepts will gain traction that leads to dissemination and implementation. This research agenda is extremely ambitious. Many different professions will need to collaborate to evaluate it in different clinical conditions, patient groups, and practice settings.

Inclusion

Inclusion is a human right and as such needs no empirical validation. However, specific practices to introduce or support inclusion can be tested using research methods. For example, the research foundation for inclusive education processes remains very limited. There are few studies comparing outcomes of young children who attend inclusive preschool settings versus segregated classes (Rafferty, Piscitelli, & Boettcher, 2003). The topic is difficult to tackle because of the wide variation in the nature and intensity of inclusive practices. Inclusion can mean anything from minimal participation in a regular classroom with pullouts for therapy to a total time in the regular classroom with push-ins for therapy. Variations also include the use of personal aides versus classroom aides versus no specific support person. Given the variation in children and education programs, health (or in this case, education) services research methods may be the most appropriate methodology to study the question. Moreover, given possible differences in which practices are best for which children, a research network, perhaps composed of schools or school districts, would allow an adequate sample size to evaluate subgroups.

Another issue of major importance relates to recommended restrictions on school attendance in the aftermath of medical illness or surgical procedures. For example, many clinicians restrict a child's participation in school or the community after heart surgery. The physicians and their team justify their recommendations on the basis of the child's increased susceptibility to infection or injury. However, if a child has siblings or friends who visit, it is not clear how much additional risk it might be to go to school. The issue is further complicated by family beliefs, values, and preferences. Some families want their child to return quickly to a full and active life, whereas others are concerned about safety and healing. To establish whether early reintroduction to school and community compromises health status, it might be possible to study medication use or rehospitalization rates for those children who reintegrated quickly versus those who remained at home for a longer period of time, equating for their health status at the conclusion of the treatment.

Contribution

Children achieve contribution when they can participate; remain involved; and give back to their families, schools, and communities. An important part of a research agenda is to establish what health care practices and delivery systems support and encourage contribution. The specific nature of the contribution may vary in relation to the child's age, developmental stage, abilities, interests, and preferences. Because of the heterogeneity of contributions, especially across ages or clinical conditions, determining the appropriate outcome measures for a research study may be challenging. It is particularly important to choose outcome measures that demonstrate change that is meaningful for the individual or family. Standardized measures may not match the individual's target objectives for treatment, and changes may be missed when they are slow or within a stable context.

Goal Attainment Scaling Goal attainment scaling is a measurement strategy to overcome the limitations of choosing a single set of measures for a diverse population or for diverse outcomes of a single population. It measures the extent to which explicit individual goals or target outcomes are met. Those target outcomes can vary widely and yet be included within the same analysis (Steenbeek, Gorter, Ketelaar, Galama, & Lindeman, 2011). Reporters can include therapists, family members, or individuals. The goals must be clearly defined and measurable and should also be highly related to the individual's contribution. The original design for the measure was a 5-point scale, with zero indicating no change, negative scores reflecting deterioration or less progress than anticipated, and positive scores indicating greater achievement than was anticipated. The number of points on the ordinal scale can vary if more precision is desirable and measurable. This measurement approach has been found to be sensitive to detecting change in activity and participation, two of the major components of function in the International Classification of Functioning, Disability and Health (ICF) (Steenbeek, Ketelaar, Galama, & Gorter, 2007). However, the psychometric properties of goal attainment scaling, particularly for children with disabilities, needs further research (Steenbeek et al., 2007)

Functional Measures Another approach to the assessment of contribution is to measure function. In fact, a report to the President and to Congress on comparative effectiveness research related to disability emphasized that functional abilities and quality of life should be included as outcome measures in all research studies (Federal Coordinating Council for Comparative Effectiveness Research, 2009). As discussed in Chapter 7, many functional measures are currently available. They have been studied from a psychometric perspective and have met high standards for reliability and validity. They include measures such as the Vineland Adaptive Behavior Scales, Second Edition (Sparrow, Cicchetti, & Balla, 2005) and the Pediatric Evaluation of Disability Inventory (Haley, Coster, Ludlow, Haltiwanger, & Andrellos, 1992). As discussed in Chapter 7 from a clinical perspective, these measures have the advantage of evaluating a child's performance in the real world and therefore have distinct advantages over IQ and other standardized, norm-referenced measures.

Patient-Reported Functional Measures The National Institutes of Health promotes a new approach to assessment, designed to reduce the fragmentation that results from discipline-specific clinical and outcome measurement. The concept is to promote the use of common, publicly available, patient-reported outcomes that address a range of functional areas ("Promis: Dynamic Tools," n.d.). This initiative builds and validates instruments to measure function, as well as emotions and perceptions applicable to a wide range of conditions. Pediatric measures have also been analyzed for use by older children themselves or by parents as the child's representative.

This development of patient-reported outcomes is highly welcome. First, patient-reported outcomes are consistent with patient- and family-centered care. The methodology recognizes that the individual who receives the care, or in the case of pediatrics, a representative who knows the child intimately, is in the best position to assess the outcomes of an intervention. Second, the measures are scientifically evaluated for psychometric properties, such as reliability and validity (Cella et al., 2007). Thus, the availability of the measures in the public domain saves individual researchers the time, effort, and expense of developing measures for their own studies. Importantly, the item banks allow for the comparisons of different conditions, treatments, or environments because the outcomes can be linked to common data elements. Third, the measures are scaled to cover a broad range of health outcomes (Cella et al., 2010). This feature means that researchers can use the same instruments for evaluations that cover a wide range of disorders and functional outcomes. Finally, after the rigorous scientific evaluation, the measures are placed in the public domain so that multiple researchers, clinicians, and patients can use them within their practices ("Promis: Dynamic Tools," n.d.). This approach, using common measures and item banks to assess functional outcomes and quality of life, is catching on for specific issues, such as the outcomes of neurological disorders ("Neuro-QOL: Quality of Life," n.d.). Because they free researchers from the obligation to create and evaluate outcome measures for each study, these common functional measures should prove a boon to health services research.

Primacy of Participation Among all of the potential functional domains that could be measured, the most important fall under the heading of participation in the ICF. Within that domain are interpersonal interactions and relationships; major life areas (education and employment); and community, social, and civic life. Children with disabilities may have strengths or difficulties in their abilities to learn, handle tasks, communicate, get around, or take care of themselves. They may differ in their general or specific cognitive abilities. However, if they can enter into meaningful relationships, progress through school, get a job they want, enjoy leisure, attend a place of worship if desired, and vote as they choose, they have achieved inclusion and participation. Therefore, in the design of research studies, the most important outcome measures, whether assessed by professionals or patient-reported, are indices of participation. Here are some examples:

- *Spina bifida*: Studies to evaluate the care of children with spina bifida might compare the early use of wheelchairs versus prolonged use of braces and crutches. One potential outcome would be children's mobility; which method allows them to navigate through home, school, or community most effectively? However, participation measures might also include interpersonal interactions with peers, progress through school, and success at obtaining employment.
- *Hearing impairment*: Studies to evaluate the education of children with hearing impairment could evaluate strictly oral versus oral–sign combination

approaches on ultimate abilities of the child to communicate verbally and nonverbally. Again, what is critical is the child's ability to make and keep friends and his or her academic or occupational success.

Function-Focused Care and Multiaxial Plans

The evaluation of the recommended practices in the earlier chapters (Chapters 7 and 8) is also appropriate for rigorous research efforts. Here one important question would be whether explicit attention on function changes health care practices. Would the health care team that created a multiaxial plan (MAP) and had it available at visits be more likely to identify community-based services than a team without benefit of the plan? Another question would be whether use of MAPs led to attention to diverse health care issues that would have been missed otherwise. Research questions like these are often addressed at the process level; the focus is on whether the MAPs were implemented and how satisfied clinicians or families and children were with their implementation. The next steps are to evaluate the approach in relation to functional outcomes of the child and family.

DISSEMINATION OF RESEARCH RESULTS

Completing high-quality research studies may be a necessary step in the evolution of improving health care and health care delivery for children with disabilities and their families. However, to meet the goals of changing health care delivery, research findings must be disseminated to the appropriate audiences, and these audiences must then change as a function of what they learn. Dissemination has its own challenges. It is a complex process to get information to all of the appropriate stakeholders, including other scientists, clinicians, public health officials, public policy makers, and the public at large (Rabin, Brownson, Kerner, & Glasgow, 2006).

Commentary
Dissemination of Findings from the Child Development/Otitis Media Studies

The results of the randomized trial of tympanostomy tubes for otitis media were published in the New England Journal of Medicine, *a highly prestigious and highly read journal (Paradise et al., 2001, 2005, 2007). In the aftermath, practice guidelines for the management of otitis media with effusion were modified to recommend a delay with watchful waiting before the placement of tympanostomy tubes (American Academy of Family Physicians, American Academy of Otolaryngology—Head and Neck Surgery, & American Academy of Pediatrics Subcommittee on Otitis Media with Effusion, 2004). However, many opinion leaders remained unconvinced (Ruben, 2008) and offered weak arguments to denigrate the findings (Paradise, 2009). We frequently hear about children who had tympanostomy tubes placed for the purposes of improving their developmental outcomes, despite a plethora of data indicating that the surgical procedure does not alter outcomes in otherwise healthy children. This experience has reinforced the importance of addressing how to disseminate findings in order to change clinical practices explicitly rather than waiting for the field to come around on its own.*

(See the commentary on p. 219.) Three pathways for the dissemination and diffusion of information have been proposed (Owen, Glanz, Sallis, & Kelder, 2006):

1. Direct to practice: In this approach tool kits and other exportable packages support the new approach. Opinion leaders promote the use of the tool kits with practitioners.
2. Policy to practice: Evidence-based practices are embedded in health improvement policies within a system or community.
3. Diffusion research: The diffusion of information to various audiences can itself become the focus of experimental study: What methods accelerate the diffusion process and persuade stakeholders to try new approaches to adopt evidence-based practices? Studies address the impact of different dissemination efforts on the diffusion of the concepts, contributing further knowledge to the scientific and public community.

Research groups and networks are now considering the dissemination and diffusion of information simultaneously with the research studies they conduct. At the time of this writing, it remains to be seen whether a focus on dissemination indeed speeds progress in health care and health care delivery for children with disabilities.

CONCLUSIONS

Scientific research has become, over the last century, the foundation of medicine, health care practices, and health care delivery. The gold standard for research studies has been the RCT, in which participants who meet rigorous inclusion and exclusion criteria are randomly assigned to receive treatments or a treatment and a placebo but are treated in every other way as similarly as possible. Because of the design features of the RCT, researchers can readily interpret differences in the outcomes of the treatment groups, positive or negative, as a function of their treatment. Although this study design may be ideal for evaluating efficacy, it does not describe how the treatment works in the real world. In addition, it is challenging in many clinical situations and impractical for many other situations, especially to study health care delivery or financing, to use the clinical trial methodology. Health services research is a broad term that encompasses many different experimental designs that allows researchers to evaluate treatments and health care delivery in the real world. These studies must be rigorously designed and carefully interpreted because they are more susceptible to bias than other designs. Nonetheless, they propel the field toward evidence-based practice.

Research networks, including DBPNet, have coalesced to speed up the process of scientific evaluation of treatment and health care delivery. The research agenda for the future must evaluate health care treatments and approaches from the perspective of inclusion and contribution. Functional measures are preferable to standardized assessments to capture contribution or function. The National Institutes of Health have further encouraged and facilitated research by making available to the public banks of outcome measures from the patient perspective that have been evaluated for their psychometric properties. With the networks in place and the tools in hand, researchers interested in improving the care of children with disabilities are poised to make important contributions. While they conduct high-quality studies, they must also pay attention to how the results will be disseminated in order to make the most of their findings.

Exercises

1. Design a study to address the controversies surrounding the use of sensory integration therapy for young children with autism. What study design would you choose? What are the advantages and disadvantages of an RCT? How could the issue be addressed using health services methods? Who should be the participants or subjects? What is the best outcome measure? How would you ensure that the treatments offered in different sites are comparable?
2. Critique a study that compared physical therapy and infant stimulation in the care of children with the spastic diplegia variant of cerebral palsy (Palmer et al., 1988). The study found that routine use of physical therapy in these children conferred no advantages over infant stimulation. What are the strengths and the weaknesses of the study design? How would you design a study to follow up on this report?
3. Investigate research networks for your discipline. How many do you find? Who are members? How many are interdisciplinary in nature?
4. Evaluate the Neuro-QOL measure banks for pediatrics. The banks include questions on social relations with peers and adults, pain, fatigue, depression, applied cognition, anxiety, and anger. How do these domains map to the ICF? If you wanted to choose three of these measures to document outcomes of a new educational program for children with fragile X syndrome, which domains would you choose and why?
5. The National Center on Shaken Baby Syndrome (www.dontshake.org) wants to disseminate information about babies crying as a strategy to reduce the prevalence of traumatic head injury in infancy and the resulting disability. Who do you think they should target as their audience? What methods have they used? How effective do you think those methods are for getting the message to the target audience? What other possibilities may be available to get information to public health officials and to the public at large?

13

Public Policy

> ### State Child Health Insurance Plan
>
> *In 1993, during the presidency of Bill Clinton, Congress once again decided against universal health insurance for Americans. Many of the individuals who lacked health insurance were children of the working poor whose family income precluded eligibility for Medicaid. For many working adults, converting from an individual to a family insurance plan was too costly, even though a serious illness in one of the children could bankrupt the family. Massachusetts had initiated a successful program to enroll such children into health insurance plans. Senator Ted Kennedy from Massachusetts decided to push a federal initiative to do the same, paying for the increased coverage with a tax on tobacco. First Lady Hillary Clinton had a similar proposal that had been part of the failed effort at universal health insurance. Senator Kennedy, a staunch Democrat, was able to entice Orrin Hatch, a Republican senator from Utah, to cosponsor the legislation. In line with conservative principles, they designed the program as a block grant to the states rather than as an entitlement. The first effort to get the bill passed was defeated in part because the president failed to support it, citing an agreement with Republicans to maintain a balanced budget. However, Kennedy and Hatch revived their efforts with increased public support. The bill, the State Children's Health Insurance Act, passed in both houses of Congress as part of the Balanced Budget Act of 1997 (PL 105-33) and was signed into law by President Clinton.*

Public policy has been a necessary tool in the evolution toward inclusion, contribution, and health for children and adults with disabilities. Public policy becomes an appropriate strategy for change when issues or problems cannot be satisfactorily addressed at the individual, community, or systems level. The challenge to addressing problems through public policy is that any changes in laws or regulations require a consensus about the problem to be addressed and the remedies to be applied to that problem. Achieving that consensus within the political process is itself an arduous task, and the remedies available for addressing problems are limited. Government can fund programs, issue regulations, and penalize infractions. Such approaches, although effective, do not necessarily change attitudes, engender confidence, or identify improved solutions. And then, if politicians choose the funding mechanism, they must forge a consensus on how to raise those funds! (See the commentary below.)

The opening vignette demonstrates the challenges of creating public policy in the establishment of the State Children's Health Insurance Act. It might seem that reaching consensus that all children should have access to health insurance and health care would be easy and straightforward. However, various constituencies put different values on the relative importance of children's access to health care and limited interference with private insurance markets. Creating the consensus in that instance required an agreement between Ted Kennedy, Democratic senator from Massachusetts, and Orrin Hatch, Republican senator from Utah. Even after the two cosponsored the bill, additional political considerations delayed its passage. The bill was ultimately ratified as part of the Budget Reconciliation of 1997 rather than as a stand-alone act because of the dynamic push and pull of different constituencies.

This chapter includes a sampling of the public policies that have promoted inclusion, contribution, and health of individuals with disabilities. Some of these policies have been mentioned in previous chapters. Here, they are included to illustrate the role of policy in transforming our society and health care system. In each case, I offer a simplified statement of the problem the law addresses and the

Commentary
National Defense

To appreciate the role of public policy, consider an entirely different arena: national defense. When it comes to defending the country from threats beyond our border, it is not difficult to create a consensus that the federal approach is more appropriate than an individual, community, or state solution. Beyond that simple agreement, however, controversy arises. Different constituencies define the problems differently, often in relation to their own interests as well as to the general good. Some consider that the greatest threat to U.S. security comes from our Cold War enemies, like Russia, and therefore advocate for conventional and nuclear weapons. Others consider the greatest threat to be from terrorist organizations operating outside of governmental controls and therefore advocate for small weapons and strategies to reduce the influence of the terrorists in the countries where they live. These two constituency groups thus have very different solutions to addressing the same problem, national defense. The competing constituencies debate how much to spend and how to balance spending among expensive conventional weapons, surveillance equipment, personnel, and strategies for isolating terrorists. To be responsible, they must also indicate how they will raise the necessary funds to pay for national defense. Because the circumstances are apt to change, policies need frequent review and updating. The defense budget before September 11, 2001, was very different from the defense budget in the following years.

solutions it offers. (See the commentary below.) Limitations of the legislation itself or unforeseen consequences of implementation have, in some instances, led to subsequent efforts to amend and improve the legislation. The final legislation discussed is the Patient Protection and Affordable Care Act of 2010 (PL 111-148) because of its important implications for health and health care of children and adults with disabilities. However, many of the provisions have yet to be enacted, and their ultimate impact cannot yet be evaluated.

The chapter concludes with policy recommendations to encourage a new model of care for children with disabilities and their families. Readers should consider what problems remain despite these policies and how the remaining issues could be appropriately handled. Are we doing enough to promote a welcoming inclusive society? If not, how could policy improve the situation? Are we actively supporting individuals of all ages to make contributions to family, school, work, and community? If not, what else could be done? Can we shift the priorities of health care delivery from institutions to individuals? How can we integrate health and social support?

POLICIES LEADING TO INCLUSION

In the 19th and early- to mid-20th centuries, some U.S. states were in the business of segregation. They ran large state hospitals for individuals with severe mental and emotional disorders and for individuals with intellectual and developmental

Commentary
Combating Autism Act and Its Reauthorization

Beginning in the late 1990s and escalating in 2000s, public attention was transfixed on the skyrocketing rates of autism in the United States. All of the major weekly magazines featured cover stories about children with autism and their families. The Centers for Disease Control and Prevention had dramatic graphs documenting the increase. At the time, a lingering worry was that autism was caused by vaccinations given routinely to children between birth and 4 years of age. Advocacy groups for children with autism, such as Autism Speaks, were extremely effective at transmitting a sense of urgency to understanding increasing prevalence of the condition and the challenges of raising a child with the condition.

Congress responded. Senator Christopher Dodd, a Democrat from Connecticut, and Senator Rick Santorum, a Republican from Pennsylvania, introduced a bill into the Senate, which passed unanimously. In the House of Representatives, Congresswomen Mary Bono, a Republican from California, and Diana DeGette, a Democrat from Colorado, introduced similar legislation. President George W. Bush signed the bill into law, and it remains the largest investment in a single condition in U.S. history.

The Combating Autism Act (PL 109-416) allocated approximately $950 million to autism programs over 5 years. The funding addressed multiple aspects of the issue: public awareness and education, research into screening measures, training of professionals to screen and diagnose autism, increased spending for biomedical research in autism, and reliance on evidence-based treatments. To accomplish these objectives, the Secretary of Health and Human Services directed funds to existing government agencies and programs rather than create new agencies or programs.

disabilities. Although these institutions may have originated with good intentions, to protect people with disabilities from a cruel and unforgiving society, they later evolved to protect society from those individuals with disabilities.

Several factors occasioned a total reevaluation and repudiation of these policies. In the mid-20th century, the prevailing philosophy began to shift as families, educators, and professionals came to recognize that it was better to treat individuals with severe mental illness or disability near their families, employment opportunities, and natural communities than in removed and segregated settings (Talbot, 2004). The introduction of psychotropic medications reduced many of the symptoms of severe mental illness, particularly of schizophrenia, and supported the shifting philosophy. The leadership of President John F. Kennedy and his family, notably Eunice Kennedy Shriver (Chapter 4), was essential in this shift in approach. As siblings of an individual with a disability, they intimately understood the needs of individuals with these disorders.

Mental Retardation Facilities and Community Mental Health Centers Construction Act of 1963

The Mental Retardation Facilities and Community Mental Health Centers Construction Act of 1963 (PL 88-164) was passed under the leadership of President Kennedy shortly before his assassination. Its main goal was to provide alternatives to institutionalization for both individuals with intellectual and developmental disabilities and with severe mental health disorders. In the words of the legislation, the purpose of the act was

> To provide assistance in combating mental retardation through grants for construction of research centers and grants for facilities for the mentally retarded and assistance in improving mental health through grants for construction of community mental health centers, and for other purpose. (Mental Retardation Facilities and Community Mental Health Centers Construction Act of 1963, p. 1)

Centers of research and training about intellectual and developmental disabilities began to build an infrastructure and workforce to support individuals with disabilities in community settings. Facilities were indeed constructed, and funding continued in support of research, education, and service programs. Major programs that are the direct descendants of the original statute include the following:

1. The University Centers for Excellence in Developmental Disabilities Education, Research, and Service (UCEDD) programs share a vision that all Americans, including those with disabilities, should participate fully in their communities. They design programs and projects to encourage independence, productivity, and community inclusion for individuals from childhood through adulthood. There is a UCEDD in every state and territory, and they are associated with universities in that region (http://www.aucd.org).

2. Leadership Education in Neurodevelopmental Disabilities (LEND) programs focus on providing graduate level interdisciplinary training to improve the health of infants, children, and adolescents with disabilities. The focus shifted from strictly clinical to leadership training in 1995, in recognition that once a large cadre of professionals from a wide range of disciplines had been successfully

prepared for clinical roles, leadership would be required to maintain a dynamic and responsive approach to disabilities.

3. Developmental Disabilities Councils were created in every state by the amendments of 1970, which required states to create an advisory council to describe and assess the quality and extent of services and to recommend how funds could be used to augment available services.
4. The amendments of 1975 required the establishment of protection and advocacy programs to protect the rights of individuals with disabilities and pursue legal, administrative, and other remedies for that purpose.

The funding for community mental health centers was designed to stimulate the process of transferring individuals from segregated state hospitals and institutions into community settings. This policy did not bring immediate success; the aftermath of the initial waves of deinstitutionalization was chaotic. Many communities lacked the resources and expertise to assist individuals who had not lived outside of the institutions for most of their lives. The results included a rise in homelessness; arrests of former institution residents; and transfers of former state hospital patients to nursing homes, smaller but nonetheless segregated settings at the other extreme (Talbot, 2004). These unfavorable results revealed the lack of planning and research to guide the deinstitutionalization process, as well as the fragility of the consensus that state hospitals could be closed without incident (Talbot, 2004). Unfortunately, the communities to which the former patients went did not naturally create the range and variety of services and supports that would have been essential for support of individuals with severe long-term conditions. The services and supports that were available were highly fragmented and difficult to navigate, particularly for individuals with intellectual and emotional problems. In addition, attitudes within the community, an arena not readily changed through public policy, were not uniformly supportive of deinstitutionalization. Negative attitudes and limiting stereotypes provide a logic that sustains discrimination by treating individuals with disabilities as unwanted. (See the commentary below.)

Commentary
State Laws

State laws, like their federal counterparts, are key to securing the rights of children and adults with disabilities. In California, the Lanterman Developmental Disabilities Services Act (AB 846), now known simply as the Lanterman Act, passed in 1969. Recognizing the profound impact on the lives of individuals, family members, and community, and determining that disability represents a social, medical, economic, and legal problem of high importance, the law establishes an entitlement for individuals with disabilities. It states that "people with developmental disabilities and their families have a right to get the services and supports they need to live like people without disabilities" (http://www.lanterman.org/lanterman_act).

The act established the Department of Developmental Services, a statewide department within the Health and Welfare Agency. The Department of Developmental

Services established 21 regional centers, nonprofit corporations that contract with the Department of Developmental Services to provide or coordinate services and supports for individuals with developmental disabilities. These regional centers are the local resources to help individuals with disabilities and their families find and access services and supports.

It is possible to see the problems with the current system of care for individuals with disabilities. However, the Lanterman Act protections are so strong that most advocates shy away from any discussions about reforming the law.

Americans with Disabilities Act

The Rehabilitation Act of 1973, Section 504 played a critical role in enhancing rights for individuals with disabilities by banning discrimination on the basis of disability. This act was a prelude to the more expansive law in support of inclusion, the Americans with Disabilities Act (ADA), originally passed in 1990, and the cornerstone of public policy in support of inclusion. In the wake of the Civil Rights Movement, the Disability Rights Movement linked inclusion to human rights and stimulated a consensus that individuals with disabilities could live and thrive in communities. This act was designed to address the many barriers that limited their full participation. (See the commentary below.)

The purpose of the law as stated in it is as follows (http://www.ada.gov):

1. To provide a clear and comprehensive national mandate for the elimination of discrimination against individuals with disabilities

Commentary
The Work of Ed Roberts

Ed Roberts is affectionately remembered as the father of the disability rights movement. He contracted polio in 1953 at the age of 14. After 18 months in the hospital, he returned home with flaccid paralysis of his whole body, save some movement in two fingers of his left hand. He used an iron lung to breathe at night and learned to swallow air into his lungs if he got into trouble during the day. Rather than acquiesce to social restrictions, prejudice, and limiting stereotypes, rather than commit suicide though he considered it actively, he found the will to fight for a high school diploma and for admission to the University of California at Berkeley. He was the first student with severe disabilities to earn a B.A. at Cal and then went on to earn an M.A. Mr. Roberts assumed leadership for the fledgling Berkeley Center of Independent Living, the first independent living service and advocacy program run by and for people with disabilities. Under his leadership, the center went through a period of rapid growth and emerged as the model for a community organization designed to support and advocate for individuals with a wide range of disabilities. His personal message was that individuals, regardless of the severity of their health condition or disability, could take control of their lives, far more so than most people think they can. This ability to guide one's own life is in turn life sustaining (Ed Roberts: 60 Minutes *Segment with Harry Reasoner, n.d.). To learn more about this movement, read* No Pity: People with Disabilities Forging a New Civil Rights Movement *(Shapiro, 1993).*

2. To provide clear, strong, consistent, enforceable standards addressing discrimination against individuals with disabilities
3. To ensure that the Federal Government plays a central role in enforcing the standards established in this chapter on behalf of individuals with disabilities
4. To invoke the sweep of congressional authority, including the power to enforce the fourteenth amendment and to regulate commerce, in order to address the major areas of discrimination faced day-to-day by people with disabilities

The act "prohibits discrimination on the basis of disability in employment, state and local government, public accommodations, commercial facilities, transportation, and telecommunications," and it "also applies to the United States Congress" (U.S. Census Bureau, 2010). By targeting discrimination, the act attempts to change lingering negative attitudes and beliefs about disability.

The act has been responsible for substantial improvements in education attainment and political participation of individuals with disabilities. However, it has not closed the large gaps between people with and without disabilities with regard to employment, household income, access to transportation, health care, socializing, and satisfaction with life (Taylor, Krane, & Orkis, 2010). In addition, the Supreme Court has rendered decisions that limit who is covered under ADA. Individuals whose functional impairment can be eradicated by medication, for example, had been deemed not eligible for protections from the ADA by the courts. Reauthorization of the ADA took place in 2008. In an effort to restore the original intent of the law, the definition of disability was changed. Under the amendments that became effective on January 1, 2009, the determination of whether a person has an impairment that substantially limits a major life activity (a disability in the legal sense under the ADA) must be made without regard to the beneficial effects of a mitigating action, such as taking medication. In addition, the amendments require that the disability has to limit only one major life activity.

As of this writing, the full impact of these amendments is not yet clear. One important reason is that since the mid-2000s, the United States has been experiencing a major recession. The state of the economy has affected individuals with and without disabilities. However, the recession has had particular negative impacts on individuals with disabilities and their families. High unemployment creates additional barriers to individuals with disabilities finding good paying jobs. Decreasing state support for education has meant increasing tuitions for higher education, and other safety net programs are under threat. Nongovernmental supports and services have been strained to keep up with the increased demand for food, housing, clothing, and other supports. The changing socioeconomic context and its differential impact on different sectors of the society is a stark reminder that public policy must be constantly evaluated to achieve the desired effects.

POLICIES PROMOTING CONTRIBUTION

How can public policy promote the ability of individuals with disabilities to make meaningful contributions to their community? One approach is to support employment opportunities for individuals with disabilities and the vocational training or rehabilitation that prepares them for that employment. Two additional approaches that are pertinent to children are to 1) ensure that all children with disabilities get an appropriate education that provides them with opportunities as students and prepares them for contribution as adults, and 2) ensure that the appropriate services and supports are available to allow individuals with disabilities to live and work in their home community.

Individuals with Disabilities Education Act (PL 94-142 and Amendments)

This groundbreaking federal legislation was stimulated by many problems that were articulated in section 601 of the original act (20 U.S.C. 1401 89 STAT 774), using language that we now find unacceptable:

1. There are more than eight million handicapped children in the United States today.
2. The special educational needs of such children are not being fully met.
3. More than half of the handicapped children in the United States do not receive appropriate educational services which would enable them to have full equality of opportunity.
4. One million of the handicapped children in the United States are excluded entirely from the public school system and will not go through the educational process with their peers.
5. There are many handicapped children throughout the United States participating in regular school programs whose handicaps prevent them from having a successful educational experience because their handicaps are undetected.
6. Because of the lack of adequate services within the public school system, families are often forced to find services outside the public school system, often at great distance from their residence and at their own expense.
7. Developments in the training of teachers and in diagnostic and instructional procedures and methods have advanced to the point, given appropriate funding, state and local educational agencies can and will provide effective special educational and related services to meet the needs of handicapped children.
8. State and local educational agencies have a responsibility to provide education for all handicapped children, but present financial resources are inadequate to meet the special educational needs of handicapped children.
9. It is in the national interest that the federal government assists state and local efforts to provide programs to meet the educational needs of handicapped children in order to assure equal protection of the law.

On the basis of this need, the purposes of the Education for All Handicapped Children Act of 1975 were as follows (U.S. Department of Education, 2007):

(1) "to assure that all children with disabilities have available to them...a free appropriate public education which emphasizes special education and related services designed to meet their unique needs"
(2) "to assure that the rights of children with disabilities and their parents...are protected"
(3) "to assist States and localities to provide for the education of all children with disabilities"
(4) "to assess and assure the effectiveness of efforts to educate all children with disabilities"

So, the strategies used in this legislation included establishing standards and providing funding.

The act has been amended on multiple occasions and was reauthorized as the Individuals with Disabilities Education Act (IDEA) in 1990. One of the major amendments in 1986 lowered the age of eligibility for special education from 6 to 3 years old. In addition, that amendment offered states funding for the provision of early intervention services to children from birth to 3 years of age. In many ways, it was a transformational act. (See the commentary below.)

As a result of IDEA, approximately 200,000 infants and toddlers and their families receive early intervention services, and close to 6 million children and youth receive special education and related services (U.S. Department of Education, 2007). Other accomplishments are as follows (U.S. Department of Education, 2007):

- The majority of children with disabilities are now educated in their neighborhood schools in regular classrooms with peers who have no apparent disabilities.

Commentary
Differences Among States in the Provision of Early Intervention

Federal law established early intervention services for children from birth to 3 years of age in 1986. However, the law provided only broad standards. It gave states the responsibility for determining the lead agency for the process, the eligibility criteria, and the nature of services. States vary widely in all of those features of early intervention. These features make a difference in the utilization of the services (McManus et al., 2009; Rosenberg, Zhang, & Robinson, 2008). Moreover, vast differences in procedures may even affect providers whose role it is to refer children to early intervention.

When I lived in Allegheny County, Pennsylvania, I had a close relationship with the early intervention providers. If I identified a child I considered eligible for services on the basis of developmental delays in domains of function, I picked up the telephone and called the local agency. They accepted my referral and proceeded to contact the family for an official intake. As far as I know, almost all of those referrals resulted in services to the child and family. I certainly received a call when there were problems, such as when the agency could not contact the referred family.

When I arrived in Santa Clara County, California, I was struck by the differences in the organization and tone of early intervention. In California, the agency overseeing the process, the regional centers, required a written form and a medical record to initiate the process. They had on staff physicians and psychologists who reviewed and often redid the evaluations. I received many calls and complaints that children failed to meet the eligibility criterion. In one case, I was incredulous. I asked the early intervention intake administrator whether they found that that child was in fact normal. Oh no, she explained, the child had a 31% delay where the eligibility criterion was a 33% delay. I don't think that she took into account the standard error of the mean on developmental testing. In another case the physician challenged my diagnosis of autism because the child had qualitative impairments in social interactions and communication, but according to the doctor, no repetitive behaviors. I noted that I reported the child obsessively opened and shut doors. The physician dismissed this behavior as typical.

- High school graduation rates and employment rates among youth with disabilities have increased dramatically. For example, graduation rates increased by 14% from 1984 to 1997. Postschool employment rates for youth served under IDEA are twice those of older adults with similar disabilities who did not have the benefit of IDEA.
- Postsecondary school enrollment rates among individuals with disabilities receiving IDEA services have increased. For example, the percentage of college freshmen reporting disabilities has more than tripled since 1978.

The challenge of providing special education remains inadequate funding. The difference in per-student expenditures varies by state and by special education category. On average, it costs about twice as much to provide special education to children with disabilities as it does to provide general education to children with no apparent disabilities (Parrish, 2006). Although the federal government originally promised to support up to 40% of the expenses of special education, its contribution is actually below 10%. The rest of the funding comes from local and state sources; the proportions vary by location (Parrish, 2006). Since the original passage of the legislation, enrollment in special education has risen sharply, and this increase has put strain on education budgets across the nation. The economic downturn of the late 2000s resulted in decreased state revenues and corresponding high pressure on states to reduce their education budgets. Teachers have been laid off in many states and communities, and class size has risen as a result. The rules for eligibility and service provision have been modified in many locations. (See the commentary below.)

The economic events of the last few years are likely to occasion another re-evaluation of federal and state education law. Ongoing policy evaluations are necessary to establish whether short-term reductions in education expenses are associated with adverse long-term consequences, such as reductions in state tax revenues or increased demand for other state services, including juvenile justice. It will be interesting to see whether the public defines inadequate or unpredictable funding for education as a problem worthy of new public policy.

Commentary
Changes in Eligibility and Programming for Children with Disabilities in California Since 2009

In the summer of 2009, after Jerry Brown was elected Governor of California, the state remained in dire financial trouble. Early intervention programs came on the chopping block to reduce state expenses. While the state remained in compliance with IDEA Part C, the scope of services became restricted. Here is a summary of the changes:

1. *Children at risk on the basis of biomedical factors such as birth weight less than 1,500 grams or central nervous system injury were no longer deemed eligible.*
2. *The criterion for significant delay for children less than 24 months of age became 33% delay in one or more areas whereas previously it had been 33% in one area or 25% delay in two or more areas.*

3. *The criteria for children between 24 and 36 months of age became 50% delay in one area or 33% in two or more areas. This standard means that a child who at age 2 can speak only two or three words may not meet eligibility criteria for service.*
4. *Parents are required to apply their private health insurance for all medical services other than evaluation and assessment. Only after they exhaust their coverage is the child eligible to receive funding through the regional center.*

The long-term impact of these changes has yet to be determined. However, the net result is to delay or deny services to the very children who are most likely to benefit quickly, those with mild delays. It will take several years to evaluate whether high eligibility criteria for early intervention leads to higher enrollment in special education services, a service more costly to the state.

Community Living Assistance Services and Supports Act

For many individuals with severe disabilities, the possibility of becoming a contributing member of their community requires that they receive appropriate supports and services. Medicaid has traditionally had a bias toward funding institutions. The problem is that this bias is a barrier to individuals who would prefer to live and work in their communities with the needed support rather than in nursing homes or other institutional settings. Institutions are also a more expensive option than community-based services. Title III, Subsection E of the Patient Protection and Affordable Care Act includes many provisions related to improving long-term services and supports for people with disabilities of all ages to allow home-and community-based services to replace institutional care (Association of Centers of Excellence on Disabilities, 2010). These provisions increase the individual's ability to live in the community and thereby encourage contribution and independence. On the basis of the specific provisions that a state chooses to implement, it either assumes responsibility for providing these supports and services or oversees their provision. In any case, the state reaps the benefits of reduced expenditures.

The act also includes a Title VIII that creates a new national long-term care insurance program, the Community Living Assistance Services and Supports (CLASS) Act. The purpose of this provision is to help adults who have or develop functional impairments to remain independent, employed, and engaged in their community. The impact of these provisions must be evaluated once the full act is implemented.

POLICIES IMPROVING ACCESS AND QUALITY OF HEALTH CARE

Access to health care requires adequate health insurance. Health insurance is simply a contract in which people pay regular premiums with the expectation that should they become ill, the insurer will pay their health care costs. In the United States, the debate about compulsory, universal health insurance has been raging for almost a century. During that time, health care has changed substantially in terms of what it offers and how much it costs. Because of the shifting conditions, the debate goes on.

Origins of Health Insurance

In the late 19th and early 20th centuries, health insurance in America originated from "sickness insurance" (Thomasson, 2003). At that time, health care costs were relatively modest, as physician capacity was limited and health care was delivered primarily in the home. However, wages lost as a result of illness could be substantial. Sickness insurance provided supplementary income to the insured individual, similar to modern disability insurance. The name changed to health insurance when the British coined the term in their National Insurance Act of 1911.

In the early 20th century, efforts to introduce compulsory, universal health insurance coverage never took root in the United States because health care costs were low and organizations, such as the American Medical Association, strongly resisted any efforts to interfere with physician salaries and doctor–patient relationships. As the century progressed, the demand for medical care increased, the site of care shifted to hospitals, and the costs of care skyrocketed.

In 1929, the beginning of the Great Depression, a group of Dallas-based teachers formed a partnership with an area hospital to provide a set amount of sickness and hospitalization days in exchange for a fixed, prepaid fee. This model became popular during the Great Depression because it was mutually beneficial to patients and to hospitals during difficult economic times. The American Hospital Association encouraged other hospitals to develop similar plans in order to provide a steady source of income. However, individual hospitals and community care organizations then began competing with one another for such plans. To avoid the corrosive effect of competition, the American Hospital Association assisted hospitals in joining together to create Blue Cross (Thomasson, 2003). Subsequently, physicians organized their own prepaid plans, under the label of Blue Shield. Under voluntary health insurance and Blue Shield, doctors retained the ability to require patients to pay the difference between their costs and what they were reimbursed from Blue Shield. Fueling the development of these private insurance plans was the decision to exempt employer and employee contributions to health plans from income tax under the 1954 Internal Revenue Code (Thomasson, 2003). By 1960, approximately 75% of Americans had voluntary health insurance. For most Americans, employers provide health insurance to their employees and their dependents, whereas in other industrialized countries, the government guarantees health care or health insurance.

Medicare and Medicaid

In the 1960s, Congress recognized that two groups who did not benefit from employer-provided health insurance were the elderly and the poor. In 1965, following the landslide victory of President Lyndon Johnson and an overwhelmingly Democratic Congress, Congress enacted two health insurance plans: Medicare and Medicaid. Medicare provides compulsory hospital insurance for people over the age of 65, as well as subsidized medical insurance. Medicaid provides care for low-income people, although the federal–state program varies across state lines according to each state's relative per-capita income.

Medicaid provides health insurance to approximately 60 million Americans, of whom 30 million are children. It insures 40% of all births and one in three children (Kaiser Commission, 2011). The benefits package for children includes early periodic screening, diagnosis, and treatment. This comprehensive approach encourages screening for health and developmental disabilities, preventive and early intervention services for conditions detected through screening, diagnostic services, and treatments to correct or improve acute and long-term physical and mental health conditions. For children with disabilities, Medicaid covers therapies, such as physical and occupational therapy; personal care services; and durable medical equipment, such as wheelchairs, walkers, and hearing aids.

Medicaid also covers approximately 8 million people with disabilities. Most of these individuals would be unable to obtain private health insurance in the private market for one of several reasons: they may not work and therefore are unable to access employer-based health insurance or they may be rejected by insurance plans because of their condition. Insurance companies actively try to avoid adding beneficiaries for whom the cost of care is high. Even when individuals with disabilities are able to obtain private health insurance, the plans often do not cover the services they need, including long-term services and supports, such as personal care assistance, transportation, or durable medical equipment. The services Medicaid covers enable many individuals with disabilities to work.

Medicaid is an important safety net for Americans. It is the major funder for health centers and public hospitals that serve the poor and uninsured (Kaiser Commission, 2011). Because it covers one third of children, it is a major source of income for children's hospitals. It provides a substantial proportion of funding for mental health services for children and adults. Physician participation in Medicaid is voluntary. Physician reimbursement rates in Medicaid are poor, far lower than the rates of Medicare. Therefore, many clinicians in private practices choose not to (or cannot afford to) participate in Medicaid, thereby reducing access to services, leading to disparities in outcomes. Medicaid and Medicare are now substantial components of the federal budget.

Even after passage of Medicaid, many children who lived near the poverty line and were ineligible for Medicaid lacked health insurance. The child-specific health program, described in the opening vignette, was an effort to rectify this situation. It lowers the financial eligibility threshold for publicly funded health insurance for children. States were given the latitude in how to achieve the goals, financial eligibility criteria, and program characteristics. Some states chose to create new insurance programs rather than expand Medicaid because of low clinician participation in the Medicaid programs.

Patient Protection and Affordable Care Act

Unlike the situation in the early 20th century, in the beginning of the 21st century, health insurance is essential to American families; it is almost impossible to afford health care without it. A visit to the emergency room may cost hundreds to thousands of dollars. The birth of a baby may cost thousands of dollars, and if the baby is born by Cesarean section, tens of thousands of dollars. Operations and hospitalizations in intensive care might cost tens to hundreds of thousands of dollars. In the United States, medical expenses are a major cause of personal bankruptcy. As a result of the rising costs of health care, the cost of health insurance premiums has also increased dramatically. Many individuals who do not have an employer contribution and need to buy health insurance on their own cannot afford the premiums.

They then go without preventive health maintenance and seek care when a condition is so advanced that care is unavoidable and more costly.

These problems again put the debate over health care and health insurance at the foreground of public policy discussions after the election of Barack Obama in 2008. The problems included high rates of uninsured individuals and high costs of care without concomitant quality. The following were some of the specifics:

1. Over 40 million Americans, including many working people and their dependents, were uninsured. The reasons included that a substantial proportion of small employers failed to offer health insurance, individuals were denied health insurance because of preexisting conditions, and some individuals reached lifetime caps on health care expenditures.
2. Surprisingly, though the United States spent more on health care than any other industrialized nation, Americans did not enjoy the best health outcomes in the world. Basic indicators, such as life expectancy and infant mortality rates, were less favorable in the United States than in other developed and developing countries, including the United Kingdom, Australia, Scandinavia, Singapore, France, Italy, and Japan. What made the situation even more alarming is that those other countries had some form of nationalized health care coverage available to 100% of their total populations.
3. U.S. health care had evolved to ensure rapid access for most elective health procedures and yet had not guaranteed access to preventive measures.
4. The uninsured depended on high-cost emergency room care and then received no follow-up care.
5. Navigating health insurance plans as an individual or representative of a family was extremely challenging. The lack of transparency about what would and would not be covered made it difficult to make sensible decisions for an individual or a family.

The Patient Protection and Affordable Care Act is complex legislation that is designed to address many of these issues. Several provisions that were enacted soon after passage of the law were particularly important to children with disabilities and their families.

- The law provided rules to prevent insurance companies from denying health care insurance coverage to children less than 19 years old on the basis of preexisting conditions. This provision restores health insurance to many children with disabilities.
- The law prohibits insurance companies from imposing limits on the number of dollars an individual receives. Because children with disabilities are likely to accumulate considerable lifetime health care expenses, this provision protects them from reaching an end to their coverage.
- Insurance companies were also banned from rescinding care when people got sick. This provision restored the integrity of the implied contract between the

insurance provider and the enrollee, who anticipated coverage precisely at the time that he or she became sick.

The law also has several provisions to improve the quality of health care for all Americans (Commonwealth Fund, 2011). At the time of this writing, these provisions have yet to be implemented.

- New payment and delivery approaches will encourage payment on the basis of quality rather than volume.
- Medicare is to launch programs that encourage providers to organize into accountable care organizations (Chapter 10), an antidote to the fragmentation and poor coordination among the various health care providers that serve individuals with long-term conditions. They are coalitions of clinicians, hospitals, long-term care facilities, and other health care providers that primarily serve individuals with long-term conditions. Improving communication and coordination of care across the interdisciplinary team and across settings will hopefully reduce errors, lower costs, and improve care (Chapter 8). These organizations will be tested under the new law within Medicare and are likely then to become standards for the health care industry.
- A state option in the Medicaid program is to implement "health homes" for Medicaid beneficiaries with chronic conditions. The health home is an extension of the patient- and family-centered medical home construct discussed in Chapter 9. The model relies on enhanced integration and coordination of primary care, mental and behavioral health, and long-term services and supports. Rather than fees for service, the providers are reimbursed through a per-patient-per-month mechanism (Kaiser Commission, 2012).
- Health care companies and insurers must simplify administrative processes and information exchange to reduce costs. This provision will assist individuals and families in making wise decisions about the health insurance plan for them.
- Benefits packages of essential services are to be defined and available for purchase in statewide exchanges, the equivalent of large group plans that are set up by government rather than by companies. The exchanges will allow individuals or families to buy health insurance at affordable rates, far lower than individual rates in the current commercial insurance market. The packages may have different tiers of benefits and different degrees of cost sharing. Grouping a wide range of individuals and families together in an exchange will allow individuals who otherwise cannot receive employer-based insurance to afford health insurance.
- An independent board is to review payments to identify waste and find savings, particularly in Medicare, although not to approve or deny specific services to individuals.
- Individuals are to be required to carry health insurance, and premium subsidies will help those on limited incomes to afford it.

POLICY ADJUSTMENTS NEEDED FOR THE CARE OF CHILDREN WITH DISABILITIES

In the face of a growing population of children with disabilities and increasing costs for health care for this potentially vulnerable group, the health care system needs a major transformation. What is critical is that these changes improve the quality of care while achieving substantial cost savings. The Affordable Care Act includes many provisions designed to address this pressing public policy issue.

It would take enormous time and space to advocate for a specific mechanism or program. In this section, I articulate principles that should guide any changes in health care insurance and health care delivery rather than propose specific programs. The National Council on Disability has articulated many of these principles in a position paper titled, Successfully Enrolling People with Disabilities in Managed Care Plans: Guiding Principles (National Council on Disability, 2012). The principles derive from the positions proposed throughout this book.

- The focus of health care for children and for adults with disabilities should be their inclusion in community life and should support their contribution to homes, families, schools, and communities (Chapter 4 and 5).
- Health care reform initiatives must ensure family- and person-centered care. The hospital and institutional focus of health insurance from the last century has led to approaches that may or may not meet with individual choice. Health services must be integrated with long-term supports to achieve the outcomes of an individualized family- or person-centered plan.
- Given the critical role of family members in the care of children with disabilities, family members should receive the tools they need to carry out their responsibilities, including information, counseling, training, and support.
- States should be highly prepared before embarking on any major changes, based on a detailed assessment of their capacity and with the active input of representatives of the groups who will be most significantly affected, explicitly including people with disabilities and parents of children with disabilities. The lessons of the deinstitutionalization movement of the 1970s highlight the need for well-designed and efficient community health services. Now that most individuals with developmental disabilities live in the community, any changes should ensure that they remain in their homes and communities.
- In order to achieve savings, institutional care and home- and community-based care should be financed by the same system. Otherwise, provider groups may be tempted to exclude individuals who have the highest care and support costs, leaving as their only recourse being cared for within institutions that would be funded through a different mechanism. This situation throws the system back at least 50 years.

The design of a transformed health care system must find the right balance between hospital and institutional care and among medical costs, habilitation or rehabilitation services, and long-term supports and services. For any given individual, the form and ratio of services and supports must be customized to their needs.

It may be possible, as we improve care delivery, to reduce institutional care to virtually zero. At the same time, the system should not encourage volume through fee-for-service provisions or compromise health by denying or delaying care. Rather, as the Affordable Care Act is attempting, payment must take health outcomes into account.

Care coordination must be a centerpiece to help individuals and families navigate through the system and make wise choices. Chapter 10 emphasized the importance of care coordination for children and families. There is another benefit. In the current arrangement, professionals have an implicit or explicit conflict of interest when they recommend their own services to children and families. A surgeon who recommends an operation benefits financially if the family accepts this recommendation. A physical therapist who evaluates and treats children has a conflict of interest when recommending more physical therapy. Care coordination, if done right, may serve as a check on this conflict of interest. The care coordinator, properly educated about disabilities and their impact, can help families and individuals to evaluate these recommendations. To achieve this role, organizing care coordination within the medical home or health home as opposed to a distinct care coordination structure means that medical considerations and personal preferences can be integrated in the decision-making process. It must be clear that the care coordinators work independently from care organizations, that their role is to serve clients and not to save funds. It also means that the practitioners in the medical or health home may need education about disability in order to effectively discharge this responsibility effectively (Chapters 10 and 11). Education must include the benefits of inclusion and the promises of contribution and must rise beyond the strict medical model of disability (Chapter 3)

The final principle that must be followed in health care reform is that we need to pay for what we value. If we value care coordination, then professional engagement in it must be reimbursed. If we recognize the importance of interdisciplinary team conferences, then these activities, too, need to be reimbursed. If families want to receive time-intensive counseling before making health care decisions, then the time it requires must be reimbursed. If families want to use modern information technology rather than face-to-face visits to connect with clinicians, including telephone, e-mail, and texting, then the time taken for this communication must also be reimbursed. Managed care provides payments to providers in a per-patient-per-month fashion rather than fee-for-service model. This method encourages providers to choose low-cost strategies whenever possible. For managed care to work for individuals with disabilities, reimbursement must also take into account health outcomes and family satisfaction. Without the counterweight of outcomes and satisfaction, providers have no incentive to improve quality, only to reduce costs. A new conflict of interest substitutes for the old.

OPPORTUNITIES FOR ADVOCACY

Health care clinicians from all professional backgrounds should consider becoming advocates for health care reform. *Advocacy* is a broad term that includes representing a group or a position, defining or defending actions, and intervening in ways that support that group or position. Advocacy takes place at the individual level; for example, many clinicians write letters to insurance companies on behalf of children in their practice. Advocacy also takes place at the systems level; for example, clinicians promote changes in their profession or organization to benefit a group of children. Advocacy at the public policy level is important for fashioning the right laws and regulations in support of children with disabilities and their families. Professionals who work with children with disabilities and their families often feel a deep passion about their work. They have accumulated a comprehensive understanding of the issues that this constituency faces. They are committed to contribute to change and may even have creative ideas for reducing barriers and burdens. Their energy and expertise are therefore extremely valuable in systems redesign and new public policies.

A key to successful advocacy in the public policy arena is to work with other individuals, or more importantly, groups and organizations that share the same vision for the future. The coalition is far more powerful than the individual. Because of its size and breadth, the coalition is more likely than the individual to be able to exercise multiple strategies for getting the point of view out.

Several organizations currently speak for children with disabilities and their families. Three different models are as follows:

- *The professional organization*: The American Academy of Pediatrics (AAP) speaks loudly for children and families as well as advocating for pediatricians. Thirty-five pediatricians broke away from the American Medical Association (AMA) in 1930 to form the AAP. The issue that divided the two organizations was their profound differences in the approach to advocacy. The AMA focused narrowly on the doctors, whereas the AAP focused broadly on the patients. The AAP has since grown to a membership of 60,000 pediatricians and has a long track record of championing public policy that benefits the health and welfare of children.
- *Interdisciplinary professional organization*: The Association of University Centers on Disabilities is a network of federally funded programs regarding disabilities, including the LENDs and UCEDDs described earlier. It also includes the developmental-behavioral pediatrics fellowship training programs funded by the Maternal and Child Health Bureau. Its mission is to "advance policy and practice for and with people with developmental and other disabilities, their families, and their communities by supporting our members in research, education, and service activities that achieve our vision" (www.aucd.org).
- *Families and consumers*: Family Voices is an organization that is designed to "to achieve family-centered care for all children and youth with special health care needs and/or disabilities" (Family Voices, 2008). The organization evolved in the aftermath of the introduction of Medicaid waivers to support health and related services for children and adults with disabilities living at home, rather than provide support directly to large, expensive institutions. Family Voices developed a network of experts on Medicaid waivers to train families and professional partners in applying for waivers. The mission then expanded to provide families with "tools to make informed decisions, advocate for improved public and private policies, build partnerships among professionals and families, and serve as a trusted resource on health care" (Family Voices, 2008).

These coalitions and many others like them serve several roles in the public policy arena. They incubate new ideas and approaches in line with their vision for the future, closely monitor public policy to weigh in on the ideas floated by others, and provide information to their membership and galvanize activity as needed.

For emerging professionals either in their preservice phase or early in practice, it may seem difficult to engage in advocacy regarding public policy. However, membership in groups that share a vision for the future allows the student and young clinician to get involved at the level they think possible. Experienced clinicians who serve as teachers and mentors make strong advocates because their clinical, research, or educational experience contributes to their credentials for speaking out on behalf of their patients or clients.

Federal legislation attracts the most attention in the world of public policy. However, it is possible to work at many different levels and stages in the process. Even after federal legislation is passed, regulations must be written and implemented. Therefore, many opportunities for input remain even after passage of a bill. In addition, state-level policies are extremely important, especially for education and social services. Medicaid regulations and implementation occur at the state level, with federal legislation providing only a framework. Counties also have responsibility for many important functions, such as the administration of offices for individuals with intellectual and developmental disabilities and for child abuse and neglect. Opportunities for participation in public policy are vast; the important issue is to get involved.

SUMMARY

Public policy has played a major role in promoting the inclusion of individuals with disabilities within communities and has become a key mechanism for reforming the health care system with goals of improving outcomes while reducing costs. The most recent federal legislation to address health care is the Patient Protection and Affordable Care Act of 2010, a very long and complicated piece of legislation because it addresses two major problems: 1) the large proportion of Americans who lack health insurance in an era in which health insurance buys access to health care, and 2) a mismatch between high expenditures for health care in the United States and mediocre health outcomes in terms of life expectancy, infant mortality, and other basic public health indicators. As of this writing, the full impact of this law has not yet been felt, as the provisions are rolling out gradually.

I encourage the readers of this book to get involved in advocacy efforts that benefit children with disabilities and their families. Although advocacy may involve considerable personal time and effort, that effort is likely to reap benefits for children and families and to engender a sense of personal satisfaction through acting consistently on one's deeply held values. To amplify a message, it makes sense to become a member of an organization or coalition with shared vision and effective organization. The organization may be a professional organization; a network of organizations; or a consortium of families, consumers, and professionals. The ability of like-minded groups to collaborate increases the likelihood that their point of view prevails. The individuals who are affected by these advocacy efforts must be front and center. Disability rights advocates say, "Nothing about me without me."

Well-intentioned professionals and citizens have made many mistakes by deciding what was best for others.

The need to ensure inclusion, contribution, and health for children with disabilities is our shared responsibility.

Exercises

1. Contrast early intervention programs in two states. How do the eligibility criteria compare? What services are provided? What would happen if a child moved from one state to another? What are the implications of different programs in different locations from a social justice perspective?
2. Review the history of managed care organizations from the 1990s. What were the forces that led to their introduction? In what ways were they successful? What happened to them and why?
3. Learn about the advocacy arm of the main professional organization of your discipline. What issues has it made central to its efforts? How would you classify those issues in relation to patient/client/child needs versus professional interests? How might you add new issues to the organization's agenda?
4. What has the governor of your state said about implementation of the Affordable Care Act? How do you feel about your governor's stance? How would you work to challenge that stance if you disagree?
5. Find an organization in your state or community that represents children with disabilities and investigate their vision and mission. Why would you consider joining this organization? Why might you decide not to join?

References

Accreditation Council for Graduate Medical Education. (2007). *ACGME program requirements for graduate medical education in family medicine.* Retrieved from http://www.acgme.org/acgmeweb/Portals/0/PFAssets/ProgramRequirements/120pr07012007.pdf

Ad Hoc Task Force on Definition of the Medical Home. (1992). The medical home. *Pediatrics, 90,* 774.

Adams, K., & Corrigan, J.M. (Eds.). (2003). *Priority areas for national action: Transforming health care quality.* Washington, DC: National Academies Press.

Adams, K., Greiner, A.C., & Corrigan, J.M. (Eds.). (2004). *1st annual Crossing the Quality Chasm Summit: A focus on communities.* Washington, DC: National Academies Press.

Ainbinder, J.G., Blanchard, L.W., Singer, G.H., Sullivan, M.E., Powers, L.K., Marquis, J.G., & Santelli, B. (1998). A qualitative study of Parent to Parent support for parents of children with special needs. Consortium to evaluate Parent to Parent. *Journal of Pediatric Psychology, 23*(2), 99–109.

American Academy of Family Physicians, American Academy of Otolaryngology—Head and Neck Surgery, & American Academy of Pediatrics Subcommittee on Otitis Media with Effusion. (2004). Otitis media with effusion. *Pediatrics, 113,* 1412–1429.

American Academy of Pediatrics. (2003). *Caring for children with ADHD: A resource toolkit for clinicians.* Washington, DC: Author.

American Academy of Pediatrics. (2005). *What is a family-centered medical home?* Retrieved from http://www.medicalhomeinfo.org

American Academy of Pediatrics. (2011). *Caring for children with ADHD: A resource toolkit for clinicians* (2nd ed.). Evanston, IL: Author.

American Association of Intellectual and Developmental Disabilties. (2010). *Definition of intellectual disability.* Retrieved from http://www.aaidd.org/content_100.cfm?navID=21

American Psychiatric Association. (1980). *Diagnostic and statistical manual of mental disorders* (3rd ed.). Philadelphia, PA: Author.

American Psychiatric Association. (1994). *Diagnostic and statistical manual of mental disorders* (4th ed.). Washington, DC: Author.

American Psychiatric Association. (2000). *Diagnostic and statistical manual of mental disorders* (4th ed., text revision). Washington, DC: Author.

American Recovery and Reinvestment Act of 2009, Pub. L. No. 111-5, H.R. 111th Congress (2009).

Americans with Disabilities Act of 1990, Pub. L. No. 101-336, § 2, 104 Stat. 328 (1991).

Anderson, D., Dumont, S., Jacobs, P., & Azzaria, L. (2007). The personal cost of caring for a child with a disability: A review of the literature. *Public Health Reports, 122,* 3–16.

Antonelli, R.C., Stille, C.J., & Antonelli, D.M. (2008). Care coordination for children and youth with special health care needs: A descriptive, multisite study of activities, personnel costs, and outcomes. *Pediatrics, 122,* e209–e216. doi:10.1542/peds.2007-2254

Association of Centers of Excellence on Disabilities. (2010). *Patient Protection and Affordable Care Act: New options for long-term services and supports.* Retrieved from http://www.aucd.org/docs/policy/health_care/Section%20by%20Section%20summary%20of%20LTSS%20in%20HCR%20law%205-5-10.pdf

Association of University Centers on Disabilities. (2011). *History.* Retrieved from http://www.aucd.org/template/page.cfm?id=156

Aylward, G.P. (2002). Cognitive and neuropsychological outcomes: More than IQ scores. *Mental Retardation & Developmental Disabilities Research Reviews, 8*(4), 234–240.

Bailey, D.B., Jr., Golden, R.N., Roberts, J., & Ford, A. (2007). Maternal depression and developmental disability: Research critique. *Mental Retardation & Developmental Disabilities Research Reviews, 13*(4), 321–329.

Baker, D.P., Salas, E., King, H., Battles, J., & Barach, P. (2005). The role of teamwork in the professional education of physicians: Current status and assessment recommendations. *Journal on Quality and Patient Safety, 31*(4), 185–202.

Balanced Budget Act of 1997, Pub. L. No. 105-33, 111 Stat. 251 (1997).

Beach, M.C., Saha, S., & Cooper, L.A. (2006). *The role and relationship of cultural competence and patient-centeredness in health care quality: The Commonwealth Fund.* Retrieved from http://www.commonwealthfund.org/Publications/Fund-Reports/2006/Oct/The-Role-and-Relationship-of-Cultural-Competence-and-Patient-Centeredness-in-Health-Care-Quality.aspx

Beck, A.H. (2004). The Flexner Report and the standardization of American medical education. *Journal of the American Medical Association, 291*, 2139–2140.

Behrman, R.E., Butler, A.S., & Committee on Understanding Premature Birth and Assuring Healthy Outcomes (Eds.). (2007). *Preterm birth: Causes, consequences, and prevention.* Washington, DC: The National Academies Press.

Bender, J. (2012). *Message from the CEO.* In Bender Consulting Services, Inc. Retrieved from http://www.benderconsult.com/about-us/message-ceo

Bhutta, A.T., Cleves, M.A., Casey, P.H., Cradock, M.M., Anand, K.J., Adnan, T., ... Anand, K.J.S. (2002). Cognitive and behavioral outcomes of school-aged children who were born preterm: A meta-analysis. *Journal of the American Medical Association, 288*, 728–737.

Blesch, P., & Fisher, M.L. (1996). The impact of parental presence on parental anxiety and satisfaction. *AORN Journal, 63*, 761–768.

Blum, N.J., Feldman, H.M., Barbaresi, W.J., Schonfeld, D.J., Hansen, R.L., & Forrest, C.B. (2012, July/August). Research priorities for developmental-behavioral pediatrics: A DBPNet consensus study. *Journal of Developmental & Behavioral Pediatrics, 33*(6), 509–516.

Bogdan, R., & Taylor, S.J. (1989). Relationships with severely disabled people: The social construction of humanness. *Social Problems, 36*(2), 135–148.

Boyle, C.A., Boulet, S., Schieve, L.A., Cohen, R.A., Blumberg, S.J., Yeargin-Allsopp, M., ... Kogan, M.D. (2011). Trends in the prevalence of developmental disabilities in US children, 1997–2008. *Pediatrics, 127*(6): 1034–1042.

Bradford Dementia Group. (2012). *Dementia partnerships.* Retrieved from http://www.dementiapartnerships.org.uk/

Brault, M. (2008). *Americans with disabilities: 2005 current population reports.* Washington, DC: U.S. Census Bureau.

Brewer, E.J., McPherson, M., Magrab, P.R., & Hutchins, V.L. (1989). Family-centered, community-based, coordinated care for children with special health care needs. *Pediatrics, 83*, 1055–1060.

Bull, M.J., & the Committee on Genetics. (2011). Health supervision for children with Down syndrome. *Pediatrics, 128*, 393–406. doi:10.1542/peds.2011-1605

Camilleri, J.M. (2003). *Born again: A personal journey towards the social model of disability.* Retrieved from http://www.knpd.org/pubs/opus/bornagain.pdf

Camp, B.W., Gitterman, B., Headley, R., & Ball, V. (1997). Pediatric residency as preparation for primary care practice. *Archives of Pediatrics & Adolescent Medicine, 151*, 78–83.

Campinha-Bacote, J. (2002). The process of cultural competence in the delivery of healthcare services: A model of care. *Journal of Transcultural Nursing, 13*, 181–184.

Casey, P.H., Lyle, R.E., Bird, T.M., Robbins, J.M., Kuo, D.Z., Brown, C., ... Burns, K. (2011). Effect of hospital-based comprehensive care clinic on health costs for

Medicaid-insured medically complex children. *Archives of Pediatrics & Adolescent Medicine*, *165*, 392–398.

Cella, D., Riley, W., Stone, A., Rothrock, N., Reeve, B., Yount, S., ... on behalf of the PROMIS Cooperative Group. (2010). The Patient Reported Outcomes Measurement Information System (PROMIS) developed and tested its first wave of adult self-reported health outcome item banks: 2005–2008. *Journal of Clinical Epidemiology*, *63*, 1179–1194.

Cella, D., Yount, S., Rothrock, N., Gershon, R., Cook, K., Reeve, B., ... on behalf of the PROMIS Cooperative Group. (2007). The Patient Reported Outcomes Measurement Information System (PROMIS): Progress of an NIH roadmap cooperative group during its first two years. *Medical Care*, *45*(5), S3–S11.

Center for Mental Health Services. (2010). *Shared decision-making in mental health: Practice, research, and future directions*. Rockville, MD: Substance Abuse and Mental Health Services Administration.

Centers for Disease Control and Prevention. (n.d.). *Disability and health. Data & statistics*. Retrieved from http://www.cdc.gov/ncbddd/disabilityandhealth/data.html

Children's Charter. (1930). *Children and youth in history, Item #124*. [Government Document]. Retrieved from http://chnm.gmu.edu/cyh/primary-sources/124

Children's Health Insurance Program Reauthorization Act of 2009, Pub. L. No. 111-3, 123 Stat. 8 (2009).

Children's Oncology Group. (n.d.). Retrieved from http://www.childrensoncologygroup.org

Clardy, A. (2006). Andragogy: Adult learning and education at its best? *Human Resources Development Program*. Towson, MD: Towson University.

Cohen, E., Jovcevska, V., Kuo, D.Z., & Mahant, S. (2011). Hospital-based comprehensive care programs for children with special health care needs: A systematic review. *Archives of Pediatrics & Adolescent Medicine*, *165*, 554–561.

Combating Autism Act of 2006, Pub. L. No. 109-416, Senate Bill 843 (2006).

Committee on Genetics. (2001). Health care supervision for children with Williams syndrome. *Pediatrics*, *107*, 1192–1204.

Committee on Hospital Care, American Academy of Pediatrics, & Institute for Family-Centered Care. (2003). Family-centered care and the pediatrician's role. *Pediatrics*, *112*, 691–696.

Commonwealth Fund. (2011). *Major provisions of the Affordable Care Act*. Retrieved from http://www.commonwealthfund.org/Health-Reform/ /media/Files/Publications/Other/2010/CMWF_Overview_Timeline_20102018.pdf

Cooper, W.O., Habel, L.A., Sox, C.M., Chan, K.A., Arbogasi, P.G., Cheetham, T.C. ... Ray, W.A. (2011). ADHD drugs and serious cardiovascular events in children and young adults. *New England Journal of Medicine*, *365*, 1896–1904.

Data Resource Center for Child & Adolescent Health. (2009). Influence of survey design on medical home prevalence. In *Measuring medical home for children and youth: A resource manual for child health program leaders, researchers and analysts* (pp. 42–51). The Child and Adolescent Health Measurement Initiative. Retrieved from http://www.childhealthdata.org/docs/medical-home/mhmanual_withappendices-updated-12-7-10-pdf.pdf

Department of Health and Ageing, Australian Government. (2011). *MBS primary care items: History of key MBS primary care initiatives 1999–2010*. Retreived from http://www.health.gov.au/internet/main/publishing.nsf/Content/mbsprimarycare-History

DeVoe, J.E., Ray, M., Krois, L., & Carlson, M.J. (2010). Uncertain health insurance coverage and unmet children's health care needs. *Health Services Research*, *42*(2), 121–132.

Disability Rights California. (2011). *GOP lawmakers stand with Democrats, unions to protest cuts to in-home care*. Retrieved from http://www.disabilityrightsca.org/news/2011_newsaboutus/2011-01-27-sfgate.html

Dollaghan, C.A. (2007). *The handbook for evidence-based practice in communication disorders*. Baltimore, MD: Paul H. Brookes Publishing Co.

Douvanis, G., & Hulsey, D. (2002). The least restrictive environment mandate: How has it been defined by the courts? *ERIC Digest*. Arlington, VA: ERIC Clearinghouse on Disabilities and Gifted Education. ERIC ID: ED469442. Retrieved from http://www.ericdigests.org/2003-3/courts.htm

Dunst, C.J., & Trivette, C.M. (1996). Family matters. Empowerment, effective helpgiving practices and family-centered care. *Pediatric Nursing, 22*(4), 334–337.

Ed Roberts, activist: 60 Minutes segment with Harry Reasoner (n.d.). Retrieved from http://www.mnddc.org/ed-roberts/sixtyminutes.html

Education for All Handicapped Children Act, Pub. L. No. 94-142, 94th Congress (1975).

Ellingsen, K.M., & Simeonsson, R.J. (2011). *ICF-CY Developmental Code Set for children six through twelve years* (6-12). Retrieved from http://www.icf-cydevelopmentalcodesets.com/Page_3_KXVK.html

Family Voices. (2008). *Family-Centered Care Self-Assessment Tool: Provider tool.* Retrieved from http://www.familyvoices.org/admin/miscdocs/files/fcca_ProviderTool.pdf

Farmer, J.E., Clark, M.J., Drewel, E.H., Swenson, T.M., & Ge, B. (2011). Consultative care coordination through the medical home for CSHCN: A randomized controlled trial. *Maternal & Child Health Journal, 15*, 1110–1118.

Federal Coordinating Council for Comparative Effectiveness Research. (2009). *Report to the President and the Congress.* Washington, DC: U.S. Department of Health and Human Services.

Feldman, H.M., Ploof, D., & Cohen, W.I. (1999). Physician-family partnerships: The adaptive practice model. *Journal of Developmental & Behavioral Pediatrics, 20*(2), 111–116.

Ferner, R., Huson, S., Thomas, N., Moss, C., Willshaw, H., Evans, D., ... Kirby, A. (2007). Guidelines for the diagnosis and management of individuals with neurofibromatosis 1. *Journal of Medical Genetics, 44*(2), 81–88.

Fina, D.K., Lopas, L.J., Stagnone, J.H., & Santucci, P.R. (1997). Parent participation in the postanesthesia care unit: Fourteen years of progress at one hospital. *Journal of Perianesthesia Nursing, 12*, 152–162.

Fitz, D. (2011). Why does health care in Cuba cost 96% less than in the US? *Links International Journal of Socialist Renewal.* Retrieved from http://links.org.au/node/2082

Flexner, A. (1910). *Medical education in the United States and Canada: A report to the Carnegie Foundation for the Advancement of Teaching, Issue 3.* [Google eBook] New York, NY: Carnegie Foundation for the Advancement of Teaching.

Forest, M., & Pearpoint, J. (2001). *Common sense tools: MAPS and CIRCLES for inclusive education.* Retrieved from http://www.inclusion.com/artcommonsensetools.html

Fujiura, G.T., & Yamaki, K. (2000). Trends in demography of childhood poverty and disability. *Exceptional Children, 66*(2), 187–199.

Ganz, M.L., & Tendulkar, S.A. (2006). Mental health care services for children with special health care needs and their family members: Prevalence and correlates of unmet needs. [Erratum appears in *Pediatrics.* 2006 Oct;118(4):1806-7]. *Pediatrics, 117*, 2138–2148.

General Assembly of the United Nations. (n.d.). *The universal declaration of human rights.* Retrieved from http://www.un.org/en/documents/udhr/index.shtml

Gever, J. (2012). *DSM-5*: What's in, what's out. *MedPage Today.* Retrieved from http://www.medpagetoday.com/MeetingCoverage/APA/32619

Glessner, J.T., Wang, K., Cai, G., Korvatska, O., Kim, C.E., Wood, S., ... Hakonarson, H. (2009, May 28). Autism genome-wide copy number variation reveals ubiquitin and neuronal genes. *Nature, 459*, 569–573.

Goldman, R., & Fristoe, M. (2000). *Goldman-Firstoe Test of Articulation* (2nd ed.). Circle Pines, MS: American Guidance Service, Inc.

Grimby, G., & Smedby, B. (2001). ICF approved as the successor of ICIDH. *Journal of Rehabilitation Medicine, 33*(5), 193–194.

Haley, S.M., Coster, W.J., Ludlow, L.H., Haltiwanger, J.T., & Andrellos, P.J. (1992). *Pediatric Evaluation of Disability Inventory (PEDI).* San Antonio, TX: Pearson.

Hay, P., Katsikitis, M., Begg, J., Da Costa, J., & Blumenfeld, N. (2003). A two-year follow-up study and prospective evaluation of the DSM-IV axis V. *Psychiatric Services, 54*, 1028–1030.

Head, L.S., & Abbeduto, L. (2007). Recognizing the role of parents in developmental outcomes: A systems approach to evaluating the child with developmental disabilities. *Mental Retardation & Developmental Disabilities Research Reviews, 13*(4), 293–301.

Health Professions Network, Nursing & Midwifery, Human Resources for Health. (2010). *Framework for action on interprofessional education & collaborative practice.* Geneva, Switzerland: World Health Organization. Retrieved from http://whqlibdoc.who.int/hq/2010/WHO_HRH_HPN_10.3_eng.pdf

Hill, K., Freeman, L., Yucel, R., & Kuhlthau, K. (2008). Unmet need among children with special health care needs in Massachusetts. *Maternal Child Health Journal, 12*, 650–661.

Hilsenroth, M.J., Ackerman, S.J., Blagys, M.D., Baumann, B.D., Baity, M.R., Smith, S.R., ... Holdwick, D.J., Jr. (2000). Reliability and validity of DSM-IV axis V. *American Journal of Psychiatry, 157*, 1858–1863.

Hintz, S., Kendrick, D., Vohr, B., Poole, W., Higgins, R., & National Institute of Child Health and Human Development (NICHD) Neonatal Research Network. (2008). Community supports after surviving extremely low-birth-weight, extremely preterm birth: Special outpatient services in early childhood. *Archives of Pediatrics & Adolescent Medicine, 162*(8), 748.

Hofmarcher, M.M., Oxley, H., & Rusticelli, E. (2007). Improved health systems performance through better care coordination. *OECD Health Working Papers* (Vol. 30). Paris, France: Directorate for Employment, Labour and Social Affairs.

Honberg, L.E., Kogan, M.D., Allen, D., Strickland, B.B., Newacheck, P.W., Honberg, L.E., ... Newacheck, P.W. (2009). Progress in ensuring adequate health insurance for children with special health care needs. *Pediatrics, 124*, 1273–1280.

Honeycutt A., Dunlap, L., Chen, H., al Homsi, G., Grosse, S., & Schendel, D. (2004, January 30). Economic costs associated with mental retardation, cerebral palsy, hearing loss, and vision impairment—United States, 2003. *Morbidity and Mortality Weekly Report*, pp. 53, 57–59. Retrieved from http://www.cdc.gov/mmwr/preview/ mmwrhtml/mm5303a4.htm#tab

Hoover, J., & Stenhjem, P. (2003). Bullying and teasing youth with disabilities: Creating positive school environments for effective inclusion. *Issue Brief: Examining Current Challenges in Secondary Education and Transition, 2*(3), 1–6.

Hudson, K.M., & Giardino, A.P. (1996). Child abuse and neglect. In L.A. Kurtz, P.W. Dowrick, S.E. Levy, & M.L. Batshaw (Eds.), *Handbook of developmental disabilities* (pp. 542–554). Gaithersburg, MD: Aspen Publishers.

Huffman, L.C., Sutcliffe, T.L., Tanner, I.S.D., & Feldman, H.M. (2011). Management of symptoms in children with autism spectrum disorders: A comprehensive review of pharmacologic and complementary-alternative medicine treatments. *Journal of Developmental & Behavioral Pediatrics, 32*(1), 56–68.

ICF Research Branch. (2010). *ICF core set projects.* Retrieved from http://www.icf-research-branch.org/icf-core-sets-projects.html

IGDA Workgroup & World Psychiatric Association. (2003a). 7: Standardized multi-axial diagnostic formulation. *British Journal of Psychiatry, 182*(Suppl. 45), s52–s54.

IGDA Workgroup & World Psychiatric Association. (2003b). 8: Idiographic (personalized) diagnostic formulation. *British Journal of Psychiatry, 182*(Suppl. 43), s55–s57.

Improving Chronic Illness Care. (2011). *The chronic care model.* Retrieved from http://www.improvingchroniccare.org/index.php?p=The_Chronic_Care_Model&s=2

Individuals with Disabilities Education Act of 1990, Pub. L. No. 101-476, 104 Stat. 1142.

Institute for Patient- and Family-Centered Care. (2010). *Frequently asked questions.* Retrieved from http://www.ipfcc.org/faq.html

Institute for Patient- and Family-Centered Care. (2012). *Free downloads: Tools/checklists.* Retrieved from http://www.ipfcc.org/tools/downloads-tools.html

Institute of Medicine, Committee on Quality of Health Care in America. (2001). *Crossing the quality chasm: A new health system for the 21st century.* Washington, DC: National Academies Press.

Ireys, H.T., Chernoff, R., DeVet, K.A., & Kim, Y. (2001). Maternal outcomes of a randomized controlled trial of a community-based support program for families of children with chronic illnesses. *Archives of Pediatrics & Adolescent Medicine, 155*, 771–777.

Johnson, A.H. (2001). The Balint movement in America. *Family Medicine, 33*(3), 174–177.

Kaiser Commission. (2011). *Medicaid and the uninsured.* Washington, DC: Kaiser Family Foundation.

Kaiser Commission. (2012). *Medicaid and the uninsured: Medicaid health homes for beneficiares with chronic conditions.* Washington, DC: Kaiser Family Foundation.

Kaiser Family Foundation. (2012). *Oral health and Medicare beneficiaries: Coverage, out-of-pocket spending, and unmet need:* Menlo Park, CA: Author.

Kaiser Family Foundation. (2013). *The U.S. government and international family planning & reproductive health.* Menlo Park, CA: Author.

Kanner, L. (1964). *A history of the care and study of the mentally retarded.* Springfield, IL: Charles C Thomas.

Kaye, H.S. (2013). Disability rates for working-age adults and for the elderly have stabilized, but trends for each mean different results for costs. *Health Affairs, 32*(1), 127–134.

Kleinman, A., Eisenbery, L., & Good, B. (1978). Culture, illness, and care: Clinical lessons from anthropologic and cross-cultural research. *Annals of Internal Medicine, 88*(2), 251–258.

Kohn, L.T., Corrigan, J.M., & Donaldson, M.S. (Eds.). (1999). *To err is human: Building a safer health system.* Washington, DC: National Academies Press.

Koop, C.E. (1987). *Surgeon General's report: Children with special health care needs—Campaign 87—Commitment to family-centered, coordinated care for children with special health care needs.* Washington, DC: U.S. Department of Health and Human Services.

Kussman, B.D., Wypij, D., Laussen, P.C., Soul, J.S., Bellinger, D.C., DiNardo, J.A., ... Newburger, J.W. (2010). Relationship of intraoperative cerebral oxygen saturation to neurodevelopmental outcome and brain magnetic resonance imaging at 1 year of age in infants undergoing biventricular repair. *Circulation, 122*(3), 245–254.

The Lanterman Developmental Disabilities Services Act, California Assembly Bill 846 (1969).

Lawson, K.A., Bloom, S.R., Sadof, M., Stille, C.J., & Perrin, J.M. (2011). Care coordination for children with special health care needs: Evaluation of a state experiment. *Maternal & Child Health Journal, 15*, 993–1000.

Lerner, S., Magrane, D., & Friedman, E. (2009). Teaching teamwork in medical education. *Mount Sinai Journal of Medicine: A Journal of Translational and Personalized Medicine, 76*(4), 318–329.

Lewis, C.W. (2009). Dental care and children with special health care needs: A population-based perspective. *Academic Pediatrics, 9*(6), 420–426.

Limperopoulos, C., Tworetzky, W., McElhinney, D.B., Newburger, J.W., Brown, D.W., Robertson, R.L., Jr., ... du Plessis, A.J. (2010). Brain volume and metabolism in fetuses with congenital heart disease: Evaluation with quantitative magnetic resonance imaging and spectroscopy. *Circulation, 121*(1), 26–33.

Lobato, D.J., & Kao, B.T. (2005). Brief report: Family-based group intervention for young siblings of children with chronic illness and developmental disability. *Journal of Pediatric Psychology, 30*, 678–682.

Loe, I.M., & Feldman, H.M. (2007). Academic and educational outcomes of children with ADHD. *Journal of Pediatric Psychology, 32*, 643–654.

Lucile Packard Foundation for Children's Health. (2009) *The importance of integrated services.* Retrieved from http://www.lpfch.org/nationalmodels/financing.pdf

Maag, E. (2000). *Supportive health services needs for children with disabilities.* Retrieved from http://aspe.hhs.gov/daltcp/reports/2000/suphsnd.htm

Martin, D.P. (2008). *Health Services Research Core Competencies: Final Report: Agency for Healthcare Research and Quality.* Rockville, MD: Agency for Healthcare Research and Quality.

Martin, J.C., Avant, R.F., Bowman, M.A., Bucholtz, J.R., Dickinson, J.R., Evans, K.L., ... Future of Family Medicine Project Leadership Committee. (2004). The future of family medicine: A collaborative project of the family medicine community. *Annals of Family Medicine, 2*(Suppl. 1), S3–S32.

Mayer, M. L., Skinner, A.C., & Slifkin, R.T., Slifkin, R.T. (2004). Unmet need for routine and specialty care: Data from the National Survey of Children with Special Health Care Needs. *Pediatrics, 113*(2), e109–e115.

McColl, M.A., Forster, D., Shortt, S.E., Hunter, D., Dorland, J., Godwin, M., & Rosser, W. (2008). Physician experiences providing primary care to people with disabilities. *Health Policy, 4*(1), e129–e147.

MCH Training Grantee Network. (2011). *MCH leadership competencies.* Retrieved from http://leadership.mchtraining.net/

McManus, B., McCormick, M.C., Acevedo-Garcia, D., Ganz, M., Hauser-Cram, P., McManus, B., … Hauser-Cram, P. (2009). The effect of state early intervention eligibility policy on participation among a cohort of young CSHCN. *Pediatrics, 124*(Suppl. 4), S368–S374.

McPherson, M., Arango, P., Fox, H., Lauver, C., McManus, M., Newacheck, P.W., … Strickland, B. (1998). A new definition of children with special health care needs. *Pediatrics, 102*(1), 137–139.

Medical Outcomes Trust. (n.d.). *SF-36. org.* Retrieved from http://www.sf-36.org/wantsf.aspx?id=1

Mental Retardation Facilities and Community Mental Health Centers Construction Act of 1963, Pub. L. No. 88-164, 1576 Stat. 282 (1963).

Markel, H. (2008, January 1). When hospitals kept children from parents. *The New York Times.* Retrieved from http://www.nytimes.com/2008/01/01/health/01visi.html?_r=0

Middlebrooks, J.S., & Audage, N.C. (2008). *The effects of childhood stress on health across the lifespan.* Atlanta, GA: Centers for Disease Control and Prevention.

Milstein, A., Kothari, P.P., Fernandopulle, R., & Helle, T. (2009). Are higher-value care models replicable? *Health Affairs Blog.* Retrieved from http://healthaffairs.org/blog/2009/10/20/are-higher-value-care-models-replicable/

Minnesota Governor's Council on Developmental Disabilities. (n.d.). *Marc Gold: "Try another way" overview.* Retrieved from http://www.mnddc.org/extra/marc-gold1.html

Moderators and mediators of treatment response for children with attention-deficit/hyperactivity disorder: The multimodal treatment study of children with attention-deficit/hyperactivity disorder. (1999). *Archives of General Psychiatry, 56*, 1088–1096.

Molina, B.S.G., Hinshaw, S.P., Swanson, J.M., Arnold, L.E., Vitiello, B., Jensen, P.S., …, MTA Cooperative Group. (2009). The MTA at 8 years: Prospective follow-up of children treated for combined-type ADHD in a multisite study. *Journal of the American Academy of Child & Adolescent Psychiatry, 48*(5), 484–500.

Mont, D. (2007, March). *Measuring disability prevalence.* SP Discussion Paper No. 0706. Washington, DC: The World Bank.

Nageswaran, S. (2009). Respite care for chidlren with special health care needs. *Archives of Pediatrics & Adolescent Medicine, 163*, 49–54.

National Center for Cultural Competence. (n.d.). *Rationale for self-assessment.* Retrieved from http://nccc.georgetown.edu/orgselfassess.html

National Center for Cultural Competence. (n.d.). *Self-assessments.* Retrieved from http://nccc.georgetown.edu/resources/assessments.html

National Council on Disability. (2012). *Successfully enrolling people with disabilities in managed care plans: Guiding principles.* Washington, DC: Author.

National Dissemination Center for Children with Disabilities. (2011). *Categories of disability under IDEA.* Retrieved from http://nichcy.org/disability/categories

Neisworth, J.D., & Bagnato, S.J. (2004). The mismeasure of young children: The authentic assessment alternative. *Infants and Young Children, 17*(3), 198–212.

Newacheck, P.W., Halfon, N., & Inkelas, M. (2000). Commentary: Monitoring expanded health insurance for children: Challenges and opportunities. *Pediatrics, 105*(Suppl. 3), 1004–1007.

Newacheck, P.W., Hughes, D.C., Hung, Y., Wong, S., & Stoddard, J.J. (2000). The unmet health needs of America's children. *Pediatrics, 105*(4), 989–997.

Newacheck, P.W., Inkelas, M., & Kim, S.E. (2004). Health services use and health care expenditures for children with disabilities. *Pediatrics, 114*, 79–85.

Newacheck, P.W., & Kim, S.E. (2005). A national profile of health care utilization and expenditures for children with special health care needs. *Archives of Pediatrics & Adolescent Medicine, 159*, 10–17.

Newburger, J.W., Jonas, R.A., Soul, J., Kussman, B.D., Bellinger, D.C., Laussen, P.C., … Wypij, D. (2008). Randomized trial of hematocrit 25% versus 35% during hypothermic cardiopulmonary bypass in infant heart surgery. *Journal of Thoracic & Cardiovascular Surgery, 135*(2), 347–354.

NICHD Neonatal Research Network. (n.d.). Retrieved from https://neonatal.rti.org

Office of Minority Health. (2005). *What is cultural competency?* Retrieved from http://minorityhealth.hhs.gov/templates/browse.aspx?lvl=2&lvlID=11

Ogonowski, J.A., Kronk, R.A., Rice, C.N., & Feldman, H.M. (2004). Inter-rater reliability in assigning ICF codes to children with disabilities. *Disability and Rehabilitation, 26*, 353–361.

Omnibus Budget Reconciliation Act of 1989, Pub. L. No. 101-239, 103 Stat. 2106 (1989).

Orlander, J.D., Barger, T.W., & Fincke, B.G. (2002). The Morbidity and Mortality Conference: The delicate nature of learning from error. *Academic Medicine, 77*, 1001–1006.

Owen, N., Glanz, K., Sallis, J.F., & Kelder, S.H. (2006). Evidence-based approaches to dissemination and diffusion of physical activity interventions. *American Journal of Preventive Medicine, 31*(Suppl. 4), S35–S44.

P2P USA: Parent to Parent USA. (2012). Retrieved from http://www.p2pusa.org

Palfrey, J.S., Sofis, L.A., Davidson, E.J., Liu, J., Freeman, L., & Ganz, M.L. (2004). The Pediatric Alliance for Coordinated Care: Evaluation of a medical home model. *Pediatrics, 113*(Suppl. 4), 1507–1516.

Palisano, R., Rosenbaum, P., Walter, S., Russell, D., Wood, E., & Galuppi, B. (1997). Development and reliability of a system to classify gross motor function in children with cerebral palsy. *Developmental Medicine & Child Neurology, 39*(4), 214–223.

Palmer, F.B., Shapiro, B.K., Wachtel, R.C., Allen, M.C., Hiller, J.E., Harryman, S.E., … Capute, A.J. (1988). The effects of physical therapy on cerebral palsy. *New England Journal of Medicine, 318*, 803–808.

Palsbo, S.E., Mastal, M.F., & O'Donnell, L.T. (2006). Disability care coordination organizations: Improving health and function in people with disabilities. *Lippincotts Case Management, 11*(5), 255–264.

Paradise, J.L. (2009). Generalizability of randomized trial results: Tympanostomy-tube insertion and tonsillectomy. *Otolaryngology—Head & Neck Surgery, 140*(3), 439–440; author reply 440–431.

Paradise, J.L., Campbell, T.F., Dollaghan, C.A., Feldman, H.M., Bernard, B.S., Colborn, D.K., … Smith, C.G. (2005). Developmental outcomes after early or delayed insertion of tympanostomy tubes. *New England Journal of Medicine, 353*, 576–586.

Paradise, J.L., Feldman, H.M., Campbell, T.F., Dollaghan, C.A., Colborn, D.K., Bernard, B.S., … Smith, C.G. (2001). Effect of early or delayed insertion of tympanostomy tubes for persistent otitis media on developmental outcomes at the age of three years. *New England Journal of Medicine, 344*, 1179–1187.

Paradise, J.L., Feldman, H.M., Campbell, T.F., Dollaghan, C.A., Rockette, H.E., Pitcairn, D.L., … Pelham, W.E., Jr. (2007). Tympanostomy tubes and developmental outcomes at 9 to 11 years of age. *New England Journal of Medicine, 356*, 248–261.

Parrish, T.D. (2006). *National and state overview of special education funding: Kansas association of special education administrators*. Lawrence, KS: American Institutes for Research.

Patient Protection and Affordable Care Act of 2010, Pub. L. No. 111-148, 124 Stat. 119 through 124 Stat. 1025 (2010).

Peck, C.A., Carlson, P., & Helmstetter, E. (1992). Parent and teacher perceptions of outcomes for typically developing children enrolled in integrated early childhood programs: A statewide survey. *Journal of Early Intervention, 16*(1), 53–63.

Peter, S., Chaney, G., Zappia, T., Van Veldhuisen, C., Pereira, S., & Santamaria, N. (2011). Care coordination for children with complex care needs significantly reduces hospital utilization. *Journal of Special Pediatric Nursing, 16*(4), 305–312.

Plucker, J. (2012). Jean-Marc Gaspard Itard. *Human Intelligence*. Retrieved from http://www.indiana.edu/ intell/itard.shtml

PROMIS. (n.d.).: *Dynamic tools to measure health outocmes from the patient perspective*. Retrieved from http://www.nihpromis.org

Pruitt, L.J. (2012). Living with spina bifida: A historical perspective. *Pediatrics, 130*, 181–183.

Rabin, B.A., Brownson, R.C., Kerner, J.F., & Glasgow, R.E. (2006). Methodologic challenges in disseminating evidence-based interventions to promote physical activity. *American Journal of Preventive Medicine, 31*(Suppl. 4), S24–S34.

Rafferty, Y., Piscitelli, V., & Boettcher, C. (2003). The impact of inclusion on language development and social competence among preschoolers with disabilities. *Exceptional Children, 69*, 467–479.

Reed, G.M., Lux, J.B., Bufka, L.F., Trask, C., Peterson, D.B., Stark, S., . . . Hawley, J.A. (2005). Operationalizing the International Classification of Functioning, Disability, and Health in clinical settings. *Rehabilitation Psychology, 50*(2), 122–131.

Rehabilitation Act of 1973, Pub. L. No. 93-112, 87 Stat. 355 (1973).

Resnick, B., Galik, E., Gruber-Baldini, A.L., & Zimmerman, S. (2010). Perceptions and performance of function and physical activity in assisted living communities. *Journal of the American Medical Directors Association, 11*, 406–414.

Resnick, B., Galik, E., Gruber-Baldini, A.L., & Zimmerman, S. (2011). Testing the effect of function-focused care in assisted living. *Journal of the American Geriatrics Society, 59*, 2233–2240.

Rieser, R. (2000). *Together we are better.* Retrieved from http://www.worldofinclusion.com/res/edeqhr/Together_We_are_Better.doc

Rosenberg, S.A., Zhang, D., & Robinson, C.C. (2008). Prevalence of developmental delays and participation in early intervention services for young children. *Pediatrics, 121*, e1503–e1509.

Ruben, R.J. (2008). Randomized controlled studies and the treatment of middle ear effusions and tonsillar pharyngitis: How random are the studies and what are their limitations? *Otolaryngology Head and Neck Surgery, 139*, 333–339.

Sackett, D.L., Rosenberg, W.M.C., Gray, J.A.M, Haynes, R.B., & Richardson, W.S. (1996). Evidence based medicine: What it is and what it isn't. *British Medical Journal, 312*, 71–72.

Saigal, S., & Doyle, L.W. (2008). An overview of mortality and sequelae of preterm birth from infancy to adulthood. *The Lancet, 371*, 261–269.

Saigal, S., & Streiner, D. (2009). Socio-economic achievements of individuals born very preterm at the age of 27 to 29 years. *Developmental Medicine & Child Neurology, 51*, 848–850.

Schoen, C., Osborn, R., Squires, D., Doty, M., Pierson, R., & Applebaum, S. (2011). New 2011 survey of patients with complex care needs in eleven countries finds that care is often poorly coordinated. *Health Affairs (Millwood), 30*, 2437–2448.

Scott, I., & Campbell, D. (2002). Health services research: What is it and what does it offer? *Internal Medicine Journal, 32*, 91–99.

Section on Complementary and Integrative Medicine and Council on Children with Disabilties. (2012). Sensory integration therapies for children with developmental and behavioral disorders. *Pediatrics, 129*, 1186–1189.

Shapiro, J.P. (1993). *No pity: People with disabilities forging a new civil rights movement.* New York, NY: Random House.

Shea, S.E., Gordon, K., Hawkins, A., Kawchuk, J., & Smith, D. (2000). Pathology in the Hundred Acre Wood: A neurodevelopmental perspective on A.A. Milne. *Canadian Medical Association Journal, 163*, 1557–1559.

Shelton, T.L., & Stepanek, J.S. (1994). *Family-centered care for children needing specialized health and developmental services.* Bethesda, MD: Association for the Care of Children's Health.

Simeonsson, R.J. (2003). Classification of communication disabilities in children: Contribution of the International Classification on Functioning, Disability and Health. *International Journal of Audiology, 42*(Suppl. 1), S2–S8.

Simeonsson, R.J., Leonardi, M., Bjorck-Akesson, E., Hollenweger, J., Lollar, D., Martinuzzi, A., & TenNapel, H. (2006, October 29–November 4). *ICF-CY: A universal tool for practice policy and research. World Health Organization.* Report presented at the Meeting of the WHO Collaborating Centres for the Family of International Classifications, Tunis, Tunisia.

Simpson, L.A. (1999, June 26). *Children's health services research: An overview.* Paper presented at Improving Children's Health Through Health Services Research, Chicago.

Singer, G.H.S., Marquis, J., Powers, L.K., Blanchard, L., Divenere, N., Santelli, B., ... Sharp, M. (1999). A multi-site evaluation of parent to parent programs for parents of children with disabilities. *Journal of Early Intervention, 22*(3), 217–229.

Slora, E.J., Harris, D.L., Bocian, A.B., & Wasserman, R.C. (2010). Pediatric clinical research networks: Current status, common challenges, and potential solutions. *Pediatrics, 126*, 740–745.

Sneed, R.C., May, W.L., & Stencel, C.S. (2000). Training of pediatricians in care of physical disabilities in children with special health needs: Results of a two-state survey of practicing pediatricians and national resident training programs. *Pediatrics, 105*, 554–561.

Snow, K. (2009). *Disability is natural.* Retrieved from http://www.disabilityisnatural.com

Social Security Act of 1935, Pub. L. No. 74-271, 49 Stat.620 (1935).

Social Security Administration. (2011). *What we mean by disability.* Retrieved from http://www.ssa.gov/dibplan/dqualify4.htm

Sparrow, S.S., Cicchetti, D.V., & Balla, D.A. (2005). *Vineland Adaptive Behavior Scales, Second Edition (Vineland-II).* San Antonio, TX: Pearson.

Spitz, R.A. (1945). Hospitalism—An inquiry into the genesis of psychiatric conditions in early childhood. *Psychoanalytic Study of the Child, 1,* 53–74.

Steenbeek, D., Gorter, J.W., Ketelaar, M., Galama, K., & Lindeman, E. (2011). Responsiveness of Goal Attainment Scaling in comparison to two standardized measures in outcome evaluation of children with cerebral palsy. *Clinical Rehabilitation, 25,* 1128–1139.

Steenbeek, D., Ketelaar, M., Galama, K., & Gorter, J.W. (2007). Goal attainment scaling in paediatric rehabilitation: A critical review of the literature. *Developmental Medicine & Child Neurology, 49,* 550–556.

Stephens, J., Levine, R., Burling, A.S., & Russ-Eft, D. (2011). *An organizational guide to building health services research capacity. A final report.* Rockville MD: Agency for Healthcare Research and Quality.

Strickland, B., McPherson, M., Weissman, G., van Dyck, P., Huang, Z.J., & Newacheck, P. (2004). Access to the medical home: Results of the National Survey of Children with Special Health Care Needs. *Pediatrics, 113*(Suppl. 5), 1485–1492.

Subcommittee on Attention-Deficit/Hyperactivity Disorder, Steering Committee on Quality Improvement and Management. (2001). Clinical practice guideline: Treatment of the school-aged child with attention-deficit/hyperactivity disorder. *Pediatrics, 108,* 1033–1044.

Subcommittee on Attention-Deficit/Hyperactivity Disorder, Steering Committee on Quality Improvement and Management. (2011). ADHD: Clinical practice guideline for the diagnosis, evaluation, and treatment of attention-deficit/hyperactivity disorder in children and adolescents. *Pediatrics, 128,* 1007–1022.

Talbot, J.A. (2004). Deinstutionalization: Avoiding the disasters of the past. *Psychiatric Services, 55,* 1112–1115.

Taylor, H., Krane, D., & Orkis, K. (2010). *The ADA, 20 years later: Executive summary: Kessler Foundation/National Organization on Disability.* New York, NY: Harris Interactive. Retrieved from http://www.2010disabilitysurveys.org/pdfs/surveyresults.pdf

Taylor, S.J. (2002). *Disabled workers deserve real choices, real jobs.* Syracuse, NY: The Center for an Accessible Society, Center on Human Policy, Syracuse University.

Tervalon, M., & Murray-Garcia, J. (1998). Cultural humility versus cultural competence: A critical distinction in defining physician training outcomes in multicultural education. *Journal of Health Care for the Poor and Underserved, 9*(2), 117–125.

The American Balint Society. (2012). Retreived from http://americanbalintsociety.org/

The Arc. (2012). *History of the Arc.* Retrieved from http://www.thearc.org/page.aspx?pid=2338

The Medical Home. (2002). *Pediatrics, 110,* 184–186.

The MTA Cooperative Group. Multimodal Treatment Study of Children with ADHD. (1999). A 14-month randomized clinical trial of treatment strategies for attention-deficit/hyperactivity disorder. *Archives of General Psychiatry, 56,* 1073–1086.

Thomasson, M. (2003). Health insurance in the United States. *EH.Net Encyclopedia.* Retrieved from http://eh.net/encyclopedia/article/thomasson.insurance.health.us

Trute, B., Benzies, K.M., Worthington, C., Reddon, J.R., & Moore, M. (2010). Accentuate the positive to mitigate the negative: Mother psychological coping resources and family adjustment in childhood disability. *Journal of Intellectual & Developmental Disability, 35*(1), 36–43.

United Nations, Department of Economic and Social Affairs, Division for Social Policy and Development. (2006). *United Nations enable: Background and current needs.* Retrieved from http://www.un.org/esa/socdev/enable/dissre01.htm#Background

United Nations, Department of Economic and Social Affairs, the Office of the United Nations High Commissioner for Human

Rights, & Inter-Parliamentary Union. (n.d.). Chapter Six: From provisions to practice: Implementing the Convention. In *Handbook for Parliamentarians on the Convention on the Rights of Persons with Disabilities.* Retrieved from http://www.un.org/disabilities/default.asp?id=240

United Nations Secretary Generals Report on Violence against Children & Thematic Group on Violence against Disabled Children. (2005). *Violence against disabled children: Summary report.* New York, NY: UNICEF.

United Nations Web Services Section, Department of Information. (2006). *Convention on the rights of persons with disabilities.* Retrieved from http://www.un.org/disabilities/convention/conventionfull.shtml

U.S. Bureau of Labor Statistics, Division of Current Employment Statistics. (2012). *Economic news release.* Washington, DC: U.S Department of Labor.

U.S. Census Bureau. (2000). *Census 2000. Washington*, DC: Author: Retrieved from http://www.census.gov/people/disability/methololology/decennial.html

U.S. Census Bureau. (2010). 20th Anniversary of Americans with Disabilities Act: July 26. *Facts for Features and Special Editions.* Retrieved from http://www.census.gov/newsroom/releases/archives/facts_for_features_special_editions/cb10-ff13.html

U.S. Department of Education, Office of Special Education Programs, Data Analysis System (DANS). (2006). *OMB# 1820-0043: Children with disabilities receiving special education under part B of the Individuals with Disabilities Education Act, 1996–2005.* Retrieved from https://www.ideadata.org/tables29th-5Car_1-9.htm

U.S. Department of Education. (2007). *History: Twenty-five years of progress in educating children with disabilities through IDEA.* Retrieved from http://www2.ed.gov/policy/speced/leg/idea/history.html

U.S. Department of Health and Human Services. (2012). *Key features of the Affordable Care Act, by year.* Retrieved from http://www.healthcare.gov/law/timeline/full.html

U.S. Department of Health and Human Services, Health Resources and Services Administration, Maternal and Child Health Bureau. (2008). *The National Survey of Children with Special Health Care Needs Chartbook 2005–2006.* Rockville, MD: U.S. Department of Health and Human Services.

U.S. Equal Employment Opportunity Commission. (2009). *Section 902 definition of the term disability.* Retrieved from http://www.lb5.uscourts.gov/ArchivedURLs/Files/07-20661%283%29.pdf

Weschler, D. (2002). *Wechsler Preschool and Primary Scale of Intelligence* (3rd ed.). San Antonio TX: The Psychological Corporation.

Wikman, A., Marklund, S., & Anderson, K. (2005). Illness, disease, and sickness absence: An empirical test of concepts of ill health. *Journal of Epidemiology and Community Health, 59*, 450–454.

Wisconsin Education Association Council. (2007). *Special education inclusion.* Retrieved from http://www.weac.org/Issues_Advocacy/Resource_Pages_On_Issues_one/Special_Education/special_education_inclusion.aspx

Wolfensberger, W., & Thomas, S. (1998). *A history of human services: Universal lessons, and future implications.* Retrieved from http://www.mnddc.org/wolfensberger/index.html

Wolraich, M.L., Felice, M.E., & Drotar, D.D. (1996). The classification of child and adolescent mental conditions in primary care. In *Diagnostic and statistical manual for primary care (DSM-PC), child and adolescent version* (pp. 32–53). Elk Grove Village, IL: American Academy of Pediatrics.

Woolf, S.H., Grol, R., Hutchinson, A., Eccles, M., & Grimshaw, J. (1999). Potential benefits, limitations, and harms of clinical guidelines. *British Medical Journal, 318*, 527–530.

World Health Organization. (1946). WHO definition of health. *Preamble to the Constitution of the World Health Organization.* Retrieved from http://www.who.int/about/definition/en/print.html

World Health Organization. (2002). *Towards a common language for functioning, disability and health: ICF.* Geneva, Switzerland: Author.

World Health Organization. (2004). *ICF—Children and youth version.* Retrieved from http://www3.who.int/icf/onlinebrowser/icf.cfm?undefined&version=7

World Health Organization. (2010). *Third Geneva conference on person-centred medicine.* Retrieved from http://www.who.int/mediacentre/events/meetings/2010/geneva_conference_20100503/en

World Health Organization. (2011a). *Disability, including prevention, management and rehabilitation.* Retrieved from http://www.who.int/nmh/a5817/en/

World Health Organization. (2011b). *International statistical classification of diseases and related health problems, 10th revision, 2010 edition, volume 2, instruction manual.* Geneva, Switzerland: World Health Organization. Retrieved from http://apps.who.int/classifications/icd10/browse/2010/en

World Health Organization. (2012). *Patients for patient safety.* Retrieved from http://www.who.int/patientsafety/patients_for_patient/en

World Health Organization Workgroup for Developmental of version of ICF for Children & Youth. (2007). *International classification of functioning, disability and health—Version for children and youth: ICF-CY.* Geneva, Switzerland: World Health Organization.

Wright, P.W.D., & Wright, P.D. (2011). Wrightslaw game plan: *Writing good IEP goals & objectives.* Retrieved from http://www.wrightslaw.com/info/iep.goals.plan.htm

Yin, H.S., Johnson, M., Mendelsohn, A.L., Abrams, M.A., Sanders, L.M., & Dreyer, B.P. (2009). The health literacy of parents in the United States: A nationally representative study. *Pediatrics, 124*(Suppl. 3), S289–S298.

Yu, S.M., Singh, G.K., Yu, S.M., & Singh, G.K. (2009). Household language use and health care access, unmet need, and family impact among CSHCN. *Pediatrics, 124*(Suppl. 4), S414–S419.

Zimmerman, I.L., Steiner, V.G., Pond, M.A. (2002). *Preschool Language Scale* (4th ed.) (PLS-4). San Antonio, TX: The Psychological Corporation.

Index

Tables and figures are indicated by *t* and *f*, respectively.